Fundamentals of
FORENSIC NURSING
&
Introduction to
INDIAN LAWS

Fundamentals of
FORENSIC NURSING
& Introduction to
INDIAN LAWS

Gautam Biswas
MBBS MD (Forensic Medicine)
Professor and Head
Department of Forensic Medicine and Toxicology
Dayanand Medical College and Hospital
Ludhiana, Punjab, India

Triza Jiwan
BSc (Nursing) MSc (Nursing) PhD
Principal and Professor and Head (Psychiatry)
Department of Psychiatric Nursing
College of Nursing, Dayanand Medical College and Hospital
Ludhiana, Punjab, India

Foreword
Virginia A Lynch

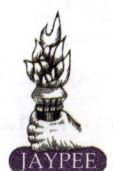

JAYPEE BROTHERS MEDICAL PUBLISHERS
The Health Sciences Publisher
New Delhi | London

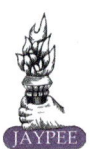 **Jaypee Brothers Medical Publishers (P) Ltd.**

Headquarters
Jaypee Brothers Medical Publishers (P) Ltd
EMCA House
23/23-B, Ansari Road, Daryaganj
New Delhi - 110 002, India
Landline: +91-11-23272143, +91-11-23272703
+91-11-23282021, +91-11-23245672
Email: jaypee@jaypeebrothers.com

Corporate Office
Jaypee Brothers Medical Publishers (P) Ltd
4838/24, Ansari Road, Daryaganj
New Delhi 110 002, India
Phone: +91-11-43574357
Fax: +91-11-43574314
Email: jaypee@jaypeebrothers.com

Overseas Office
J.P. Medical Ltd
83 Victoria Street, London
SW1H 0HW (UK)
Phone: +44 20 3170 8910
Fax: +44 (0)20 3008 6180
Email: info@jpmedpub.com

Website: www.jaypeebrothers.com
Website: www.jaypeedigital.com

© 2024, Jaypee Brothers Medical Publishers (P) Ltd

The views and opinions expressed in this book are solely those of the original contributor(s)/author(s) and do not necessarily represent those of editor(s) and publisher of the book.

All rights reserved. No part of this publication may be reproduced, stored or transmitted in any form or by any means, electronic, mechanical, photocopying, recording or otherwise, without the prior permission in writing of the publishers.

All brand names and product names used in this book are trade names, service marks, trademarks or registered trademarks of their respective owners. The publisher is not associated with any product or vendor mentioned in this book.

Medical knowledge and practice change constantly. This book is designed to provide accurate, authoritative information about the subject matter in question. However, readers are advised to check the most current information available on procedures included and check information from the manufacturer of each product to be administered, to verify the recommended dose, formula, method and duration of administration, adverse effects and contraindications. It is the responsibility of the practitioner to take all appropriate safety precautions. Neither the publisher nor the author(s)/editor(s) assume any liability for any injury and/or damage to persons or property arising from or related to use of material in this book.

This book is sold on the understanding that the publisher is not engaged in providing professional medical services. If such advice or services are required, the services of a competent medical professional should be sought.

Every effort has been made where necessary to contact holders of copyright to obtain permission to reproduce copyright material. If any have been inadvertently overlooked, the publisher will be pleased to make the necessary arrangements at the first opportunity.

Inquiries for bulk sales may be solicited at: jaypee@jaypeebrothers.com

Fundamentals of Forensic Nursing and Introduction to Indian Laws

First Edition: **2024**

ISBN: 978-93-5696-269-9

Printed at: Sterling Graphics Pvt. Ltd. India

Dedication
To all our students...
Past, Present and Future

Reviews

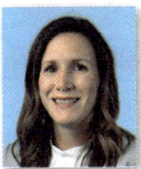

Kelly Berishaj DNP RN
ACNS-BC AFN-C SANE-A

"This book will make significant contributions towards educating forensic nurses in India in regard to the unique health and legal considerations of patients who have been victims of sexual violence."

"Since forensic nursing subject is new to nursing curriculum, authors have made an effort to write it as per the INC syllabus, the attempt is made to keep the book simple and brief while covering the whole syllabus in its sequential order."

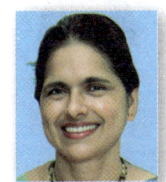

Molly Saldanha MSc
(Cardiothoracic Nursing)

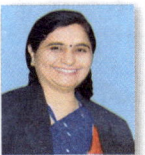

Jyoti Sarin MSc
(Pediatric Nursing) PhD

"The content is comprehensive and parallel to the learning objectives. MCQs and case studies are very well framed."

"This book provides the nursing students with the best information regarding concepts of Forensic Nursing and various other topics about Indian Laws related to that."

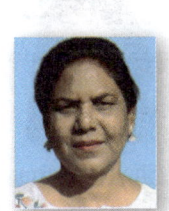

Usha Singh MSc
(Psychiatric Nursing) MSc
(Counselling and Family therapy) PhD (Psychology)

Reviews

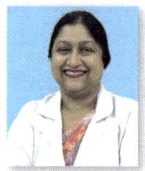

Swapna Melchisedec MSc
(Psychiatric Nursing) PhD

"All the chapters have distinct features, such as learning objectives, chapters outline, tables, flowcharts, MCQs, SAQs and LAQs, as well as excellent pictorial illustrations make this book different from other books."

"The case studies included will help the students to understand the concepts more clearly."

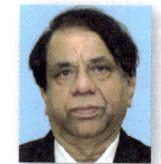

Shridhar KV MSc
(Medical Surgical) PhD
Scholar

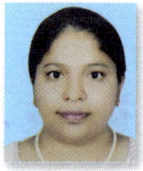

Charlotte Ranadive MSc
(Psychiatric Nursing)

"In spite of using terms and terminologies related to legal/law, the authors have made an effort to simplify the language for easy understanding which will help nursing students to develop a comprehensive understanding about the subject and to practice with confidence."

"Authors have carefully highlighted the main aspects of forensic nursing along with the forensic nurse roles and responsibilities in this book."

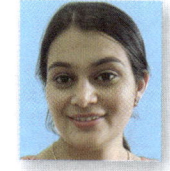

Sukhbir Kaur MSc
(Psychiatric Nursing)

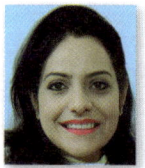

Shailza Sharma MSc
(Psychiatric Nursing)

"I admire the efforts of the authors to organize the content in an understandable manner for nursing students as this is a new subject in the curriculum. The book contains all the aspects of forensic nursing with needed figures and diagrams."

Contributors and Reviewers

Abey Varughese PhD MBA
Professor-cum-Principal
Sharbati College of Nursing
Mahendragarh, Haryana, India

Akbar Nawaz MSc(N)
Vice-Principal
Graphic Era College of Nursing
Dehradun, Uttarakhand, India

Anil Kumar Purvia PhD
Principal
Siddhartha Nursing Education and
Research Institute
Dehradun, Uttarakhand, India

Anjana Williams PhD
Principal
Himalaya College of Nursing
Patna, Bihar, India

Ankur Pathania MSc(N)
Principal
DRD College of Nursing and Pharmacy
Rajbagh, Kathua, Jammu and Kashmir, India

Anoop Sandhu PhD
Professor-cum-Principal
SBDS College of Nursing
Ratia, Haryana, India

Anureet MSc(N)
Nursing Tutor
College of Nursing
Dayanand Medical College and Hospital
Malakpur, Ludhiana, Punjab, India

Arti MSc(N)
Assistant Professor
Amity College of Nursing
Gurugram, Haryana, India

Asha Chacko PhD
Principal
Sunrise College of Nursing
Udaipur, Rajasthan, India

Baba Vajrala PhD
Principal
Birender Singh College of Nursing
Jind, Haryana, India

Balbir Yadav PhD
Associate Professor
Government College of Nursing
Safidon, Jind, Haryana, India

S Balamani Bose MSc(N) PGDCA
Principal
Government College of Nursing
LLRM Medical College
Meerut, Uttar Pradesh, India

Bharat MSc(N)
Associate Professor
Savitri Jindal Institute of Nursing
Hisar, Haryana, India

Bhaskar Bhatt MSc(N)
Counsellor
College of Nursing
Government Medical College
Rudrapur, Uttarakhand, India

Bhuneshwari Dewangan PhD
Principal
Shri Chandra Nursing College
Bhilai, Chhattisgarh, India

Chandra Prakash Dekhawat PhD
Professor-cum-Vice Principal
Ananta College of Nursing
Rajsamand, Rajasthan, India

Contributors and Reviewers

Charlotte Ranadive MSc (Psychiatric Nursing)
Vice-Principal and Professor
Army College of Nursing
Jalandhar, Punjab, India

Deepika Khakha MSc(N) PhD
Associate Professor
College of Nursing AIIMS, New Delhi, India
Nursing Advisor
Ministry of Health and Family Welfare

Dorjee Dolker PhD
Associate Professor
Graphic Era College of Nursing
Dehradun, Uttarakhand, India

Govind Gaurav Pandey MSc(N)
Counsellor
Government Nursing College
Haldwani, Uttarakhand, India

Gurjeet Kaur MSc(N)
Associate Professor
Sukhjinder College of Nursing
Gurdaspur, Punjab, India

Gurpreet Kaur PhD
Professor-cum-Officiating Principal
Narayan Swami College of Nursing
Dehradun, Uttarakhand, India

Harleen Kaur PhD
Vice-Principal
CKD International Nursing College
Amritsar, Punjab, India

Heena MSc(N)
Associate Professor
Graphic Era College of Nursing
Dehradun, Uttarakhand, India

Hemant Tak PhD
Principal
Mass College of Nursing
Udaipur, Rajasthan, India

Imtiyaz Beg PhD
Professor/Principal
Choudhary Nursing College
Rajgarh, Churu, Rajasthan, India

Indra Devi Moza PhD
Principal
Acharya Shri Chander College of Nursing Education
Sidhra, Jammu, Jammu and Kashmir, India

Jamsheeda Zaroo PhD
Principal
Ramzaan College of Nursing and Paramedical Sciences
Galander, Pampore, Jammu and Kashmir, India

Jashandeep Kaur PhD
Professor
CKD International Nursing College
Amritsar, Punjab, India

Jasleen Kaur Brar MSc(N)
Assistant Professor
College of Nursing
Dayanand Medical College and Hospital
Malakpur, Ludhiana, Punjab, India

Jibi Sebastian MBA (Hospital Management)
Director
Sai College of Nursing
Dehradun, Uttarakhand, India

Jitendra Khatri MSc(N)
Principal
Mai Khadija Institute of Nursing Sciences
Jodhpur, Rajasthan, India

Jitendra Pujari PhD
Vice-Principal
Venkateshwara College of Nursing
Umarda, Udaipur, Rajasthan, India

Jitika Royal MSc(N)
Content Strategist
Jaypee Brothers Medical Publishers
New Delhi, India

Jyoti MSc(N)
Associate Professor
KVM Nursing College
Rohtak, Haryana, India

Jyoti Sarin MSc (Pediatric Nursing) PhD
Dean–Faculty of Nursing
Director–Principal
MM College of Nursing
Mullana, Ambala, Haryana, India

Kamlesh Kumari Sharma PhD FCRMEBM
Principal and Professor
Institute of Nursing Education and Research
College of Nursing AIIMS
Bathinda, Punjab, India

Contributors and Reviewers

Kelly Berishaj DNP RN ACNS-BC AFN-C SANE-A
Forensic Nursing Program Director
Oakland University School of Nursing
Rochester, MI, USA

Kushanpreet Kaur MSc(N)
Demonstrator
University College of Nursing
Faridkot, Punjab, India

Lalita Bhat PhD
Principal
Maharaja Agrasen Nursing College
Bahadurgarh, Haryana, India

Loyd Melwyn Mendonca MSc(N)
Associate Professor
Maharaja Agrasen Nursing College
Bahadurgarh, Haryana, India

Mahendra Kumar Yadav MSc(N) MA (Sociology)
Principal
Yamuna Institute of Nursing
Yamuna Nagar, Haryana, India

Mavitha VG MSc(N)
Assistant Professor
Maharaja Agrasen Nursing College
Bahadurgarh, Haryana, India

Meena Rani PhD
Vice-Principal
College of Nursing
RP Indraprastha Institute of Medical Sciences
Bastara, Karnal, Haryana, India

Molly Saldanha MSc (Cardiothoracic Nursing)
Principal and Professor
Kanachur College of Nursing Sciences
Deralakatte, Mangaluru, India

Monika Sangar MSc(N)
Nursing Tutor
College of Nursing
Dayanand Medical College and Hospital
Malakpur, Ludhiana, Punjab, India

Nandeibam Phajaton Chanu MSc(N) PhD Scholar
Principal
Muzaffarnagar Nursing Institute
Muzaffarnagar, Uttar Pradesh, India

Pawan Kumar MSc(N) PhD
Professor and Head
Department of Medical Surgical Nursing
Maharaja Agrasen Nursing College
Bahadurgarh, Haryana, India
TNAI-Haryana State Branch Committee Member

Praveen Kumar Arora MD MBA-HA
Professor and Head
Department of Forensic Medicine and Toxicology
Sri Aurobindo Medical College and PG Institute
Indore, Madhya Pradesh, India

Pravin Prakash MSc(N) PGDHI
Principal
Metro College of Nursing
Greater Noida, Uttar Pradesh, India

Preeti Pal MSc(N)
Assistant Professor
Maa Ambey Institute of Nursing and Paramedical Sciences
Almora, Uttarakhand, India

Priya R PhD
Principal
Savitri Jindal Institute of Nursing
Model Town, Hisar, Haryana, India

Priyanka Sharma MSc(N)
Assistant Professor
Sai College of Nursing
Dehradun, Uttarakhand, India

Priyanka Yadav BSc(N)
Assistant Nursing Superintendent
All India Institute of Medical Sciences
Rishikesh, Uttarakhand, India

Promila Pandey PhD
Principal
Maharaja Agrasen College of Nursing
Agroha, Haryana, India

Poonam Paul MSc(N)
Professor-cum-In-Charge Principal
Government Nursing College
Gandhinagar, Jammu, Jammu and Kashmir, India

Rachna Gardia MSc(N)
Principal
Oriental College of Nursing
Manikpur, Korba, Chhattisgarh, India

Contributors and Reviewers

Rahina Banoo MSc(N)
Assistant Professor
Venkateshwar College of Nursing
Udaipur, Rajasthan, India

Rajesh Kumar MSc(N) PhD INC Consortium FAIMER Fellow, Fellow Johns Hopkins, USA
Associate Professor
College of Nursing AIIMS
Rishikesh, Uttarakhand, India

Rajkumari Gunisana Devi MSc(N)
Associate Professor
Government College of Nursing
Safidon, Jind, Haryana, India

R Revanth MSc(N)
Principal
Bansal College of Nursing
Hanumangarh, Rajasthan, India

Safiya MSc(N)
Tutor
Government College of Nursing and Paramedical Sciences
Srinagar, Jammu and Kashmir, India

Shailza Sharma MSc (Psychiatric Nursing)
Associate Professor
College of Nursing
Dayanand Medical College and Hospital, Ludhiana, Punjab, India

Shivani Dhasmana MSc(N)
Associate Professor
Graphic Era College of Nursing
Dehradun, Uttarakhand, India

Shridhar KV MSc (Medical Surgical) PhD Scholar
Principal
College of Nursing
Adesh University
Bathinda, Punjab, India

Subhasankari G PhD
Principal
National College of Nursing
Barwala, Hisar, Haryana, India

Sukhbir Kaur MSc (Psychiatric Nursing)
Associate Professor
SGRD College of Nursing
Amritsar, Punjab, India

Suman Bodh MSc(N)
Principal
GNM Training School
Dr Rajendra Prasad Government Medical College
Kangra, Tanda, Himachal Pradesh, India

Sumaya Sidiqi MSc(N)
Assistant Professor
Government College of Nursing
Dewan Bagh, Srinagar, Jammu and Kashmir, India

Swapna Melchisedec MSc (Psychiatric Nursing) PhD
Principal and Professor
Mohan Dai Oswal College of Nursing
Ludhiana, Punjab, India

Upendra Veerwal MSc(N)
Lecturer
Geetanjali College of Nursing
Udaipur, Rajasthan, India

Usha Singh MSc (Psychiatric Nursing) MSc (Counselling and Family therapy) PhD (Psychology)
Principal and Professor
College of Nursing
Christian Medical College
Ludhiana, Punjab, India

Vibha Speciality-MCH
Professor
State Institute of Nursing Paramedical Sciences
Badal, Faridkot, Punjab, India

Vipin Kumar Pillai MSc(N) PhD
Principal
Udaipur College of Nursing
Udaipur, Rajasthan, India

Yassar Khan MSc(N)
Tutor
Government Nursing College
Kishtwar, Jammu and Kashmir, India

Foreword

A New Era of Nursing Practice: The Science of Forensic Nursing

Forensic Nursing Science is a body of diverse and collective knowledge drawn from the application of the forensic sciences to the nursing process in public or legal proceedings. These areas include the physiological, psychological, and behavioral sciences relevant to medico-legal matters. Forensic nurses are licensed, registered nurses, qualified in academics, and the discipline of *Forensic Nursing Science*. Forensic nurse examiners (FNE) serve as a clinical liaison to medical professionals and legal agencies supplementing the need for vital forensic services to provide fair and equal justice as questions of innocence or criminality arise. The FNE, as the first point of contact in the immediate post-trauma period, is in an ideal position to gather information, recover forensically significant evidence, and report crime-related trauma as required by law. These responsibilities are applicable to the forensic nurse in each subspecialty of the various roles within the science of forensic nursing. The sexual assault nurse examiner (SANE) has become the primary face of forensic nursing roles worldwide. However, forensic nurses within the discipline's members are active in a wide range of subspecialties including pediatric and adult forensic health, psychiatric mental health, nursing jurisprudence, forensic nurse academicians, and other areas where forensic assessments are analyzed.

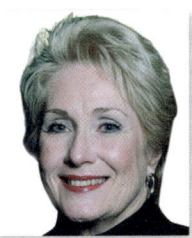

Students of forensic nursing will find this textbook *Fundamentals of Forensic Nursing and Introduction to Indian Laws* rich with insight, enlightenment, and advancement into the realms of forensic nursing roles and skills practiced at the center of human violence: sexual assault, intentional vs non-intentional trauma, interpersonal violence, child, and elder abuse, and associated deaths. Each chapter addresses issues not previously included in traditional nursing education but has become the latest state-of-the-art knowledge in contemporary nursing knowledge to prepare the forensic nurses of the future. This incisive text is strongly recommended to those who work with the FNEs to understand their role and how to form a working partnership.

I wish to express my gratitude to those of the Indian Nursing Council for formally recognizing Forensic Nursing Science as an essential discipline, to Dr RK Gorea, the *Indian Father of Forensic Nursing*, and to the authors of this significant text, Gautam Biswas and Triza Jiwan. It is an exciting point in history as these individuals bring India to the forefront of victim-centered, trauma-informed practice through the application of the forensic sciences to nursing practice in keeping with the progressive heritage of the Indian people and health of the nation.

Virginia A Lynch MSN RN FCNS DF-IAFN DF-AAFS FAAN Fulbright Scholar (Punjab, India)
Distinguished Fellow, American Academy of Forensic Sciences
Founding President, International Association of Forensic Nurses

Preface

It gives us immense pleasure to introduce the book *Fundamentals of Forensic Nursing and Introduction to Indian Laws*. This book aims to provide the forensic nurses with the basic understanding of the various aspects that this discipline offers and the fundamentals of Indian laws. This book deals with various duties of forensic nurses in the hospital and community settings in association with the law enforcement agencies. The text contains cases studies, extensive diagrams, flowcharts, images, along with MCQs and practice assessment questions at the end of the chapters that will make the readers sail through the examination and provide them with clear concepts to deal with any practical issues coming in their way. A separate section with case study worksheets provides the readers with additional opportunity to widen their horizon on this subject. For their practical aspects, few common forms and proformas have been appended.

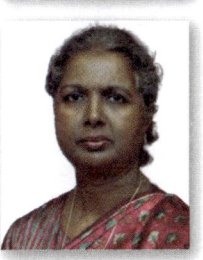

Forensic nursing is a growing field and is taking its baby steps in Indian subcontinent. With the current implementation of INC's curriculum, albeit limited, the nursing graduates will have an exposure to the various duties of a forensic nurse regarding patients involved in medico-legal cases, such as violence, trauma, death, abuses, and accidents. They will understand the importance of documentation of injuries, collecting and preserving the biological evidences from such cases because of their training and education. Forensic nursing is vital to patient care, and nurses in any clinical setting will use the forensic skills in screening, assessing and treating patients. They will also help in guiding the clinicians in cases where the evidences are required to be preserved and subsequently helping the judiciary in getting justice for the victims.

It is our sincere hope that the book will be useful for the undergraduate and postgraduate [MSc (Forensic Nursing)] nursing students.

Gautam Biswas
Triza Jiwan

Acknowledgments

Writing a book is harder than we thought and more rewarding than we could have ever imagined. This work would not have been possible without the constant support and guidance of numerous individuals.

We wish to express our sincere thanks and gratitude to all our contributors and reviewers, and in particular Ms Virginia Lynch, Dr Kelly Berishaj, Ms Molly Saldanha, Dr Jyoti Sarin, Dr Kamlesh Kumari Sharma, Dr Usha Singh, Dr Swapna Melchisedec, Dr Deepika Khakha, Ms Charlotte Ranadive, Dr Rajesh Kumar, Ms Sukhbir Kaur, Ms Shailza Sharma, Ms Jasleen Kaur Brar, Ms Monika Sangar, and Ms Anureet, for reviewing the manuscript and providing valuable suggestions.

We are thankful to Dr Rakesh K Gorea, Dr Viswakanth B and Dr Murugesa Bharathi, for their invaluable suggestions, help and advice. Dr Virendar Pal Singh, Professor, FMT, DMCH deserves special appreciation for providing positive feedback and valuable suggestions. Special thanks go to Mr Kuljeet Singh, Mr Luv Sharma and Mr Amit Kumar, for their help in typing and checking the manuscript without any complaints.

Sincere thanks and gratitude goes to Shri Bipin Gupta, Secretary, Managing Society, DMCH; Dr Sandeep Puri, Principal, DMCH; Dr GS Wander, Vice-Principal, DMCH, and Dr Sandeep Kausal, Dean Academics, DMCH, for their continuous support, motivation, encouragement and invaluable suggestions.

It is with greatest pleasure and pride we acknowledge the wholehearted encouragement, cooperation, help and support provided by Shri Jitendar P Vij (Group Chairman), Mr Ankit Vij (Managing Director) and Mr MS Mani (Group President) of M/s Jaypee Brothers Medical Publishers (P) Ltd, New Delhi, India.

We also thank Dr Madhu Choudhary (Director–Educational Publishing), Ms Pooja Bhandari [Director–Production (Books and Journals)], Ms Sunita Katla (Executive Assistant to Group Chairman and Publishing Manager), Mr Ajay Sharma [DGM–Production (Books and Journals)], Ms Jitika Royal (Content Strategist), Mr Rajesh Sharma (Production Coordinator), Ms Seema Dogra (Cover Visualizer), Mr Vakil Khan (Proofreader), and Mr Jagvir Singh Tomar (Typesetter), Mr Manoj Pahuja (Graphic Designer) of M/s Jaypee Brothers Medical Publishers (P) Ltd, New Delhi, India. Special thanks to Mr Rishi Sharma (Regional Business Development Manager).

We will be failing in our duty if we do not acknowledge the sincere support, sacrifices and contributions of our families at every step of this journey. We are eternally grateful to the Almighty God, for providing this opportunity and strength to accomplish this herculean task.

Last but not the least, we wish to offer apologies to all our colleagues and friends whose names have been omitted inadvertently, for without their constant support, encouragement and well wishes the book would not have been completed.

Contents

SECTION I: Introduction to Forensic Nursing and Indian Laws

1. **Introduction to Forensic Science 3**
   - Definitions 3
   - History of Forensic Science 4
   - Development of Forensic Science in India 5
   - Importance and Scope of Forensic Science 9
   - Forensic Science Laboratory 10

2. **Violence and Sexual Abuse 17**
   - Definition of Violence 17
   - Nature of Violence 19
   - Interpersonal Violence 19
   - Epidemiology 22
   - Sexual Violence 23
   - Child Abuse 26

3. **Introduction to Forensic Nursing and Nursing Jurisprudence 30**
   - Definition 30
   - Scope—Areas of Practice and Subspecialties 32
   - Role and Responsibilities of Forensic Nurse 34
   - Nursing Jurisprudence 35
   - Indian Nursing Council 35
   - State Nursing Council 37
   - Ethical Principles 38
   - Code of Ethics for Nurses 39
   - Code of Professional Conduct for Nurses 40
   - Code of Ethics for Forensic Nurses 41

4. **Comprehensive Forensic Nursing Care of Victim and Family 47**
   - Forensic Team Members and their Roles in Crime Scene 48
   - Comprehensive Care of Victim and Family 51

5. **Comprehensive Forensic Nursing Care of Survivor of Sexual Assault 61**
   - Comprehensive Care of Sexual Assault Survivor 62
   - Informed Consent 65
   - The Medico-legal Interview 66
   - Physical Examination 68
   - Opinion 70
   - Role of Forensic Nurse Examiner 71
   - Psychosocial Care 71
   - Cultural and Spiritual Aspects 72
   - Legal Aspects 72
   - Punishment of Rape 73
   - Expert Witness 74

6. **Collection and Preservation of Evidence 78**
   - Types of Evidence 79
   - Principle of Exchange 80
   - Consent 80
   - Guidelines for Collecting and Preserving Evidence 80
   - Collection and Preservation of Evidence 81
   - Labelling of Evidence 90
   - Chain of Custody 90
   - Documentation of Evidence 91
   - Forwarding of Biological Samples 91

7. **Fundamental Rights and Human Rights Commission** 94
   - Indian Constitution 94
   - Rights of Victim 96
   - Rights of Accused 97
   - National Human Rights Commission 99

8. **Indian Judicial System and Laws** 104
   - Sources of Laws and Law-making Powers 104
   - Indian Penal Code 106
   - Criminal Procedure Code 108
   - Indian Evidence Act 110
   - The Protection of Children From Sexual Offenses Act, 2012 111

SECTION II: Basic Forensic Medicine

9. **Legal Procedures and Nursing Jurisprudence** 119
   - Inquest 119
   - Dying Declaration 120
   - Summons 120
   - Medical Evidence 121
   - Procedure of Recording of Evidence 122
   - Professional Negligence 123
   - Consent 124
   - Acts Related to Nursing Practice 126

10. **Injuries** 129
    - Abrasion 129
    - Bruise/Contusion 130
    - Lacerated Wound/Laceration 131
    - Incised Wound 132
    - Stab Wound 133
    - Chop Wound 134
    - Hesitation Cuts 134
    - Patterned Injuries 134
    - Self-inflicted Injury/Fabricated Injuries 135
    - Firearms Injury 135
    - Thermal Burns 137
    - Electrical Injury 138

11. **Medico-legal Autopsy** 140

12. **Thanatology** 143
    - Cause of Death, Mechanism of Death, and Manner of Death 145
    - Death Certificate 145
    - Mode of Death 146
    - Sudden Death 146
    - Changes after Death 146
    - Algor Mortis 147
    - Rigor Mortis 149
    - Conditions Simulating Rigor Mortis 149
    - PM Staining 150
    - Decomposition/Putrefaction 151
    - Determination of Time Since Death 152

13. **Identification** 155
    - Examination of Skeletal Remains 155
    - Scars 160
    - Tattoo Marks 161
    - Dactylography 162
    - DNA Fingerprinting 163

14. **Forced Anal Intercourse** 165
    - Opinion 165

15. **Forensic Psychiatry** 166
    - Civil Responsibility of Insane 168
    - Criminal Responsibility of Insane 169
    - Feigned Insanity/Malingering 169

16. **Asphyxial Conditions** 171

17. **Forensic Toxicology** 176

Case Study Worksheets 181
Hint 191
Appendix 195
References and Further Reading 203
Index 207

Syllabus

PLACEMENT: V SEMESTER

THEORY: 1 Credit (20 hours)

DESCRIPTION: This course is designed to help students to know the importance of forensic science in total patient care and to recognize forensic nursing as a specialty discipline in professional nursing practice.

COMPETENCIES: On completion of the course, the students will be able to:
1. Identify forensic nursing as an emerging specialty in healthcare and nursing practice
2. Explore the history and scope of forensic nursing practice
3. Identify forensic team, role and responsibilities of forensic nurse in total care of victim of violence and in preservation of evidence
4. Develop basic understanding of the Indian judicial system and legal procedures

COURSE OUTLINE
(T – Theory)

Unit	Time (Hrs)	Learning outcomes	Content	Teaching/learning activities	Assessment methods	Page No.
I	3 (T)	Describe the nature of forensic science and discus issues concerning violence	**Forensic Science** • Definition • History • Importance in medical science • Forensic Science Laboratory **Violence** • Definition • Epidemiology • Source of data **Sexual abuse—child and women**	• Lecture cum discussion • Visit to Regional Forensic Science Laboratory	• Quiz—MCQ • Write visit report	3 17 26
II	2 (T)	Explain concepts of forensic nursing and scope of practice for forensic nurse	**Forensic Nursing** • Definition • History and development • Scope—setting of practice, areas of practice and subspecialties • Ethical issues • Roles and responsibilities of nurse • INC and SNC acts	Lecture cum discussion	• Short answer • Objective type	30

Unit	Time (Hrs)	Learning outcomes	Content	Teaching/learning activities	Assessment methods	Page No.
III	7 (T)	Identify members of forensic team and describe role of forensic nurse	**Forensic team** Members and their roles **Comprehensive forensic nursing care of victim and family** • Physical aspects • Psychosocial aspects • Cultural and spiritual aspects • Legal aspects • Assist forensic team in care beyond scope of her practice • Admission and discharge/referral/death of victim of violence • Responsibilities of nurse as a witness **Evidence preservation—role of nurses** • Observation • Recognition • Collection • Preservation • Documentation of biological and other evidence related to criminal/traumatic event • Forwarding biological samples for forensic examination	• Lecture cum discussion • Hypothetical/real case presentation • Observation of postmortem • Visit to department of forensic medicine	• Objective type • Short answer • Write report	48 51 81
IV	3 (T)	Describe fundamental rights and human rights commission	**Introduction of Indian Constitution** **Fundamental rights** **Rights of victim** **Rights of accused** **Human Rights Commission**	• Lecture cum discussion • Written assignment • Visit to prison	• Short answer • Assessment of written assignment • Write visit report	94 95 99
V	5 (T)	Explain Indian judicial system and laws	**Sources of laws and law-making powers**	Lecture cum discussion	Quiz	104
		Discuss the importance of POSCO Act	**Overview of Indian Judicial System** • JMFC (Judicial Magistrate First Class) • District • State • Apex **Civil and Criminal Case Procedures** • IPC (Indian Penal Code) • CrPC (Criminal Procedure Code) • IEA (Indian Evidence Act) **Overview of POSCO Act**	• Guided reading • Lecture cum discussion	Short answer	104 106 111

SECTION 1

Introduction to Forensic Nursing and Indian Laws

SECTION OUTLINE

1. Introduction to Forensic Science — 1
2. Violence and Sexual Abuse — 17
3. Introduction to Forensic Nursing and Nursing Jurisprudence — 30
4. Comprehensive Forensic Nursing Care of Victim and Family — 47
5. Comprehensive Forensic Nursing Care of Survivor of Sexual Assault — 61
6. Collection and Preservation of Evidence — 78
7. Fundamental Rights and Human Rights Commission — 94
8. Indian Judicial System and Laws — 104

CHAPTER 1

Introduction to Forensic Science

"Forensic scientists are not policemen. We are scientists. We deal with these matters objectively. We do not (act) on our suspicion."

— **Cyril Wecht (Forensic Pathologist)**

LEARNING OBJECTIVES

At the end of this topic, the student should be able to:
1. Define forensic science.
2. Discuss the history of forensic science.
3. Understand the importance and scope of forensic science.
4. Explain the setup of forensic science laboratory.

CASE STUDY

Mr X returned home drunk from a 12-hour shift and his wife was very angry, she started arguing for failing to deposit fees for their kids in spite of informing him thru text messages during the day. Tired and just wanting to go to sleep, he started to get irritated from the arguments. The wife got hold of a stick and attacked him all of a sudden. Mr X grabbed the stick and threw it away. She lunged forward but tripped over and injured herself. Later on, the wife came to the ER with the complaints of assault by her husband with significant injury involving her face, lip and her neck.

Q. Do you think the patient above has markers that have medico-legal implications and potential court involvement?*

*Discuss the question with your teacher/facilitator.

DEFINITIONS

Forensic science: It is the application of scientific methods and principles to questions of law.
- Any science used for the purposes of the law is considered as forensic science.
- Forensic scientists examine objects, substances (including blood/drug samples), chemicals (paints/explosives/toxins), tissue traces (hair/skin) or impressions (fingerprints/tire marks) left at the scene of crime—*a multidisciplinary subject*.

Branches of forensic science (Flowchart 1.1)

a. **Forensic nursing:** It is the application of nursing sciences to public or legal proceedings.
   - The practice of forensic nursing facilitates connections among the healthcare, social services, and criminal justice systems to assist victims, perpetrators and their families to receive assistance, services and resources.

b. **Forensic medicine (Legal medicine or State medicine):** It is the application of principle and knowledge of medical sciences

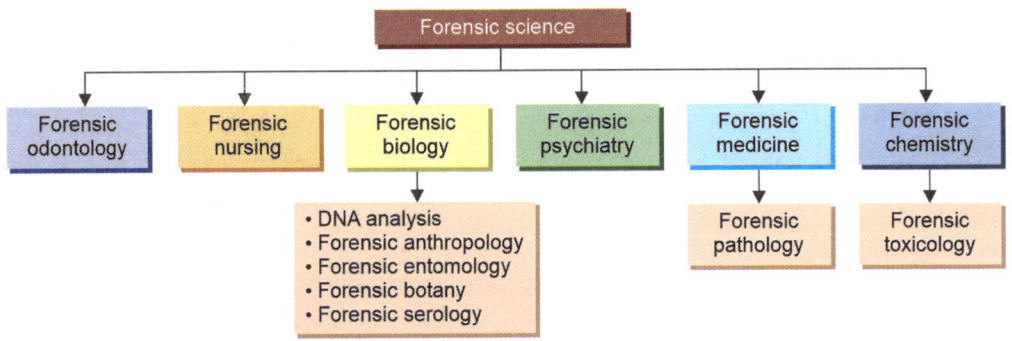

Flowchart 1.1: Forensic science—a multidisciplinary branch.

to legal purposes and legal proceedings so as to aid in the administration of justice.
- **Forensic pathology:** It is a sub discipline of forensic medicine, deals with examination of deceased persons to determine cause and manner of death (whether suicide, homicide, accident or undetermined).

c. **Forensic psychiatry:** It deals with the application of knowledge of psychiatry to aid in the administration of justice. It is subspecialty of psychiatry.

d. **Forensic odontology:** It deals with the application of dentistry to aid in the administration of justice.

e. **Forensic biology:** It is the application of biology to law enforcement. It includes sub-disciplines like forensic anthropology, forensic botany, forensic entomology, wildlife forensics and DNA forensics.
- **Forensic anthropology:** It deals with the examination of human remains or skeletons in a legal context to help determine the race, age, height, sex, and ancestry.
- **Forensic entomology:** The study of insects and other arthropods found in dead bodies to determine time since death and sometimes, cause of death.
- **Forensic serology:** Study of blood and other biological fluids in connection to the investigation of a crime. Forensic serologist may be involved in DNA analysis or bloodstain pattern analysis.

f. **Forensic chemistry:** The application of facts related to findings in chemistry to issues of law. It includes the sub-discipline forensic toxicology.
- **Forensic toxicology:** It involves analysis of body tissues and fluids to check for the presence of toxins and drugs (commonly alcohol and drugs).

g. **Forensic physics:** It is the application of physics for purposes of law. Ballistics is the sub-discipline of forensic physics.
- **Forensic ballistics:** Science which deals with the investigation of firearms, ammunition and the problems arising from their use.

> The term "forensic" is derived from the Latin word *forensic* which means "of or before the forum". In Rome, "forum" was the meeting place, where civic and legal matters used to be discussed by those with public responsibility. Thus, the origin and the very definition of "forensic science" points to its close association with the legal system.

HISTORY OF FORENSIC SCIENCE

Forensic evidence is extensively used worldwide to both convict and exonerate defendants. This is because when scientific techniques and methods are used, there is not much scope for bias or injustice. Using these techniques, crimes are detected with greater certainty and consequently, conviction rate increases. A brief history of development of forensic science is given below **(Fig. 1.1)**:
- Law-medicine problems were found written in records in Egypt, Sumer, Babylon, India and China dating 4000–3000 BC.

CHAPTER 1: Introduction to Forensic Science

- Code of Hammurabi specified by King of Babylon (about 1754 BC) is the oldest known medico-legal code.
- Hippocrates (460–377 BC), father of Western medicine discussed the lethality of wounds and contributed to the field of ethics.
- First medico-legal autopsy in history was conducted by the Roman physician Antistius who examined the body of Julius Caesar after his assassination in 44 BC.
- Chinese publication in the 13th century titled 'Hsi Yuan Lu' dealt with findings in cases of infanticide, drowning, hanging, poisoning and assault.
- Ambroise Pare (1510–1590), a French surgeon is considered the father of modern forensic pathology. He studied the effects of violent death on internal organs, and wrote *Reports in Court*, a procedure on writing of legal report in relation to medicine.
- In 1659, the Merriam-Webster Dictionary officially recognized and printed the word 'forensic'. The term has been used in medical writings for many years, but until then was not considered to be an 'official' word in English language.
- In the 18th century, Italian anatomist Giovanni Morgagni (1682–1771) dissected the dead bodies and compared the alterations in their organs with the symptoms of the diseases that had caused death.
- Swedish chemist, Carl Wilhelm Scheele, first developed a chemical test to detect arsenic in dead body in 1773.

1800s

- Tests developed for the forensic analysis of the presence of blood.
- Scotland Yard's Henry Goddard became the first in 1835 to connect a bullet to a murder weapon using physical analysis.
- In 1836, Scottish chemist, James Marsh developed a test for arsenic detection which was used successfully in a murder trial at that time.
- Teichman test used for the determination of presence of hemoglobin of blood.
- Photography used for the first time for the identification of criminals and documentation of evidence and crime scenes.
- In 1879, Alphonse Bertillon developed a scientific system of personal identification using a series of bodily measurements (anthropometry). It was later replaced by fingerprints.
- In 1885, first three-dimensional facial reconstruction made by Welcker and His from cranial remains.
- In 1890, Sir Francis Galton systemized the use of fingerprints and its use for identification.
- In 1897, the world's first fingerprint Bureau established in Kolkata.

1900s

- In 1900, Karl Landsteiner discovered the ABO blood groups.
- Calvin Goddard created the comparison microscope for bullet comparison in the 1920s.
- In 1935, Glaister and Brash used the skull superimposition technique to solve the Ruxton case.
- In 1958, Robert Borkenstein developed the Breathalyzer for alcohol tests.
- In 1971, Eva Engvall and Peter Perlman independently invented the ELISA test.
- In 1974, Saint Luke's Hospital of Kansas City (SLH) opened the first private rape treatment center in the US.
- In 1984, Alec Jeffreys pioneered the use of DNA profiling for identification.
- The polymerase chain reaction (PCR) was discovered by Kary B Mullis in 1985 (got Nobel Prize in chemistry).
- **2001:** Technology speeded up DNA profiling—from 6–8 weeks to 1–2 days.

DEVELOPMENT OF FORENSIC SCIENCE IN INDIA

- Manusmriti (3102 BC), a famous treatise where rules for marriage, punishment for adultery, incest and sexual offenses were formulated.

44 BC
Roman physician, Antistius, performed the first officially recorded autopsy on the assassinated body of Roman ruler, Julius Ceaser

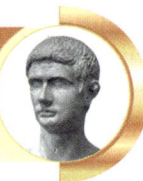

13th century
The book 'Hsi Yuan Lu' by Song Ci in China became the earliest available literature to deal with medico-legal issues

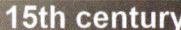

15th century
French surgeon Ambroise Paré, the father of modern forensic pathology did methodical studies on the effects of violent death on internal organs

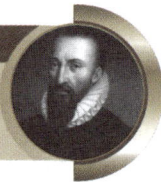

1773
Swedish chemist, Carl Wilhelm Scheele developed a chemical test to detect arsenic in dead bodies

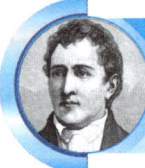

18th century
Italian anatomist Giovanni Morgagni dissected the dead bodies to find the cause of death

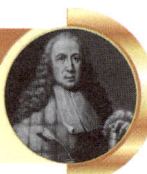

1814
Mathieu Orfila, the father of forensic toxicology, published the first scientific treatise on the detection of poison

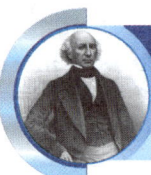

1835
Henry Goddard became the first to connect a bullet to a murder weapon using physical analysis

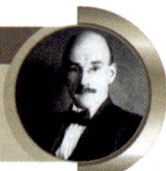

1879
Alphonse Bertillon developed a scientific system of personal identification

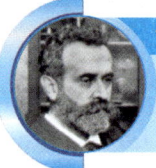

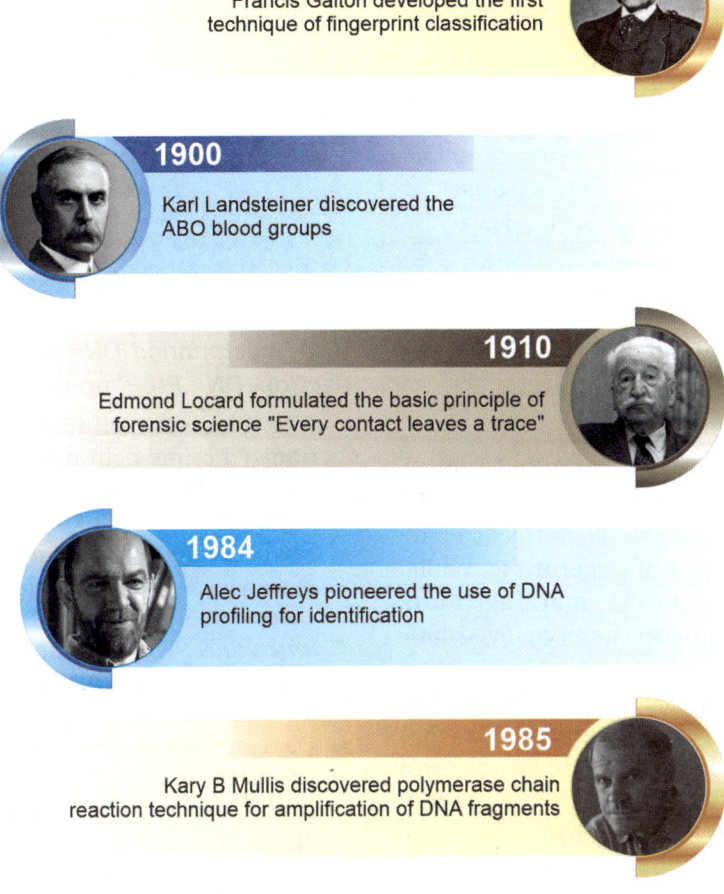

Fig. 1.1: History of forensic science.

- Kautilya's Arthashastra (2300 years ago) discussed the detection and investigation of crime and administration of justice.
- Charaka Samhita, the first treatise on Indian medicine dates back to 100–200 BC.
- The first recorded medico-legal autopsy performed in India was by Edward Buckley in 1693 at Madras (now Chennai) on a suspected case of arsenic poisoning.
- The first Chemical Examiner's Laboratory was set up at the then Madras Presidency in 1849.
- Anthropometric Bureau, for maintaining anthropometric records of criminals, was established in 1892 at Kolkata.
- Dr Jaising Modi was the first to handle cases of medico-legal nature and published the first book in India 'Forensic Medicine'.
- In 1930, a ballistic laboratory was setup under the Kolkata police to deal with the examination of firearms.
- The first Central Finger Print Bureau was established in 1905 at Shimla.
- The Indian Academy of Forensic Sciences was established in the year 1960.
- CFSL Hyderabad established the first Cyber Forensic laboratory in 2000.

Who's who in forensic science	
Mother of forensic nursing	Virginia Lynch
Father of forensic science	Bernard Spilsbury
Father of blood grouping	Karl Landsteiner
Father of forensic toxicology	Mathieu Orfila
Father of ballistics	Calvin Goddard
Father of anthropometry	Alphonse Bertillon
Father of fingerprinting	Francis Galton
Father of DNA fingerprinting	Alec Jeffreys
Father of DNA fingerprinting in India	Lalji Singh

In 1912, a woman was found murdered in her parents' house, and the prime suspect, her boyfriend had a strong alibi—four men testified that they had been playing cards with the suspect at the time of the murder. Locard analyzed the dead body and determined the cause of death to be strangulation. He then scraped under the suspect's fingernails and found a pink residue, which he identified to be women's makeup. Makeup was not mass-produced at the time, and was traced back to its vendor. Locard matched the fingernail residue to the victim's beauty shop, and the boyfriend was arrested. In his confession, he revealed that he had set the clock back an hour at the card game where the others had vouched for his presence.

Major Milestones in the History of Forensic Science

Fingerprint Analysis

- Fingerprint analysis resulted from the groundbreaking theory established by Henry Faulds and William Herschel from the uniqueness of fingerprints. William Herschel found that markings on the fingertips of a person never changed during his lifetime.
- It was Francis Galton and Edward Henry who actually implemented Herschel's fingerprinting practices in criminal investigations.
- Sir Francis Galton systematized the classification of fingerprints.
- Sir Edward Henry used the direction, flow, pattern and other characteristics in fingerprints to develop his own system of fingerprint analysis.
- A fingerprint match is widely accepted as *most reliable evidence of identification*.

Locard's Exchange Principle

- Locard is famous for his *exchange principle*, which states that whenever there is contact between two items, there will be an exchange of material i.e., "very contact leaves a trace".
- This principle now forms the basis for much of forensic science, taking into account fingerprints, blood samples, hair analysis, and other forms of trace evidence.

DNA Fingerprinting (DNA Typing, DNA Identification, DNA Profiling or Genetic Typing)

- DNA analysis techniques have revolutionized crime fighting and have helped convict the guilty and exonerate the innocent.
- DNA profiling is a technique that is capable of distinguishing every individual, with the exception of *identical/monozygotic twins and clones*. This technique identifies an individual at molecular level and is based on the principles of inheritance.
- DNA profiling has become one of the most valuable tool in modern investigation, such as human identification in mass disasters, paternity and maternity disputes, identification of victim and suspect in rape and murder cases, child swapping in hospitals, identification of deceased, organ transplantation and immigration.

- In 1984, Sir Alec Jeffreys, a British geneticist accidentally found that DNA showed both similarities and differences between family members.
- In 1986, the local police were investigating the rape and murder of two girls—one that occurred in 1983, and the other in 1986.
- Blood and saliva samples were collected from more than 4,000 men in the area, but the method identified only one match for both crime scenes—the DNA of Colin Pitchfork. But more importantly, it exonerated Richard Buckland, a man who had been the prime suspect till then (having falsely confessed) and would have served life in prison if not for DNA fingerprinting.
- Colin Pitchfork was found guilty of the rape and murder of two girls, and became the first person to be convicted of a crime based on DNA profiling.

IMPORTANCE AND SCOPE OF FORENSIC SCIENCE

Importance of Forensic Science

- Forensic science is the use of scientific methods or expertise to investigate crimes or examine evidence that might be presented in a court of law so as to prosecute the perpetrators of crime or acquit/free an innocent person charged of a crime.
- Forensic science plays a pivotal role in the legal system. Without the application of forensic science, conviction of criminals would have been impossible, unless an eyewitness is present.
- A diverse pool of forensic scientists and forensic tools go into the investigation of a criminal act. For instance, forensic medicine specialists are skilled at determining the cause of a death by performing autopsies. An autopsy helps establish the cause and manner of death through the crime scene examination, examination of body, weapons found at the scene, body fluids and tissues.
- Forensic scientists analyze evidence (fingerprints, blood, hair, etc.) collected from the crime scene to identify suspects. Additionally, forensic professionals use image modification tools to search for criminals absconding from the law for a long time. This tool enables them to digitally age a photograph to understand how the individual would look at aging.
- Forensic scientists play an important role in the justice delivery system because their opinion is given more weightage and consideration by the judges. They must be accurate and honest when reporting their analysis results, even if errors have occurred.

> **Legal aspects**
> a. If it is proved that the forensic scientist caused disappearance of evidence or gave false evidence with the intention of protecting the accused, then punishment is imprisonment up to 7 years depending upon the nature of offense (**Sec 201 IPC**). In this case, the onus of proving a nondeliberate omission would lie on the forensic scientist.
>
> Contd....

> Contd....
> b. If he conceals the information, he is liable to be prosecuted under **Sec. 202 IPC** (imprisonment up to 6 months with/without fine).
> c. If he gives false information during judicial proceedings, he is liable to be charged under **Sec. 193 IPC** (punishment for false evidence—imprisonment up to 7 years and fine).
>
> **Real life forensics**
> - Ted Bundy from Florida, US, a serial killer who kidnapped and killed many women was convicted by his distinctive bite mark (due to his crooked teeth) on one of his victims. Fabric threads from his car were also found on another victim.
> - Bruno Hauptmann from New Jersey, US kidnapped Charles Lindberg's baby in 1932 and was paid a ransom of $50,000. The baby was found dead shortly thereafter. Police tracked the numbers on the money paid in the ransom to find Hauptmann, then matched his handwriting to the ransom note to convict him.
> - In another case, 'snarge' (which is crushed bird gut resulting from collision of an airplane and a bird) was sent for analysis. Deer DNA was identified on the plane that had a strike at 1,500 ft which is not possible. Forensic feather analysis identified the bird as a black vulture which may had eaten a deer remains seen in its stomach.

Scope of Forensic Science

- There are several career options in the area of forensic science. Most of the forensic science candidates are hired by government agencies. Many legal firms and private investigators also hire forensic experts to strengthen their investigations and cases. There is a lot of demand for highly qualified and trained forensic science experts in India.
- Forensic science, as discussed earlier, comprises a diverse array of disciplines, from crime scene and DNA analysis to anthropology and wildlife forensics. Some of the areas where forensic science experts are employed are:
    - Forensic science laboratories (FSLs)
    - Research and analysis
    - Police department
    - Central bureau of investigation (CBI)
    - Intelligence bureau (IB)
    - Hospitals

- Legal firms
- Universities
- Defense/army
- Private detectives
- Banks/Insurance firms

Few forensic science careers are discussed below:

a. **Forensic science laboratory:** There are many crime labs or forensic laboratories across India which employs forensic scientists to analyze evidence recovered from a crime scene.
b. **Crime scene investigators:** Crime scenes are analyzed by forensic experts who are highly trained and specialized, and whose sole duty is to investigate and process crime scenes.
c. **Death scenes investigators:** They are attended by coroners, medical examiners, or other trained death investigators, depending on jurisdiction (not in India).
d. **Forensic medicine experts:** Forensic medicine experts are specialized medical doctors who analyze the body, performing autopsies and determining cause and manner of death.
e. **Other forensic specialists:** There are many other forensic specialists including forensic nurses, anthropologists, entomologists, odontologists, engineers, botanists, artists, psychologists, psychiatrists, profilers and wildlife specialists, to name just a few.

FORENSIC SCIENCE LABORATORY

- The first forensic science laboratory (FSL) in India was set up at Kolkata in 1952.
- Currently, there are seven CFSLs in India—Hyderabad, Kolkata, Delhi, Chandigarh, Bhopal, Pune and Kamrup (Guwahati).
- The head of the laboratory is the director. He is supported by deputy directors who are specialists in a particular field and oversee the respective department. They are assisted by assistant director, joint scientific officer, assistant scientific officer, junior scientific assistant, lab assistant, and attendants **(Flowchart 1.2)**.
- FSL is divided into many departments/division viz. chemistry/toxicology, biology/serology, fingerprints, physics/ballistics, explosives, DNA, voice analysis, lie detection, narco-analysis, etc. **(Flowchart 1.2 and Fig. 1.2)**. Some of them are discussed below:

1. **DNA division (forensic genetics):** In this division, the biological samples such as blood, semen, saliva, hair, muscle and bone are analyzed for the identification of the individual. The DNA contained in these samples is purified to obtain a DNA profile that may link evidence found at the crime scene to an individual. In addition, DNA testing can establish parentage and can positively identify human remains. The polymerase chain reaction (PCR) is used to prepare large quantities of specific DNA region. However, DNA fingerprints are usually never used as a single piece of evidence in the court of law.
2. **Toxicology division:** This division examines and detects the poisons from body fluids, organs, etc. A toxicologist analyzes biological samples from the victims who have been poisoned accidentally or purposely, and is important in road traffic accidents (RTAs), poisoning, sexual violence, etc.
    - It provides analytical services in medico-legal death investigations (postmortem analysis), driving under intoxication (DUI) by alcohol and/or drugs and drug facilitated sexual assault.
    - Headspace gas chromatography–flame ionization detection (GC/FID)—detects ethanol and other volatile substances; ELISA screens for common classes of drugs; GC-MS confirms and quantifies drugs and their metabolites.
3. **Fingerprints division:** This division does the examination of fingerprints—whether it is development, lifting

CHAPTER 1: Introduction to Forensic Science

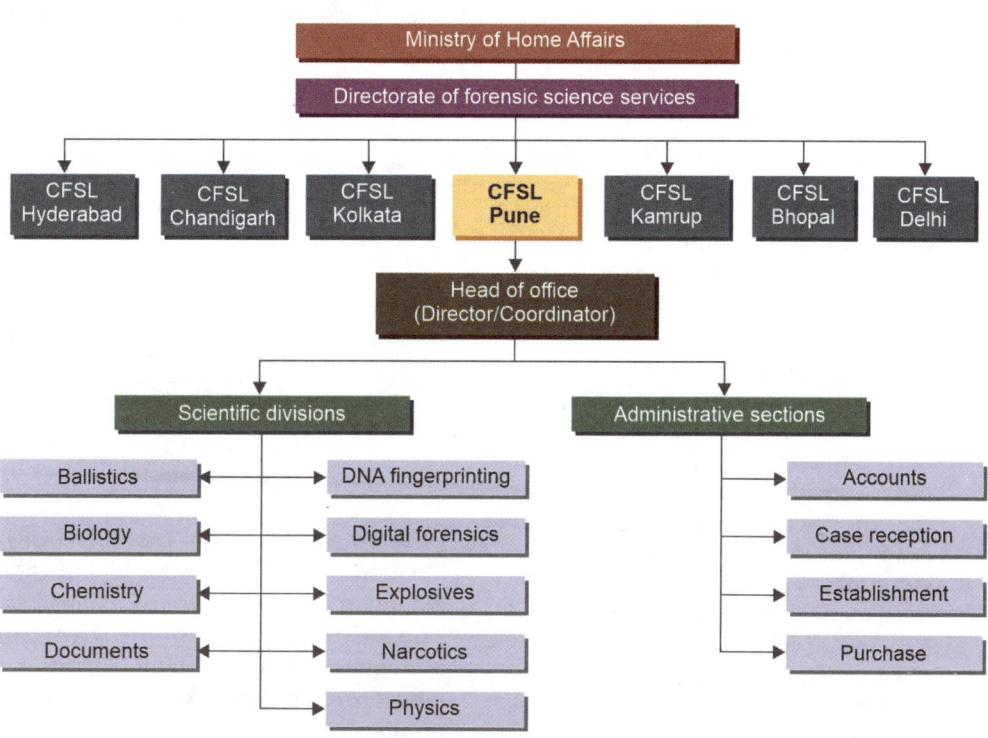

Flowchart 1.2: Various divisions of FSL lab.

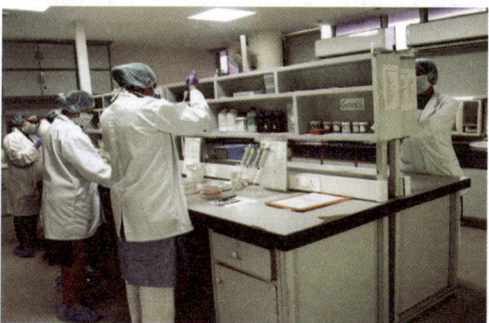

Fig. 1.2: Forensic science laboratory.
(*Courtesy:* CFSL, Chandigarh)

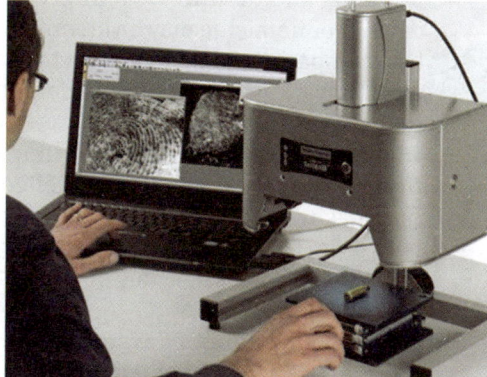

Fig. 1.3: Examination of a bullet in ballistic division.

the fingerprints from any surface for comparison, and matching.

4. **Ballistics/firearm division:** Examination of fired cartridges casings, bullets recovered from crime scene and firearm involved in gun related incident is done in this division **(Fig. 1.3)**. This department investigates incidents involving the use of a firearm, draw inferences on the exact weapon used, the distance (range of firearm, i.e., distance *from where a bullet was fired*), velocity, and angle of firing, and ultimately the shooter.

5. **Trace evidence division:** Gunshot residue analysis [done with scanning electron microscopy/energy dispersive X-ray analysis—(SEM-EDX)] for presence of lead, barium

and antimony is done in this division. Fire debris analyses for the presence of ignitable liquid residues using gas chromatography, and automotive paint analysis in hit and run cases using optical microscopy or SEM-EDX are some of the other functions.

6. **Hair and fiber analysis**: Types of trace evidence that can be analyzed for classification as to origin of the hair or the fiber, or for contents, such as use of drugs in hair analysis.
7. **Anthropology division**: In this division, examination of skeleton remains or bones is carried out for the determination of sex, race, age and other aspects. It also helps establish the time since death by identifying and examining injuries, if any.
8. **Odontology division:** Forensic odontologists aid in the comparative identification of a person by examining the development and anatomy of the teeth including any restorative dental corrections, such as filling, crowns, implants and dentures. Victims of a disaster or homicide may be identified by a comparison of their dental charts and X-rays with their previous dental records.
9. **Digital forensics:** It involves the extraction and analysis of digital evidence (such as those found in computers, hard disks, USB drives, etc.). It is mostly used in the investigation of cybercrimes.
10. **Questioned document examination:** Examination of documents, handwriting comparison, study of inks, typewriter imprints, counterfeiting, etc.

Instrumental Facilities in FSL

FSL should be equipped with SEM-EDX, PCR, skull video superimposition, XRD, FT-IR Spectrophotometer and Raman spectrophotometer, HPLC, GC-MS, LC-MS-MS, high powered microscope, photographic equipments, etc. **(Table 1.1 and Figs. 1.4A to E).**

Table 1.1: Basic instruments/equipments needed for FSL.

Division	Equipments
DNA	• Automated DNA sequencer • Real time PCR • PCR machine
Toxicology	• GC-MS • High pressure liquid chromatograph (HPLC) • High performance thin layer chromatograph (HPTLC) • UV-VIS spectrometer
Serology	• Binocular DME microscope • LEICA DMLSP microscope
Ballistic	• Ballistic comparison microscope • Atomic absorption spectrophotometer

1. **PCR:** Polymerase chain reaction (PCR) is the method of choice for the identification of human remains in forensic coursework. The PCR creates enough DNA from nanogram quantities to allow a forensic laboratory scientist to generate a DNA profile.
2. **SEM-EDX**: Scanning electron microscopy-energy dispersive X-ray analysis (SEM-EDX) provides a quick nondestructive determination of the elemental composition of the sample, such as barium, potassium, strontium and chlorine.
3. **Mass spectrometers:** Mass spectrometers are used to analyze trace evidence by determining the composition of such substances.
4. **High-powered microscope:** With the help of high-powered microscopes, the minute pieces of evidence can be viewed more clearly, and can thus be more easily identified.
5. **Various cameras and photography techniques:** Photography helps forensic nurses to document the physical injury a patient has sustained. Using alternative light, such as UV photography helps to identify cuts, scratches and bite marks found on a victim's body even before physical evidence like bruises manifest themselves on the skin.

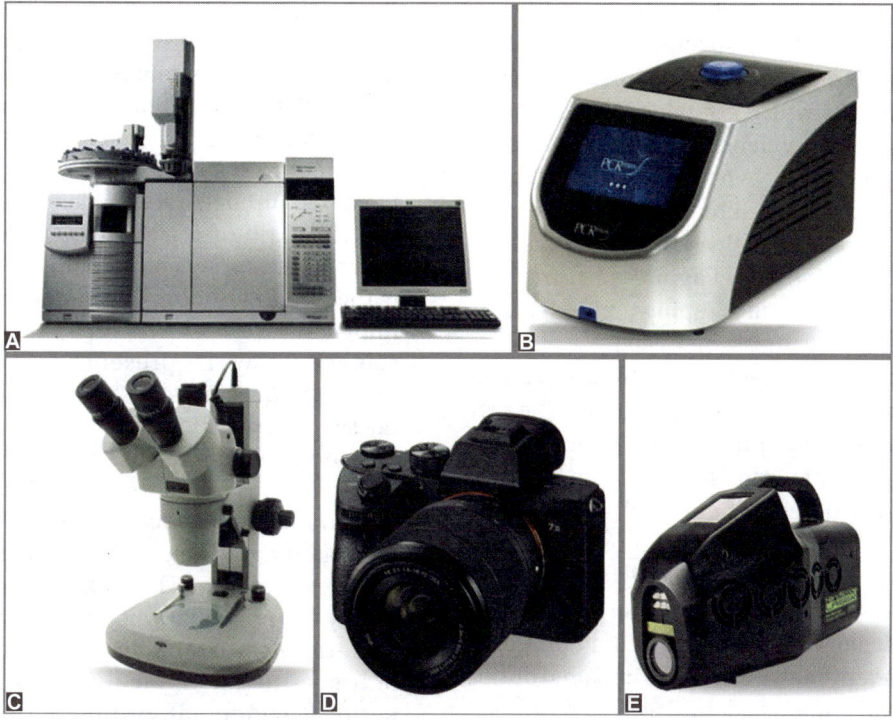

Figs. 1.4A to E: Useful tools for forensic scientists (A) GC-MS; (B) PCR; (C) High powered microscope; (D) Camera; and (E) Alternative light source.

Some recent advances of forensic science are:
a. **Artificial intelligence (AI):** AI is currently being used in digital forensics, analyze a crime scene, compare fingerprint data, and draw conclusions from photograph comparisons.
b. **Nanotechnology:** Nanosensors are utilized to examine the presence of illegal drugs, explosive materials, and biological agents at the molecular level.
c. **Carbon dot powders:** Researchers have developed a fluorescent carbon dot powder that can be applied to fingerprints, making them fluorescent under UV light and hence easier to analyze.
d. **Proteomes:** Proteomes are a complete set of proteins produced by an organism. Proteomes are found in blood, bones, and other biological materials which can be analyzed to find if a victim came in contact with otherwise undetectable venom or matching a severely degraded body fluid sample to a perpetrator.

Functions of FSL

The main functions of FSL are:
1. Analyze and provide unbiased scientific opinion on the different types of evidentiary material referred to them by the investigating authorities.
2. Provide analytical support to the investigating agencies and the judiciary.
3. Conduct research and development activities on the various problems of the forensic sciences.
4. Impart specialized training of forensic science to the forensic scientists, police officers, judicial officers and the other law enforcement officers.

Types of Evidence

Forensic evidence (physical and biological) is collected at a crime scene or in the hospital (emergency room/autopsy), analyzed in a laboratory, and often presented in court. Some of them are briefly discussed below:
1. **DNA evidence:** In forensic cases, samples are gathered from crime scene and a suspect. DNA is then extracted and analyzed for the presence of specific

DNA markers. If the sample profiles do not match, the suspect did not contribute the DNA at the crime scene. Biological evidence, which contains DNA, is a type of physical evidence. Evidence that can be subjected to DNA testing includes clothing (blood, sweat, skin cells, semen, hair), cigarette ends (saliva), bite mark (saliva), condom (semen, vaginal and/or rectal fluid), fingernail scrapings (blood, sweat, skin cells, tissue, semen) etc.

2. **Toxicology evidence:** The toxicology report can provide key information as to the type of substances present in a patient and if the amount is consistent with a therapeutic or toxic dosage. These results can be used to determine whether a substance had a potential effect on an individual's death, illness, or mental or physical impairment. Toxicology analysis is most commonly used to determine if a driver was impaired during a road traffic accident.

3. **Trace evidence:** This type of evidence is easily transferrable between objects, people or the environment during a crime. For example, blood, fibers, soil, hair, gunshot residue, wood, and pollen. Investigators can potentially link a suspect and a victim to a mutual location through trace evidence. For example, a fiber sample obtained from a deceased victim can be identified through trace-evidence analysis as originating from the coat/sweater/shawl of the suspected perpetrator. Blood is the most common, and perhaps most important form of evidence in forensic science today. Its presence will link a suspect and victim to one another and to the scene of the crime.

4. **Pathology evidence:** A forensic pathologist conducts a postmortem examination of the dead body and reconstruction the crime scene findings to determine the cause and manner of death. The pathologist may review the individual's medical history and perform histopathological examination of tissues to determine if the death was natural, accidental, or homicidal. The pathologist may recover vital evidence, such as a bullet or knife, which may help to determine the cause and manner of death.

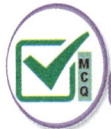

MULTIPLE CHOICE QUESTIONS

1. **Not a domain of forensic science:**
   A. Determination of cause of car skidding on the highway killing the driver
   B. Identification of skeletal remains through dental examination
   C. Verification of composition of cough syrup before it leaves the factory
   D. Identification of white powder packets found in a car during routine check by police

   Explanation: The central drugs standard control organisation (CDSCO) is the national regulatory authority of India and drug inspector visits to keeps checks and for verification of composition of drugs.

2. **Mathieu Orfila is considered the father of:**
   A. Forensic medicine
   B. Forensic toxicology
   C. Forensic serology
   D. Forensic anthropology

   Explanation: Mathieu Orfila was a Spanish toxicologist and chemist and he is considered the father of forensic toxicology. He analyzed the effects of poisons on human bodies and developed a method of detecting the presence of arsenic in suspected victims.

3. **The blood grouping system was discovered by:**
   A. Weiner
   B. Henry Faulds
   C. Lombroso
   D. Landsteiner

   Explanation: In 1900, Karl Landsteiner discovered the ABO blood grouping system.

4. **Two identical twins will not have same:**
   A. Fingerprints
   B. Iris color
   C. DNA
   D. Blood group

Explanation: Identical twins have identical genetic makeup (same DNA), iris color and blood group but distinguishably different fingerprints.

5. **First central forensic laboratory was established in:**
   A. Mumbai   B. Chandigarh
   C. Delhi   D. Kolkata

   Explanation: In 1952, the first CFSL was established in Kolkata.

6. **Assertion (A):** Hair is important to establish the link between suspect and victim and linking both with the scene of occurrence.

   Reason (R): This is as per Locard's principle of exchange.
   A. (A) is correct, but (R) is incorrect.
   B. Both (A) and (R) are incorrect.
   C. (R) is correct, but (A) is incorrect.
   D. Both (A) and (R) is correct.

   Explanation: According to principle of exchange, with every contact between two objects, there will be exchange. Hair is a form of trace evidence which may be left behind in the crime scene to establish relationship between offender, offense and victim.

7. **Causing disappearance of evidence by a forensic scientist is punishable under:**
   A. Sec. 193 IPC   B. Sec. 201 IPC
   C. Sec. 202 IPC   D. Sec. 302 IPC

   Explanation: Sec. 201 IPC deals with disappearance of evidence of offense or giving false information to screen offender.

8. **Best method to detect gunshot residue (GSR) particles can be done by:**
   A. Scanning electron microscopy
   B. Gas chromatography
   C. Atomic absorption spectroscopy
   D. Neutron activation analysis

   Explanation: Scanning electron microscopy is the only available method to confirm the presence of GSR particles; other methods, such as atomic absorption spectroscopy, only measure the amount of bulk elements present and not their individual form.

9. **Least reliable source of evidence:**
   A. Blood   B. Eye witness
   C. Fingerprints   D. DNA

   Explanation: Eyewitness testimony is the least reliable evidence because of witnesses' perceptions, prejudices, and contradictory statements.

10. **Bite marks help in personal identification using which of these types of evidence?**
    1. Saliva   2. Teeth marks
    3. DNA   4. Lip prints

    Choose the correct answer from the given options:
    A. 1, 2 and 3   B. 2, 3 and 4
    C. 1, 3 and 4   D. All of the above

    Explanation: In case of bite marks, there is very little chance of getting a legible lip print, but the examiner may be able to collect DNA, saliva and teeth marks impressions for identification.

ANSWER KEY

| 1. C | 2. B | 3. D | 4. A | 5. D | 6. D | 7. B | 8. A | 9. B | 10. A |

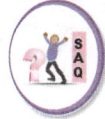

SHORT ANSWER QUESTIONS

1. Write a brief note on history of development of forensic science in India.
2. Discuss in brief the importance of forensic science.
3. Discuss briefly the scope of forensic science.
4. Discuss in brief the evidences analyzed by forensic science laboratory.
5. What are the legal issues that are of concern for the forensic scientists?

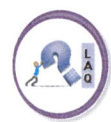

LONG ANSWER QUESTIONS

1. Define forensic science. Discuss briefly the various branches of forensic science.
2. Discuss the history of development of forensic sciences.
3. What are the major milestones in the development of forensic science?
4. Discuss the setup and functions of forensic science laboratory.

CHAPTER 2

Violence and Sexual Abuse

"Physical aggression by a man towards his partner is abuse, even it happens only once."
— **Lundy Bancroft**
(Author, and Consultant on domestic abuse and child maltreatment)

LEARNING OBJECTIVES

At the end of this topic, the student should be able to:
1. Define violence and its types.
2. Discuss the epidemiology of violence.
3. Define and explain sexual abuse of child and woman.

CASE STUDY

Patient X, a 79-year-old female comes to the ER with complaints of shoulder pain after a fall from the stairs. She lives with her divorced daughter. X cannot tell her medications or chronic conditions. On examination, she appears weak; clothes are dirty along with foul smell coming from her body. X remains quiet, not making eye contact or conversation. She does not answer questions properly and looks up to her daughter for the answers. Moreover, X has some areas of redness and bruises distributed over her lower extremities and back as shown in **figure**. When asked about it, X's daughter intervenes, stating that her mother is a bit unsteady and has a tendency to fall, which she agrees. It is noted that the daughter does not leave X's side at all during the examination. She also appears to be attentive to her mother, getting water and assisting her to use the toilet.

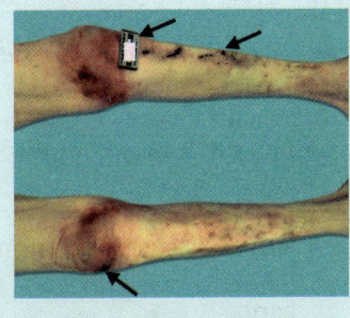

Q1. Do you think the patient's condition correlates with the description of events?
Q2. What potential signs of abuse are present in this case?
Q3. What can the forensic nurse in this situation do if she suspects abuse?*

*Discuss the questions with your teacher/facilitator.

■ DEFINITION OF VIOLENCE

The intentional use of physical force or power, threatened or actual, against oneself, another person, or against a group or community that either results in or has a high likelihood of resulting in injury, death, psychological harm, maldevelopment or deprivation (as per WHO).

Hence, violence is not only physical injury, but includes psychological harm, maldevelopment or deprivation—acts of omission or neglect, as well as commission. *This is a broad and more inclusive definition of violence.*

Flowchart 2.1: Classification of violence (from the World Report on Violence and Health).

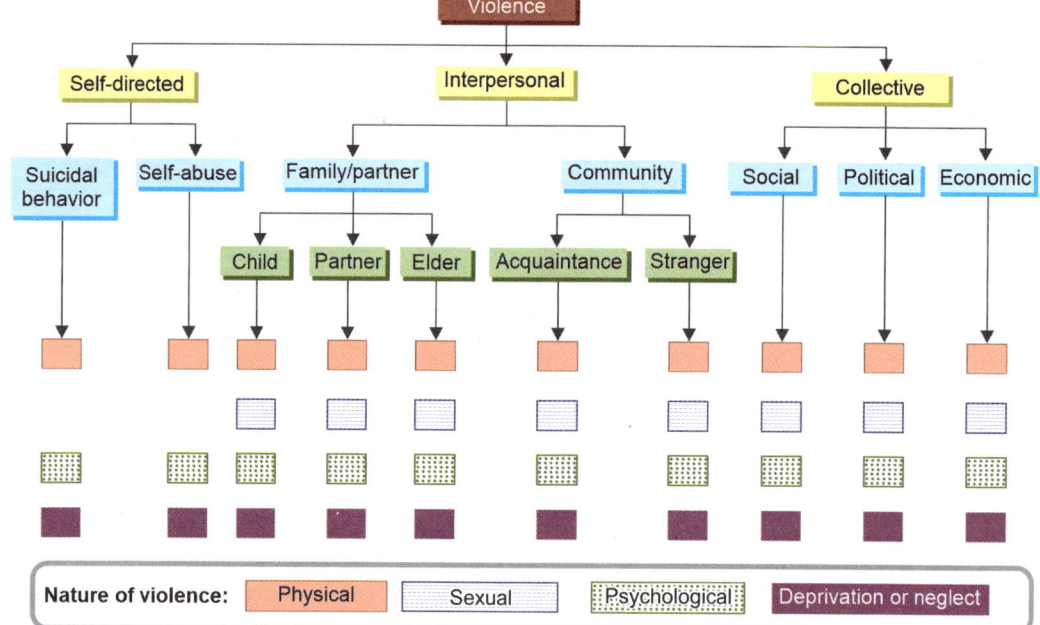

Types (Flowchart 2.1)

1. Based on *who has committed the violence*—self-directed, interpersonal or collective.
2. Based on the *nature of violence*—physical, sexual, psychological or involving deprivation or neglect.

A. **Self-directed violence**
   - Self-directed violence includes suicidal thoughts or action and forms of self-harm.
   - 'Fatal suicidal behavior' is suicidal acts that result in death. 'Nonfatal suicidal behavior', 'attempted suicide', 'parasuicide' and 'self-harm' are suicidal behaviors that do not result in death.

B. **Interpersonal violence**
   - It is behavior by persons against persons that intentionally threatens, attempts or actually inflicts physical harm. It is subdivided into:
     a. *Family violence:* Occur between family members, between intimate partners, siblings, parents, etc. This category includes child abuse, child corporal punishment, intimate partner violence and elder abuse.
     b. *Community violence:* Violence between individuals who are unrelated, and who may or may not know each other, generally taking place outside the home, e.g., random acts of violence, sexual violence, and violence in institutional settings, such as schools, workplaces, prisons and nursing homes.
   - *Intentional physical harm* also includes violence against oneself as in suicides or attempted suicides, and the use of violence by state authorities in the course of enforcing law, imposing capital punishment, etc.
   - *Unintentional physical harm* has been excluded like exposure of workers to toxic chemicals. Transport injury is also a type of unintentional violence.

C. **Collective violence**
   Collective violence is the violence by people who identify themselves as members of

a group, against another group or set of individuals, in order to achieve political, economic or social objectives, e.g., war, terrorism and violent communal riots, gang warfare, etc.
- It may include all categories of violence—physical, sexual, psychological, or neglect or discrimination.

NATURE OF VIOLENCE

a. Physical Violence
- Physical violence is an act attempting to cause or resulting in pain and/or physical injury. Some examples are hitting **(Fig. 2.1)**, slapping, pinching, punching, choking, kicking, shoving, physical restraints, burning, using weapons, beating with an object, etc.
- Physical violence occurs when someone uses a part of their body or an object to control a person's actions.
- They are intentional bodily injury.

b. Sexual Violence
- Sexual violence can occur at an interpersonal or collective level.
- Sexual violence are nonconsensual acts which can be **contact offenses**—rape, molestation, fondling, oral sex, forceful kissing, etc., or **noncontact offenses**—sexual harassment, forced pornography, exhibitionism, etc.

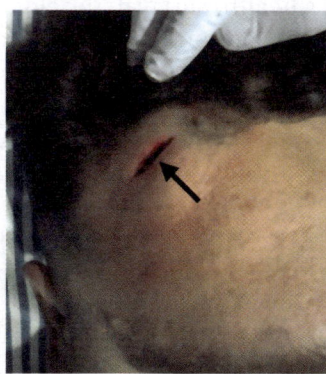

Fig. 2.1: Lacerated wound on the forehead after being hit by a "kada" (steel bangle) (arrow).

c. Psychological Violence
- Psychological violence which includes 'emotional abuse' is any intentional conduct that seriously impairs another person's psychological integrity through coercion or threats.
- It not only affects individuals' mental health and their social networks, but also deprives them of opportunities for future personal, social and economic development.
- Examples include acts, such as isolation from others, verbal aggression (including shouting or swearing), threats, intimidation, control, harassment or stalking, insults, humiliation and defamation.

d. Neglect or Deprivation
- Neglect is the failure of a parent or other person with responsibility to provide needed food, clothing, shelter, medical care or supervision to the degree that the individual's health, safety and well-being are threatened with harm.
- Neglect may happen within a person's own home or in an organization.
- Neglect can be intentional or unintentional.

INTERPERSONAL VIOLENCE

1. Gender-based Violence
- Gender-based violence is a term that recognizes that violence occurs within the context of women's and girl's subordinate status in society. Gender-based violence is sometimes used interchangeably with "violence against women".
- Gender-based violence therefore includes those occurring within the family, such as female genital mutilation, "honor killings" and dowry-related violence, forced prostitution, etc.

2. Family Violence
- Family and domestic violence represents any use of force, threats or other forms of force sufficient to injure or endanger the victim, which is committed by one family member against other person(s) with

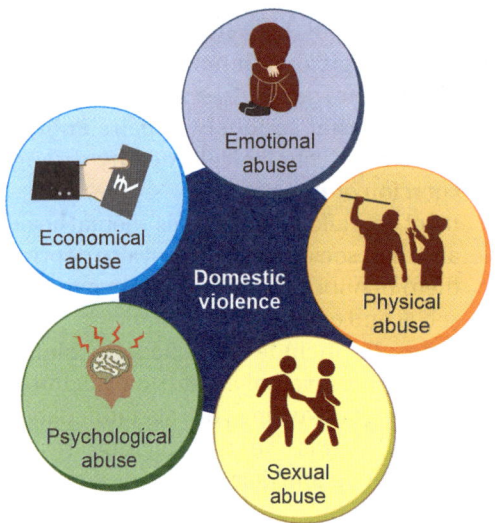

Fig. 2.2: Types of abuse in domestic violence.

whom he lives or has lived with, or with whom he is/was in an intimate relationship.
- Family violence refers to child maltreatment, sibling violence, intimate partner violence and elder abuse.
- Family violence is a common problem in India and victims may suffer physical, psychological and emotional abuse.

3. Domestic Violence

- Domestic violence takes place in the home and is characterized by physical abuse, verbal abuse, economic abuse and social abuse against a family member, such as against women (previously known as spouse abuse), child or an elder **(Fig. 2.2)**.
  - Physical and sexual violence have been described above.
  - *Economic abuse:* Making or attempting to make a victim financially dependent on the abuser, e.g., preventing or forbidding intimate partner from working or gaining education, controlling financial resources.
  - *Psychological abuse:* Intimidation, threats of harm and isolation, e.g., instilling fear through threatening behavior such as damaging property or abusing pets, constant supervision or controlling what the victim does and who they talk to.
  - *Emotional abuse:* Undermining an individual's sense of self-worth, e.g., constant criticism, name calling, embarrassing, mocking and humiliating.
- Domestic violence can be better understood as a chronic syndrome characterized not only by episodes of physical violence, but also by the emotional and psychological abuse by the perpetrators to maintain control over their partners.
- Domestic violence is often used interchangeably with intimate partner violence.

Types of Domestic Violence

1. **Intimate partner violence (IPV)**
   - It refers to physical, sexual or psychological harm by a current or former partner or spouse.
   - This type of violence can occur among heterosexual or same-sex couples and does not require sexual intimacy.
2. **Child maltreatment/child abuse:** Child maltreatment constitutes all forms of physical and/or emotional ill-treatment, sexual abuse, neglect or negligent treatment or commercial or other exploitation, resulting in actual or potential harm to the child's health, survival, development or dignity in the context of a relationship of responsibility, trust or power.
3. **Elder abuse**
   - Elder abuse may be an act of commission or omission, and may be intentional or unintentional.
   - Causes harm or distress to an aged person.
   - As with other forms of abuse, it may be physical, psychological, financial, sexual or involve neglect **(Fig. 2.3)**.

CHAPTER 2: Violence and Sexual Abuse

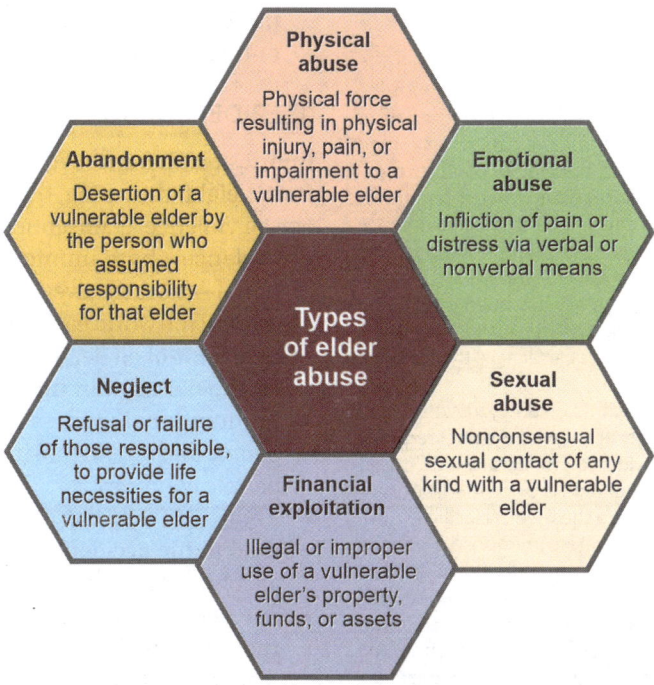

Fig. 2.3: Types of elder abuse.

Battered Wife Syndrome
- *Battered wife syndrome* is a symptom complex of repeated unwanted violent acts of physical, sexual and psychological abuse of a woman (partner) by her husband.
- **Presenting complaints:** They often present with vague somatic complaints, such as headache, insomnia, lower back pain, abdominal pain and dyspareunia. The diagnosis is usually made by asking nonthreatening open-ended questions.
- **Characteristics:** Battering men and battered women are found in all levels of society, although younger, lower income, less-educated men who have observed parental violence in their own home are at higher risk of abusing their spouses. Additionally, antisocial personality disorder, depression, and/or alcohol and drug abuse increases the risk. This violence is usually motivated by his need to control her by inducing fear and pain.
- In most cases, battering occurs in cycles comprising of a tension building phase of unpredictable length, a violent explosion, and then calm and loving respite. These contradictory behaviors cause confusion and ambivalence in battered woman; they develop a pattern of 'learned helplessness'.

The Protection of Women From Domestic Violence Act, 2005
- This Act plays a critical role in the Indian legal system vis-à-vis protecting the rights of the women, so that they can feel protected and safe within the comfort of their own house.
- It lays down the powers and duties of the various authorities, reliefs available to the victims, steps to filing a complaint regarding domestic violence, assistance provided to the victims of domestic violence, power and extent of the Indian Judiciary and the power of the Central Government to make rules.
- The Act provides civil remedies to the victims of domestic violence.

Salient Features
- The term 'domestic violence' covers all forms of physical, sexual, verbal, emotional and economic abuse that can harm, cause injury, endanger the health, safety, life, limb or well-being, either mental or physical of the aggrieved person.
- 'Aggrieved person is not just the wife, but a woman who is the sexual partner of the male irrespective of whether she is his legal wife or not. It also includes daughter, mother, sister, child (male or female), widowed relative, or any woman residing in the household who is related in some way to the respondent.

Contd....

Contd....

- 'Respondent' is any male, adult person who is, or has been, in a domestic relationship with the aggrieved person, that includes his mother, sister and other relatives; the case can also be filed against relatives of the husband or male partner.
- **Information to protection officer:** The information regarding any acts of domestic violence does not necessarily have to be lodged by the aggrieved party but by any person who has reason to believe that such an act has been or is being committed. Any medical officer, nurse, neighbors, social workers or relatives can all take the initiative on behalf of the victim.
- **Duties of medical facilities:** If an aggrieved person or a protection officer or a service provider requests the healthcare provider to provide any medical aid to the victim, he/she should provide medical aid to the aggrieved person in the medical facility.
- **Penalties:** The Magistrate can impose a penalty of up to 1 year of imprisonment with/without a fine of up to ₹ 20,000/- for an offense under this Act. The offense is also considered cognizable and nonbailable. The decision can be taken under the sole testimony of the aggrieved person; the court may conclude that an offense has been committed by the accused.
- The Act also allows the Magistrate to make the respondent pay compensation and damages for injuries including mental torture and emotional distress caused by acts of domestic violence.
- The Magistrate can impose monetary relief and monthly payments for maintenance. The respondent can also be made to meet the expenses incurred and losses suffered by the aggrieved person and can also cover loss of earnings, medical expenses, loss or damage to property.

4. Workplace Violence

- Incidents where staff are abused, threatened or assaulted in circumstances related to their work, including commuting to and from work, involving an explicit or implicit challenge to their safety, well-being or health.
- Harassment at work is any conduct based on age, disability, HIV status, gender, sexual orientation and other factors that is unreciprocated and unwanted, and affects the dignity of men and women at work.
- Within the healthcare professions, ambulance workers, nurses and workers with considerable face-to-face contact are particularly vulnerable to abusive patients or their attendants.

EPIDEMIOLOGY

Injuries result from road traffic accidents, fall from height, drowning, burns, poisoning and acts of violence against oneself or others.

- Violence—both unintentional and intentional—takes the lives of 4.4 million people around the world each year and constitutes nearly 8% of all deaths.
- Of the 4.4 million injury-related deaths, unintentional injuries cause 3.16 million people and intentional injuries 1.25 million people every year.
- About 1 in 3 of these deaths results from road traffic accidents, 1 in 6 from suicide, and 1 in 10 from homicide.
- For people age 5–29 years, 3 of the top 5 causes of death are injury-related, namely road traffic accidents, homicide and suicide. Drowning is the sixth leading cause of death for children age 5–14 years. Fall from height account for over 6 lakhs deaths each year.
- Most attention focuses upon interpersonal violence. Gender based violence is regarded as a global pandemic that effects 1 in every 3 women across their lifetime (as per WHO). An estimated 736 million women become victims of intimate partner violence or nonpartner sexual violence or both at least once in their life. In US, the number of women who ever reported experiencing domestic violence increased by 42% from 2016 to 2018.
- In India, 30% of women have experienced domestic violence at least once from when they were aged 15, and lifetime physical and/or sexual intimate partner violence is 293%. In 2022, 24% suffered physical and/or sexual intimate partner violence. According to NFHS survey report, domestic violence is highest in Karnataka (44%) and least in Lakshadweep (1.3%).

The foundation of the public health approach to violence is very similar to that

used for other diseases. From the public health perspective, to reduce violence:
1. First step is monitoring of the frequency of violence. Monitoring systems are needed to identify the number of events that occur, the victims of violence and their characteristics, as well as the outcomes of violence.
2. Second step includes an examination of the risk factors of both victims and perpetrators of crime. Much debate is there over the role of various social, environmental and genetic factors in violence.
3. Third step is the development and implementation of intervention programs to reduce violence.

Surveillance of Violence from Crime

- Death certificates
- **Police reports:** Uniform crime reports
- **Government surveys:** National criminal victimization survey
- Medical databases.

The classic epidemiologic model of understanding disease notes interactions between the host, agent, and environment. In the violence field, the model can be adapted to consider the victim (as host), the perpetrator (as agent), and the community (environment) surrounding both **(Fig. 2.4)**. With respect to injuries from violence, the perpetrator is more correctly the vehicle, and the agent is the energy transfer involved in the perpetration of violence.

SEXUAL VIOLENCE

Definition: Any sexual act, attempt to obtain a sexual act, unwanted sexual comments or advances or acts to traffic, or otherwise directed against a person's sexuality, using coercion, by any person regardless of their relationship to the victim, in any setting, including but not limited to home and work (as per WHO) **(Fig. 2.5)**.

- Acts qualify as sexual violence if they are committed against someone who is unable to consent or refuse because of age, disability, misuse of authority, violence or threats of violence etc.
- The term *'sexual assault'*, a form of sexual violence, is often used synonymously with rape[¥]. However, sexual assault could include anything from touching another person's body in a sexual way without the person's consent to forced sexual intercourse—oral and anal sexual acts, molestation, fondling, and attempted rape.

Classification of Sexual Offenses/Assault

Sexual offenses can be classified into:
1. Rape
2. Forced/nonconsensual anal sex
3. Forced/nonconsensual oral sex

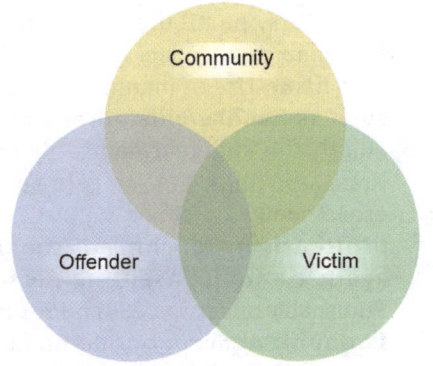

Fig. 2.4: Relation between victim, perpetrator and environment.

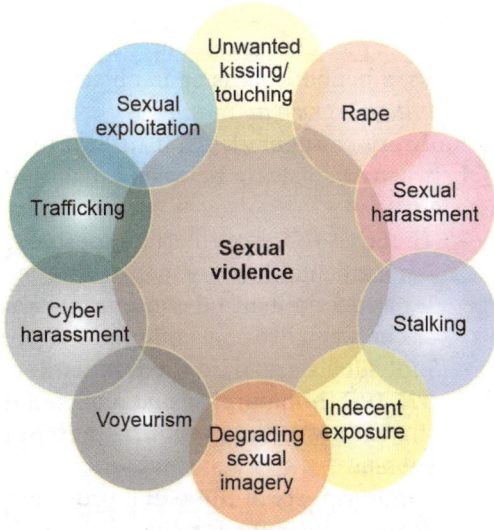

Fig. 2.5: Various types of sexual violence.

[¥] The term "sexual abuse" is mainly used to describe sexual behaviors toward children, not adults.

4. Forced/nonconsensual insertion of fingers or objects
5. Sexual acts with animals (bestiality/zoophilia—sexual attraction to animals)
6. Paraphilia*
7. Sex-linked disorders
    - **Indecent assault:** Any unwanted sexual behavior or touching of a female without her consent, with the intention or knowledge to outrage her modesty.
    - Sexual harassment

Punishments

Section	Offense
354	Punishment for **indecent** assault (1–5 years ± Fine)
354 **A**	Punishment for **sexual harassment** (frotteurism) (up to 3 years ± Fine)
354 **B**	Punishment for **disrobing a woman** (3–7 years ± Fine)
354 **C**	Punishment for **voyeurism** (1–3 years ± Fine—1st offense; 3–7 years ± Fine—2nd offense)
354 **D**	Punishment for **stalking** (up to 3 years ± Fine—1st offense; up to 5 years ± Fine—2nd offense)

Sexual Offenses

1. **Rape** is defined as physically forced or otherwise coerced penetration, even if slight, of the vulva, anus or urethra, using a penis, other body parts or an object *(legal definition is given in Chapter 5).*
2. **Sodomy (buggery):** Anal intercourse between two males or between a male and a female.
    - The SC also observed that homosexuality is not a mental illness or mental disorder. It has decriminalized consensual anal sex between two consenting adults.
    - Individuals are to be tried under **Sec. 377 IPC** (unnatural sexual offense), if the act has been *committed without consent.*
    - Other aspects of the penal provision dealing with animals remain the same.
3. **Sexual harassment** is physical contact and advances involving unwanted and explicit sexual overtures, or demanding sexual favors, showing pornography against her will or making sexually colored remarks, or any other unwelcome physical, verbal or non-verbal conduct of sexual nature.
4. **Paraphilia** *(previously known as sexual perversions):* It is any intense and persistent sexual interest other than sexual interest in genital stimulation or preparatory fondling with physically mature, consenting partners. Some examples are:
    a. **Sadism:** Inflicting pain on a person for sexual pleasure. In extreme cases of sadism, *lust murder* may be committed.
    b. **Masochism:** Receiving pain for sexual pleasure. Sexual asphyxia is seen in cases of masochism.
    c. **Transvestism:** Arousal from clothing associated with members of opposite sex.
    d. **Voyeurism:** Urges to observe an unsuspecting person who is naked, undressing or engaging in sexual activities.
        ◆ **Stalking:** Following or contacting a disinterested woman or monitoring her through internet, e-mail or any other form of electronic communication.
    e. **Exhibitionism:** Exposing one's genitals to an unsuspecting person or performing sexual acts that can be watched by others, particularly strangers. Punishable under Sec. 294 IPC.
    f. **Fetishism:** Use of inanimate objects, such as handkerchief, dress, particularly the undergarments—panties, bras, stockings, etc., to gain sexual excitement.
    g. **Frotteurism:** Touching or rubbing against a nonconsenting person. Punishable under Sec. 290 and 291 IPC.
    h. **Pedophilia:** Sexual preference for prepubescent children (9–12 years).

---

* Not all paraphilias are sexual offenses, unless done publicly or comes under any of the sections of IPC.

Long-term Effects of Sexual Assault

Medical	Psychological
Sexual dysfunctions	Anxiety
Headache	Depression
Irritable bowel syndrome	Eating disorders
Fibromyalgia	Alcohol and drug abuse
Chronic pain (pelvis, back)	Post-traumatic stress disorders
Somatoform disorders	Sleep disorders

Rape Trauma Syndrome

It is a psychological trauma and is regarded as post-traumatic stress disorder (PTSD). PTSD is an anxiety disorder marked by biological changes, as well as psychological symptoms.

It is characterized by two phases:
1. *Phase of disorganization* where there is headache, GIT complaints, immune system problems, dizziness, chest pain, discomfort, emotional imbalance, depression and feeling of guilt.
   This phase is followed by:
2. *Phase of reorganization* in which there is gradual adjustment with occasional phobia and fear state (nightmares), avoidance of thoughts, feelings and situations related to the assault, and increased arousal (e.g., difficulty in sleeping and concentrating, jumpiness, and irritability).

Treatment: PTSD is treated by psychotherapy and drug therapy. At present, cognitive-behavioral therapy (talk therapy)* appears to be somewhat more effective than drug therapy.

> **The Sexual Harassment of Women at Workplace (Prevention, Prohibition and Redressal) Act, 2013 [Prevention of Sexual Harassment (POSH) Act]**
> - The POSH Act was passed to protect women in the workplace from sexual harassment and ensure that workplaces remain safe and free from sexual harassment.
> - The Act defines sexual harassment at the work place **(Fig. 2.6)** and creates a mechanism for redressal of complaints. It also provides safeguards against false or malicious charges.
> - Every employer is required to display a notice in the organization providing details of the protection given to female employees against sexual harassment.
> - Every employer is required to constitute an Internal Complaints Committee (ICC) at office or branch with 10 or more employees to address complaints of sexual harassment.
>
> *Contd....*

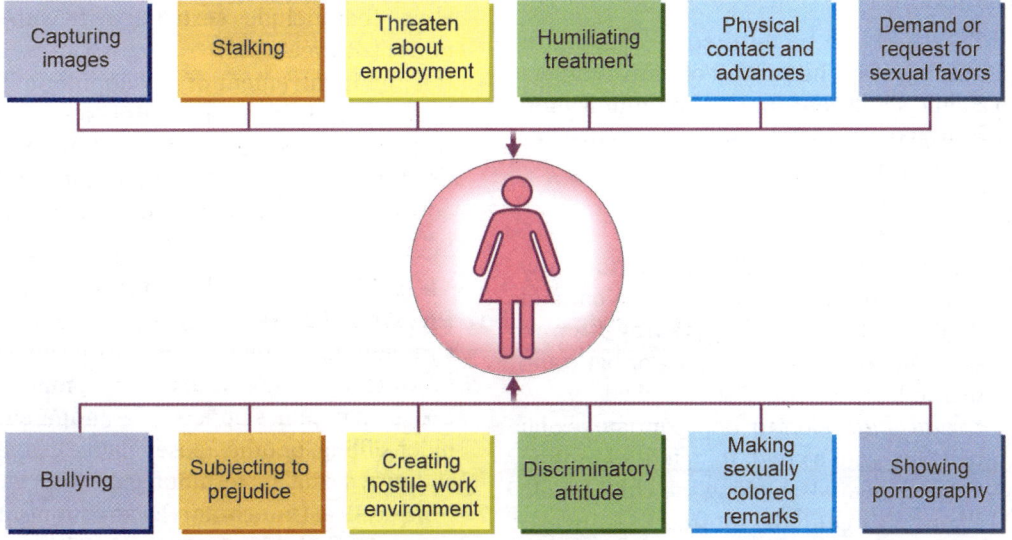

Fig. 2.6: Sexual harassment at workplace.

---
* Negative patterns of thought about self and the world are challenged in order to alter unwanted behavior patterns or treat mood disorders, such as depression.

Contd....

- A woman must head the ICC; at least half of its members should be women.
- The ICC is required to provide for conciliation before initiating an inquiry, if requested by the complainant.
- The ICC has the powers of civil courts for gathering evidence.
- Employers must take steps to prevent sexual harassment and ensure that the victims are not victimized or discriminated against.
- Penalties have been prescribed for employers. Non-compliance with the provisions of the Act shall be punishable with a fine of up to ₹50,000.
- The POSH Act only gives protection to the women—it is not a gender neutral Act. However the court has held "A person of any gender may feel threatened and sexually harassed when her/his modesty or dignity as a member of the said gender is offended by any of the acts, irrespective of the sexuality and gender of the perpetrator of the act".

CHILD ABUSE

Patient Y a 10-year-old girl is brought to the school nurse for sleeping in class. Her teacher is concerned because every Monday, she is quarrelsome, distracted, and sleepy. The school nurse learns that Y spends weekends with her uncle. Y's mother is concerned that the uncle is sexually abusing her daughter.

Definition

Child abuse can be defined as causing or permitting of any harmful or offensive contact to a child's body and/or any communication or transaction which humiliates, shames, or frightens a child.

Types of Abuse

1. *Physical abuse* of children includes any nonaccidental physical injury caused by the child's caretaker (**Caffey-Kempe syndrome**). It can be beating or battering of a child.
2. *Sexual abuse* refers to inappropriate sexual behavior with a child. It includes fondling a child's genitals, making the child fondle the adult's genitals, intercourse, incest, rape, sodomy, exhibitionism, indecent exposure and commercial exploitation through prostitution or the production of pornographic materials.
3. *Emotional abuse (verbal/mental abuse):* Acts of commission and omission which can be potentially damaging psychologically. This can include parents/caretakers using extreme and/or bizarre forms of punishment, such as confinement in a closet, washroom or dark room or being tied to a chair for long periods.
4. *Neglect* is the failure to provide for the child's basic needs. Neglect can be physical, educational or emotional. In general, neglect is an act of omission.

Reporting of Suspected Child Abuse

- In order to protect the child, the diagnosis of child abuse must be reported irrespective of the context of such assault/battery. The confidentiality of the physician-patient relationship no longer holds in cases of abuse and cruelty to child.
- In India, it is mandatory to report to the police about sexual abuse under the Protection of Children from Sexual Offenses (POCSO) Act, 2012.

Child Sexual Abuse

- Child sexual abuse (CSA) is a form of child abuse that includes sexual activity with a minor (<18 years old).
- It is the involvement of developmentally immature children and adolescents in sexual activities they do not comprehend, to which they are unable to give informed consent, or those that violate the social taboos.

CSA is divided into the following categories:
1. **Physical (contact):** Genital or oral stimulation, fondling, incest (sexual abuse in which the abuser is a family member—may be a parent, stepparent, grandparent, older sibling, or other close relative), rape, sodomy, sexual molestation etc.
2. **Nonphysical (noncontact):** Exhibitionism, voyeurism, child pornography, obscene phone calls, masturbation in the presence of a minor, or verbal sexual suggestions made to a child etc.

CHAPTER 2: Violence and Sexual Abuse

	Nightmares and sleeping problems		Resists removing clothes for bathing or changing clothes
	Regressing to younger behaviors like bedwetting and thumb sucking		Pain during urination or bowel movement
	Becoming withdrawn or very clingy, easily distracted or distant at times		Underpant soiling or bleeding unrelated to toilet training
	Becoming unusually secretive, telling lies, refusing to talk about a secret they have with an older child or adult		Sudden unexplained personality changes: rage, insecurity, anger, depression and anxiety
	New words for private body parts and no obvious source		Unaccountable or new fear of particular things, places or people, not wanting to be alone with a particular person, even someone you know and trust
	Changes in eating habits. Trouble eating or swallowing		Acting out in an inappropriate sexual way with toys or objects, playing sexual games
	Talk of new friend, and unexplained money or gifts		Self-harm cutting, burning or other harmful activities
	Changes in clothing, dressing shabbily or in some instances dressing provocatively		Physical signs, such as unexplained soreness or bruises around genitals or mouth, rashes, bleeding, hair loss and bruising or bite marks to body
	Running away from home, frequent school absences, acting out in school, not wanting to participate in physical education, sports and swimming		

Fig. 2.7: Signs and symptoms of child sexual abuse.

Identifying CSA

CSA may be difficult to identify and its presenting signs may be subtle, because children often do not provide direct disclosures. Signs and symptoms are sudden and may or may not be associated with behavioral changes **(Fig. 2.7)**.

Nonspecific Complaints: Behavior Signs

Enuresis	Encopresis	Nightmares	Withdrawal
Phobias	Sense of isolation	Temper tantrums	Sleep disturbances
Hysteria	Depression	Anxiety	Aggression
Lack of concentration at school	Increased absenteeism from school	Attempts to physically hurting herself/ himself	Increased self-stimulating behavior

In Older Children

Substance abuse	Conduct disorder	Suicidal tendencies
Sexual promiscuity	Masturbation	Absenteeism
Sexual exploration and abuse of other children	Increased attraction towards the opposite sex	Touches genitalia when in public place

Specific Complaints/Findings

a. Bloody, torn, or stained underclothes
b. Difficulty in walking or sitting
c. Pain, itching, or burning in genital area
d. Recurrent UTI, vaginitis, abdominal pain, infection of throat

When these complaints/findings are not accompanied by disclosure or other findings of sexual abuse, a close medical follow up is indicated.

Physical Findings
a. Unexplained bleeding, bruises, or swelling of genital or rectal area
b. Presence of foreign body in the vagina or rectum
c. Unexpected pregnancy
d. Presence of sexually transmitted infection (STI)

The presence of any of the above physical findings should be reported to the police.

Relationship with Perpetrator
- The majority of perpetrators are someone the child or family knows. More than 50% of victims under the age of 18 know the abuser.
- Abusers can manipulate victims to stay quiet about the sexual abuse using a number of different tactics. Often an abuser will use their position of power over the victim to coerce or intimidate the child. They might tell the child that the activity is normal or that they enjoyed it. An abuser may make threats if the child refuses to participate or plans to tell another adult.

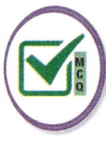

MULTIPLE CHOICE QUESTIONS

1. **Domestic violence includes all, *except*:**
   A. Stalking
   B. Child abuse
   C. Interpersonal violence
   D. Elder abuse

   Explanation: Stalking is unwanted and/or repeated surveillance by an individual of another person. Stalking is a form of sexual harassment and intimidation.

2. **Abuse ranging from emotional to sexual and other forms of physical abuse and includes financial scam is:**
   A. Elder abuse   B. Domestic violence
   C. IPV   D. Child abuse

   Explanation: Elder abuse comes in many forms, including physical, psychological, sexual abuse, as well as less obvious forms such as financial exploitation and neglect. Financial exploitation encompasses the withholding or misuse of the older adult's resources, including money, property, and other assets.

3. **Sexual assault does not include:**
   A. Forced oral intercourse
   B. Forced sexual activity that does not result in penetration
   C. Flashing one's genitalia at the victim
   D. Attempted rape

   Explanation: Flashing one's genitalia at the victim i.e., exhibitionism is a form of paraphilia. Exhibitionists (usually males) expose their genitals, usually to unsuspecting strangers, and become sexually excited when doing so.

4. **All of the following can qualify as acts of sexual assault, *except*:**
   A. Simple touching
   B. Physical intimacy
   C. Consensual sex among adults
   D. Forceful penetration

   Explanation: Consensual heterosexual/homosexual relation between adults, including pre-marital sex, is not an offense.

5. **NOT a feature of post-traumatic stress disorder (PTSD):**
   A. Hyperarousal
   B. Emotional numbing
   C. Flashbacks
   D. Hallucinations

   Explanation: Hallucinations in PTSD are *rare*; may involve auditory hallucinations and paranoid ideation. Individuals who experience auditory hallucinations may experience tinnitus, a constant ringing in one's ears, or they may hear voices that are not physically present.

6. **Any form of unwanted sexual attention is considered as:**
   A. Sexual assault   B. Sexual coercion
   C. Rape   D. Sexual harassment

   Explanation: Sexual harassment includes unwelcome sexual advances, requests for sexual favors including many types of unwelcome

verbal and physical sexual attention, such as sending intrusive letters/mails, making phone calls, touching, grabbing, cornering, etc.

7. Sexual penetration without an adult female's consent is:
   A. Sexual intimacy
   B. Rape
   C. Sexual harassment
   D. Molestation

   Explanation: Sexual activity without consent is rape. Consent means actively agreeing to be sexual with someone and let them know that sex is wanted. The term "rape" is used legally to define and specifically include sexual penetration without consent.

8. Fetishism is a paraphilia characterized by:
   A. Sexual focus on children
   B. Sexual focus on genital rubbing
   C. Sexual pleasure from getting pain
   D. Sexual pleasure from inanimate objects

   Explanation: Fetishism is a form of sexual deviance involving erotic attachment to an inanimate object or an ordinarily asexual part of the human body.

9. Deliberate, intentional acts that causes harm or threat of harm to a child is:
   A. Child abandonment B. Child neglect
   C. Child abuse   D. Child discipline

   Explanation: *Child abuse* is any intentional harm or mistreatment to a child under 18 years old. *Child abandonment* is when a parent, guardian, or person in charge of a child either deserts a child without any regard for the child's physical health, safety or welfare. *Child neglect* is failure by a child's caregiver to meet a child's physical, emotional, educational, or medical needs. *Child discipline* is the method used to prevent future unwanted behavior in children.

10. Caffey-Kempe syndrome is related to:
    A. Husband abuse   B. Child abuse
    C. Wife abuse   D. Elder abuse

    Explanation: Caffey-Kempe syndrome or battered baby syndrome is a combination of physical injuries or conditions, such as broken bones, bruises and/or burns experienced by a child as a result of gross nonaccidental violence, usually by a parent or caregiver.

ANSWER KEY

| 1. A | 2. A | 3. C | 4. C | 5. D | 6. D | 7. B | 8. D | 9. C | 10. B |

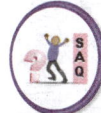

SHORT ANSWER QUESTIONS

1. Define and classify violence.
2. Write a short note on interpersonal violence.
3. Write a brief note on sexual violence.
4. Describe briefly elder abuse and its types.
5. Define and classify sexual violence.
6. What is Rape trauma syndrome? Explain briefly.
7. What are the long-term effects of sexual assault?
8. Write a brief note on indecent assault. What is the punishment for it?
9. How can you identify child sexual abuse from the non specific complaints?

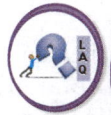

LONG ANSWER QUESTIONS

1. Describe the various forms of domestic violence and its types.
2. Define child sexual abuse. Describe the various types, signs and symptoms of child sexual abuse. What are your legal duties in dealing with such a case?
3. Describe in brief the Protection of Women From Domestic Violence Act, 2005.
4. Describe briefly the Prevention of Sexual Harassment (POSH) Act.

CHAPTER 3

Introduction to Forensic Nursing and Nursing Jurisprudence

"Forensic nursing is the future of nursing practice."

— **Anita Hufft**
(Dean College of Nursing, Valdosta State University, US)

LEARNING OBJECTIVES

At the end of this topic, the student should be able to:
1. Define forensic nursing and nursing jurisprudence.
2. Understand the history and development of forensic nursing.
3. Explain the scope—areas of practice and subspecialties.
4. Describe the roles and responsibilities of forensic nurse.
5. Understand the ethical principles concerning nursing practice.
6. Describe and discuss INC and SNC Acts.

CASE STUDY

You are a forensic nurse working in the ER when ambulance services brought in a patient who sustained a gunshot wound over the chest (arrow indicates the bullet wound in the given **figure**). Emergency healthcare providers cut the clothing off in an attempt to do a cardiopulmonary resuscitation and apply external defibrillator. The patient was declared dead 10 minutes after arrival.

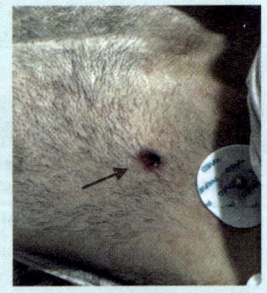

Q1. Is the death reportable to the police?
Q2. What do you do with the patient's clothing that was cut off?*

*Questions are discussed at the end of this chapter.

DEFINITION

Forensic nursing is the application of the nursing sciences to public and legal proceedings. It includes application of forensic healthcare in the scientific investigation of trauma and/or death related to abuse, violence, criminal offenses, liability, accidents, and events of nature.

- Forensic nurse is a registered nurse with additional education and training in:
  - Forensic evidence collection
  - Criminal procedures
  - Legal testimony expertise
- Forensic nursing is an evolving specialty that seeks to address issues related healthcare matter having a medico-legal component.
- Forensically trained nurses will be the bridge between healthcare and justice and will be often called to testify in legal matters.

History and Development of Forensic Nursing

- During the 13th century, the nurses played the role of forensic examiners as they examined the young girls who were about to marry royalty. The nurses at that time confirmed the girl's virginity to the monarchs, as they were required to be virgins before their marriage. Nurses also worked with sexual assault and abuse cases during this period.
- In the 1950s, forensic nurses in the United Kingdom (UK) were involved in dealing with mental health, substance use disorders and child sexual assault.
- In recent times, the role of forensic nurse evolved out of the practice of *clinical forensic medicine*—a subspecialty of forensic medicine. The need for knowledgeable nurses in the emergency departments dealing forensic cases became evident as evidences were being lost by omission or commission during trauma treatment. For this reason, it became obvious that all nurses have a responsibility to maintain the standards of practice in medico-legal cases and must have some baseline knowledge of how to assess, preserve evidence, and interface with the legal system.
- Prior to forensic nursing, sexual assault nurses were the key people who handled rape or sexual abuse cases in the United States (US). The earliest example of forensic nursing practice involved sexual assault nurse examiners (SANEs) which arose from recognizing the needs of victims of sexual assault, and how diverse and unique they were. A strong advocate for the forensic nursing specialty in the US was Virginia Lynch. She pushed to have the specialty recognized and helped to form programs for proper education.
- In the last decade, forensic nursing has developed into a high-profile nursing profession, and has evolved into collection of forensic evidence, sexual assault examination, identification of abuse, as well as reporting, investigation of deaths, mental health evaluations and expert testimony.
- The World Health Organization (WHO) and International Association of Forensic Nurses (IAFN) have urged inclusion of forensic content in both undergraduate and postgraduate nursing programs. Various institutes, death investigations agencies, and judiciary have recognized the benefits of forensic trained nurse.
- Beside US, other countries where the forensic nursing has evolved into a separate discipline are Canada, South Africa, Japan, Hong Kong, Singapore, Sweden, Switzerland, and the UK. A brief history of the development of forensic nursing is given in the **Table 3.1**.

Table 3.1: History of development of forensic nursing.

Year	Development
1970s	Nurses recognized the need of victims of sexual assault
1975	Establishment of program using registered nurse in medical examiner's death investigations in Alberta, US
1976	First SANE program was established simultaneously in Tennessee and Texas, US
1986	Virginia Lynch proposed creation of the forensic nursing specialty
Early 1990s	Development of training for nurses in sexual assaults to properly assess patients, collect evidence, document findings
1991	Forensic nursing was formally recognized by the American Academy of Forensic Sciences (AAFS)
1992	Term forensic nursing was coined, and IAFN was founded in the US
1995	American Nurses Association (ANA) recognized the Forensic Nursing Specialty
1997	Scope and standards of Forensic Nursing Practice was published by IAFN and the ANA
2002	Virginia Lynch visited Punjab, India. Rakesh Gorea played a pivotal role introducing Forensic Nursing in India
2009	Indo Pacific Academy of Forensic Nursing Science was founded
2015	One-year post-basic diploma in Forensic Nursing started at Gujarat Forensic Sciences University
2020	The Indian Nursing Council (INC) started the MSc in Forensic Nursing
2021	The INC introduced Forensic Nursing in the Undergraduate Nursing Program

Researches have validated that forensic nurse collect forensic evidence more accurately than do trained nurses or physicians which results in better evidence collection and documentation, and hence more successful prosecution.

> - Ann Burgess conducted extensive research with victims of sexual assault and interpersonal violence.
> - Virginia Lynch is considered as one of the founders of forensic nursing. While practicing as a death investigator, she advocated for the value of forensic education in nursing schools and for the role of nurses in forensic practice.

SCOPE—AREAS OF PRACTICE AND SUBSPECIALTIES

Some of the specialty areas within forensic nursing include:

1. Sexual assault nurse examiner	2. Forensic nurse death investigator
3. Forensic psychiatric nurse	4. Clinical forensic nurse specialist
5. Nurse coroner (in some countries)	6. Correctional nursing specialist
7. Legal nurse consultant and nurse attorney	8. Humanitarian forensic nurse
9. Forensic pediatric nurse examiner	10. Forensic nurse hospitalist

They may be also involved in elder maltreatment, and in the aftermath of mass disasters and community crisis situations.

Sexual Assault Nurse Examiner (SANE)

- A registered nurse who has been specially trained to provide comprehensive care to sexual assault patients and demonstrates competency in conducting a forensic examination and the ability to be an expert witness.
- SANE was the first specialized forensic role for nurses and the largest subspecialty in forensic nursing in the US.
- ER doctor is reluctant to participate in sexual assault examination (because of fear of court appearances) and many a time evidence has been lost because of their mishandling and mismanagement.
- SANE nurses are trained to address survivors' medical, psychological, legal, and forensic needs—comprehensive care to survivors of sexual assault.
- A forensic nurse examiner more readily establishes rapport with the survivors allowing them to express the true history in a frank manner and has lead to successful offender prosecution and improved healthcare.

Clinical Forensic Nurse Specialist (Emergency Department)

- Emergency department nurses are often the first to encounter a patient with forensic issues—patients who have been assaulted or involved in any accidents/assaults, or perpetrators with various types of injuries.
- Although emergency physicians are trained in forensic medicine, potential evidence such as gastric lavage, vomitus, urine samples, hair, saliva etc., linking the perpetrator to the crime are lost, discarded or destroyed resulting in wrongful convictions and exonerations.
- Forensic nurses are aware of the value of specimens, preserving as appropriate, and document them in meticulous manner for analysis.
- Hence, forensic clinical nurse specialists can provide forensic patient care while also serving as consultants, educators, and researchers.
- Forensic nurses can be of great help in the designing appropriate standards for conducting medico-legal examination, prevention programs and strategies in fighting family violence.
- In addition, the nurse has an ethical responsibility to advocate for all patients, both victims and offenders. The nurse serves as an unbiased expert who is focused on the facts and fairness of treatment and properly informing the patient of all elements of care.

Forensic Nurse Death Investigator (FNDI)

- A licensed nurse who carries out the duties of a death investigator (determine the need for autopsy, and cause and manner of death) in accordance with the standards and procedures established under the medical examiner or coroner system of death investigation (both systems are not there in India).
- FNDI serve as investigators in both coroner, as well as medical examiner jurisdictions in which a forensic pathologist who is a physician leads the team.
- Forensic nurses interpret the crime scene differently than people without medical or scientific knowledge such as the police.

Nurse Coroner

- Nurse coroner is a nurse who has experience as a death investigator and brings to the role a broad perspective when investigating circumstances that lead to death.
- Ensure appropriate measures taken to perform death investigations and certify death certificates.
- Uses nursing knowledge to identify disease process (in natural deaths) that the lay coroner may not recognize or may misinterpret as foul play.
- Utilizes communication skills when dealing with grieving families.

Forensic Correctional Nurse

- Forensic correctional nurse specializes in the care, treatment and rehabilitation of person who have been sentenced to prisons or jails.
- Goal is to maintain a safe, secure and humane environment for the inmates.

Forensic Psychiatric Nurse

- A forensic psychiatric nurse serves as direct care provider and patient advocate in caring for a most vulnerable population—those patients who suffer with mental illness and are also engaged in the legal system.
- Connects the gap between the criminal justice, legal and mental health systems.
- They are involved in competency evaluation for legal purposes—determines the intent or diminished capacity in patient's thinking at the time of incident.

Legal Nurse Consultant and Nurse Attorney

- Nurse attorneys practice law, generally specializing in civil and criminal cases involving healthcare-related issues. The nurse attorney is qualified as a nurse along with having a law degree.
- They serve as expert witnesses in nursing malpractice cases. The courts have recognized that nurses, rather than physicians, should define and evaluate the standards of nursing practice. They evaluate, analyze and provide expert opinions on the delivery of care and its outcomes.
- Nurses are uniquely qualified to assist attorneys in their medico-legal practices.

Humanitarian Forensic Nurse

- Humanitarian forensics is the branch of science involving forensic science for humanitarian purposes.
- It may be identification of victims of mass disasters/missing persons after a war or epidemics or dealing with torture victims.
- Recently, it has been understood that forensic nurses can play a vital role and should be a part of the humanitarian forensic teams.
- Attitude and communication skills can play a very important role during interviews to elicit information from the disaster and torture victims.

Forensic Pediatric Nurse Examiner

- A pediatric forensic nurse provide medico-legal examination of pediatric patients where child abuse may be suspected or confirmed and/or has been reported to child protective services and/or police.
- The forensic pediatric nurse possesses specialized knowledge of pediatric patient assessment, child developmental levels, communication, documentation, reporting

requirements, and interviewing techniques, including separating the interviewees during questioning.
- Responsibility of forensic nurse in these cases is to compare what is observed with what is obtained through the careful interview of the pediatric patient and their caretaker/guardian.

Forensic Nurse Hospitalist (FNH)

- Forensic nurse hospitalist represents one of the newest and most dynamic roles within the specialty of forensic nursing.
- FNH provides expert care, coordination of services, and leadership in the hospital setting specific to patients who have experienced intentional or unintentional trauma and have forensic implications associated with their care.
- They supplement the role of non-forensic emergency department nurses, physicians, and other healthcare providers within the hospital setting by overseeing and educating staff members in comprehensive medico-legal care of patients who have criminal or liability-related conditions and/or implications.
- The forensic nurse hospitalist leads the medical/nursing team in coordinating the hospitalized patient's clinical forensic care, provides the medico-legal management of suspected/or identified forensic cases, and guides the medical/nursing team in providing patient care that meets the forensic standards to ensure legal and ethical outcomes.
- The forensic nurse hospitalist is an advanced practice forensic nurse who has completed education and experience in the science of forensic nursing.

ROLE AND RESPONSIBILITIES OF FORENSIC NURSE

Forensic nurses are practicing in hospitals and in the community, making a difference in people's lives **(Fig. 3.1)**. Forensic nurse:
i. Identify issues that will have legal impact on the society.

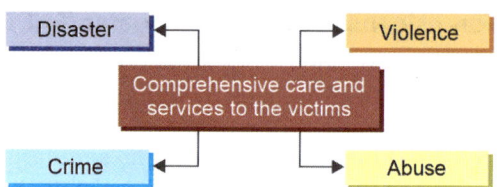

Fig. 3.1: Comprehensive care of victims.

ii. Document and photograph injuries, collect and preserve evidences, and pull communities together to address issues such as domestic violence, sexual assault, child abuse etc.
iii. Work with grieving family members when death comes unexpectedly.
iv. Care for the inmates and those in psychiatric facilities who are unable to understand the consequences of their actions.
v. Contribute to disaster planning and response.
vi. Assist lawyers to understand the medical terminology and how care was provided to the individual.
vii. Assist in development of evidence-based policies and procedures related to evidence identification, collection and preservation and photographic documentation.
viii. Develop and implement orientation and continuing education programs for the staff related to forensic nursing and forensic science techniques.
ix. Act as consultant with risk management administration.
x. Review the medical record to facilitate the legal counsel.
xi. In a school setting—identify children at risk of abuse or neglect.
xii. In law enforcement setting—provide direct evaluation and care for the victims of violence and able to collect evidence and provide referrals.
xiii. In home care settings—assess the patient for evidence of abuse or neglect; provides referral for community service agency assistance.

CHAPTER 3: Introduction to Forensic Nursing and Nursing Jurisprudence

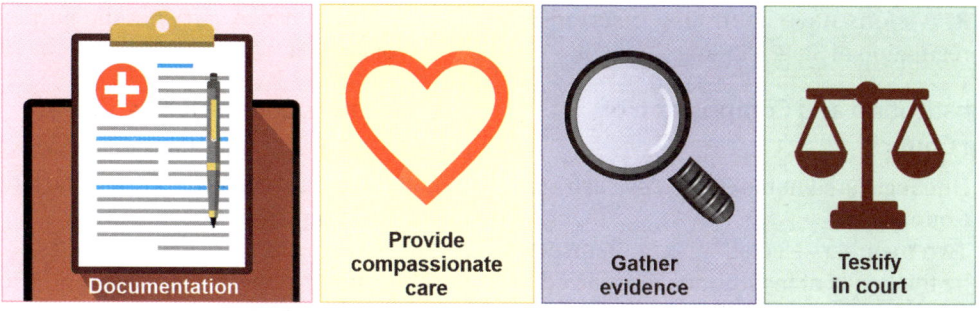

Fig. 3.2: Role of forensic nurse.

Responsibilities of Forensic Nurse in ER

- The safety of the living victim and the deceased's body remains the first priority.
- Collecting and preserving evidence should never compromise the safety or integrity of the body.

The responsibilities of forensic nurse in emergency settings may include **(Fig. 3.2)**:

- Screen patients
- Take medical history and account of the assault from the patient.
- Provide forensic examinations and nursing services for victims of violence.
- Documentation and expert testimony for victims and perpetrators in settings, such as hospitals, community clinics or crime scenes.
- Assess, collect and preserve forensic specimens while maintaining the chain of custody.
- Provide nursing care of injuries and prophylactic medications.
- Communicate with victims and their families regarding evidence collection, treatment and reporting to police (except in cases of mandated reporting).
- Meet the needs of patient experiencing violence by providing timely, comprehensive, compassionate, culturally sensitive, and expert forensic evaluation and treatment.
- Perform lab testing for patients based on the history provided by the patient.

NURSING JURISPRUDENCE

Definitions

- **Nursing jurisprudence:** The application of legal rules and principles as they relate to the practice of nursing, obligations of nurses to their patients, and to the relations of nurses with each other and other healthcare professionals. It deals with:
  - All laws, rules and regulations.
  - Legal principles and doctrines governing and regulating the practice of nursing.
  - Legal opinions and decisions of competent authority in cases involving nursing practice.
- **Ethics:** Ethics is the set of philosophical beliefs and practices concerned with the distinction between right and wrong.
- **Nursing ethics:** It is concerned with moral principles for the members of the nursing profession in their dealings with each other, their patients and the State.
  - It is a self-imposed code of conduct assumed voluntarily by nursing professionals.

INDIAN NURSING COUNCIL

The Indian Nursing Council (INC) is an autonomous and statutory body under the Government of India, Ministry of Health and Family Welfare constituted under the Indian Nursing Council Act, 1947.

- The aim of INC is to maintain uniform standards in nursing education.

- Provisions have been also inserted for regulation of State Nursing Councils.

Constitution and Composition of the Council

a. One registered nurse elected by each State Council.
b. Two members elected among themselves by the heads of institutions recognized by the Council.
c. One member elected by the heads of institutions in which health visitors are trained.
d. One member elected by the National Medical Commission.
e. One member elected by the Central Council of the Indian Medical Association.
f. One member elected by the Council of the Trained Nurses Association of India.
g. One auxiliary nurse-midwife enrolled in a State Register, elected by each of the State Councils from the four groups of States.
h. The Director General of Health Services.
i. The Chief Principal Matron, Medical Directorate, General Headquarters.
j. The Chief Nursing Superintendent, Office of the Director-General of Health Services.
k. The Director of Maternity and Child Welfare, Indian Red Cross Society.
l. The Chief Administrative Medical Officer of each State other than a Union territory.
m. The Superintendent of Nursing Services from each of the two groups of States.
n. Four members nominated by the Central Government, of whom at least two shall be nurses enrolled in the State Register and one shall be an experienced educationalist.

Officers, Committees of the Council

1. An elected or nominated President holds the office for a term of 5 years.
2. The Secretary of the Council is appointed for 3 years by the Central Government.
3. The Council shall:
   a. Elect from among its members a Vice-President.
   b. Constitute from among its members an Executive Committee and such other Committees to carry out the purposes of this Act.

The Executive Committee

1. The Executive Committee consists of nine members, of whom seven are elected by the Council from among its members.
2. The President and Vice-President of the Council remain President and Vice-President, respectively of the Committee.
3. The Executive Committee exercises and discharges powers and duties as the Council impose.

Recognition of Qualifications

1. The qualifications included in Part I of the Schedule shall be recognized qualifications, and in Part II of the Schedule shall be recognized higher qualifications.
2. The qualification only when granted after a specified date by the respective State Council shall be a recognized qualification.
3. The Council may enter into negotiations with any authority to which this Act does not extend in India or foreign country for recognition of qualification.

Functions of INC

1. **Maintain uniform standard of undergraduate and postgraduate nursing education**
   - Establish and monitor uniform standards of nursing—the Council sends inspectors for inspection of the institutions.
   - The Council prescribes minimum standards of education and training in various nursing programs, and prescribe the syllabus, course duration, training and examination for nursing programs.
2. **Recognition of nursing qualifications:** Recognize the qualification(s) under the Indian Nursing Council Act, 1947 for the purpose of registration and employment in India and abroad.

3. **Maintenance of Indian Nurses Register:** The Council maintains the Register which contains the names, address and qualifications of all registered nursing personnel. It permits title, badges and uniforms for registered nurses.
4. **Permission for establishment of new nursing college and its recognition:** It inspects any new institution recognized as a training institution, and inspectors attend examination held for the purpose of granting any recognized qualification in nursing, and then may approve or disapprove the scheme.
5. **Withdrawal of recognition of nursing institutions:** The Council may withdraw the recognition of an institution recognized by a State Council for the training of nurses, if it does not satisfy the standards and requirements of the Council.
6. **Recognition of foreign nursing qualifications under scheme of reciprocity:** The Council may enter into negotiations with any foreign University for the recognition of nursing qualifications (Degree/Diploma/Certificate) under a scheme of reciprocity.
7. **Registration of foreign qualification:** Approval for registration of Indian and foreign nurses possessing foreign qualification.
8. **Advisory powers:** Advise the State Nursing Councils, Examining Boards, State Governments and Central Government in issues regarding nursing education.
9. **Power to make regulations:** Regulate the policies of training of nursing programs to improve the quality of nursing education.
10. **Prescribe code of ethics and professional conduct:** The Council prescribes minimum standards of professional conduct, etiquette and a code of ethics for nursing professionals. It can take disciplinary actions and issue warnings in relation to unethical practices.
11. **Promote research in nursing.**

National Nursing and Midwifery Commission
- **The National Nursing and Midwifery Commission Bill** has been prepared by the government to replace the INC with a new body called National Nursing and Midwifery Commission. This body would have representatives of the Centre and the States.
- The proposed bill has the following aims and objectives:
  1. Maintenance of Central and State registers.
  2. Assessment and rating of different institutions offering courses.
  3. Regulation and maintenance of standard of nursing and midwifery education and institutions.
  4. Provide standards for nursing and midwifery faculty and clinical facility in teaching institutions.
  5. Frame policies and codes to ensure observance of professional ethics in the nursing and midwifery profession.
  6. Adoption of latest scientific advancements.
  7. Creating a system where research and development of these scientific advancements can be accessed easily.
  8. Regulation and maintenance of services rendered by nursing and midwifery professionals.

STATE NURSING COUNCIL (SNC)

- The **State Nurses and Midwives Council** was established in 1948 under the provisions of Nurses and Midwives Act with the purpose of "Better training of nurses, midwives and health visitors".
- There are many registered state-level nursing councils.
- It works as an autonomous body under the Government of respective States, Department of Health and Family Welfare.
- "State Council" means a Council constituted under the law of a State to regulate the registration of nurses, midwives or health visitors in the State.
- "State Register" means a register of nurses, midwives or health visitors maintained under the laws of a State.

Salient Features of SNC

1. Provision of an autonomous body, comprising majority of nurses, capable with decision making powers.

2. Compulsory registration for all nurses and midwives practicing within the State.
3. Provision of nurses, midwives, and public health nurses to elect their own representatives to the respective State.
4. Powers to regulate nursing education, prescribe curriculum, and frame examination policies.
5. Provision to have a nurse registrar to carry out the functions of the SNC.
6. Provision for recognition of educational institutions of nursing, and withdrawal of such recognition, if necessary.

ETHICAL PRINCIPLES

The major ethical issues of nursing practice are **(Fig. 3.3)**:

1. **Autonomy:** Autonomy refers to the right of the patient to retain control over his body. It requires that patients should have autonomy of thought, intention and action when making decisions regarding healthcare procedures, i.e., the decision-making process must be free of force or persuasion. Nurses encourage patients to make their own decision without any coercion, undue influence or compulsion. The patient has the right to reject or accept all treatments.
2. **Beneficence:** The nurse should act in the "best interest" of the patient—the procedure and treatment is provided with the intent of doing benefit to the patient.
3. **Non-maleficence:** Requires that the nurse should not intentionally create a harm or injury to the patient. It is based on the principle of *primum non nocere*—first do no harm, either through acts of commission or omission. This principle affirms the need for nursing competence.
    - The nurse must therefore consider the principles of beneficence and non-maleficence together and try to produce net benefit over harm.
4. **Justice:** The burdens and benefits of treatments must be distributed equally among all groups in society regardless of their gender, race or religion—a fair distribution of goods in society.
5. **Accountability:** It means the nurses are responsible for their actions and may be required to explain them to others. It is maintaining competency and safeguarding quality patient care outcomes and standards of the profession, while being answerable to those who are affected by the nursing practice. For example, taking care of equipment, administering medications as prescribed, and documenting any supplies used in patient.
6. **Fidelity:** The nurse should remain true to professional values, principles and standards, such as the promise to provide high-quality, competent, safe and efficient patient care. This means not engaging in any unethical behavior and following guidelines set by healthcare organizations.
7. **Veracity:** It requires that the nurse be honest in their interactions with patients (truth telling)—to never lie to patients or give them knowingly false reassurance.

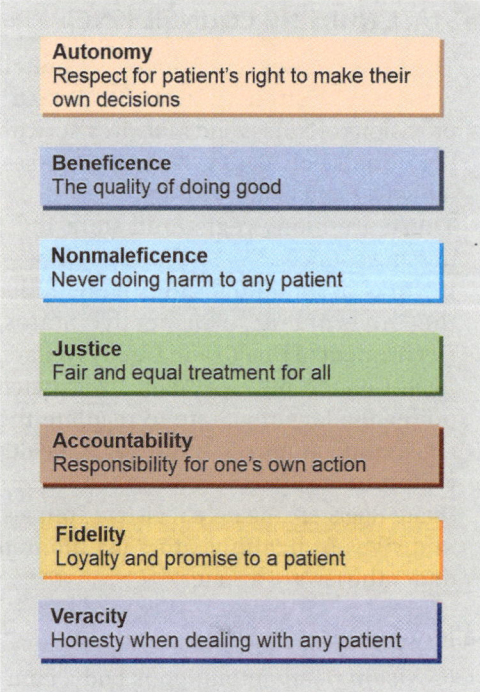

Fig. 3.3: Ethical principles for nurses.

For example, a survivor of sexual assault should be told that any evidence obtained during examination may be used in court, and that she will then be exposed to publicity and cross-examination.

CODE OF ETHICS FOR NURSES

The Code of Ethics for nurses developed by the American Nurses Association (ANA) makes explicit the primary goals, values, and obligations of the profession. An international Code of Ethics for nurses was first adopted by the International Council of Nurses in 1953. The Code of Ethics as applicable to any registered nurse are:

1. The nurse respects the uniqueness of individual in provision of care:
   - Provides care of individuals without consideration of caste, creed, religion, culture, ethnicity, gender, socio-economic and political status, personal attributes, or any other grounds.
   - Individualizes the care considering the beliefs, values and cultural sensitivities.
   - Appreciates the place of individual in the family and community, and facilitates participation of significant others in the care.
   - Develops and promotes trustful relationship with individual(s).
   - Recognizes uniqueness of response of individuals to interventions and adapts accordingly.

2. The nurse respects the rights of individuals as partner in care and help in making informed choices:
   - Appreciates individual's right to make decisions about their care, and therefore gives adequate and accurate information for enabling them to make informed choices.
   - Respects the decisions made by individual(s) regarding their care.
   - Protects public from misinformation and misinterpretations.
   - Advocates special provision to protect vulnerable individuals/groups.

3. The nurse respects individual's right to privacy, maintains confidentiality, and shares information judiciously:
   - Respects the individual's right to privacy of their personal information.
   - Maintains confidentiality of information (professional secrecy), except in life threatening situations and uses discretion in sharing information.
   - Takes informed consent and maintains anonymity when information is required for quality assurance/academic/legal reasons.
   - Limits the access to all personal records, written and computerized to authorized persons only.

4. Nurse maintains competence in order to render quality nursing care:
   - Nursing care must be provided only by registered nurse.
   - Nurse strives to maintain quality nursing care and upholds the standards of care.
   - Nurse values continuing education, initiates and utilizes all opportunities for self-development.
   - Nurses values research as a means of development of nursing profession and participates in nursing research adhering to ethical principles.

5. The nurse is obliged to practice within the framework of ethical, professional and legal boundaries:
   - Adheres to Code of Ethics and Code of professional conduct for nurses in India developed by INC.
   - Familiarizes with relevant laws and practices in accordance with the law of the State.

6. Nurse is obliged to work harmoniously with members of the health team:
   - Appreciates the team efforts in rendering care.
   - Cooperates, coordinates and collaborates with members of the health team to meet the needs of people.

7. Nurse commits to reciprocate the trust invested in nursing profession by society:
   - Demonstrates personal etiquettes in all dealings.
   - Demonstrates professional attributes in all dealings.

CODE OF PROFESSIONAL CONDUCT FOR NURSES (FIG. 3.4)

1. **Professional responsibility and accountability**
   a. Appreciates sense of self-worth and nurtures it.
   b. Maintains standards of personal conduct reflecting credit upon the profession.
   c. Carries out responsibilities within the framework of the professional boundaries.
   d. Is accountable for maintaining practice standards set by INC.
   e. Is accountable for own decisions and actions.
   f. Is compassionate.
   g. Is responsible for continuous improvement of current practices.
   h. Provides adequate information to individuals that allows them informed choices.
   i. Practices healthful behavior.
2. **Quality nursing practice**
   a. Provides care in accordance with set standards of practice.
   b. Treats all individuals and families with human dignity in providing physical, psychological, emotional, social and spiritual aspects of care.
   c. Respects individuals and families in the context of traditional and cultural practices, promoting healthy practices and discouraging harmful practices.
   d. Presents realistic picture truthfully in all situations for facilitating autonomous decision-making by individuals and families.
   e. Promotes participation of individuals and significant others in the care.
   f. Ensures safe practice
   g. Consults, coordinates, collaborates and follows up appropriately when individual's care needs exceed the nurse's competence.
3. **Communication and interpersonal relationships**
   a. Establishes and maintains effective interpersonal relationships with individuals, families and communities.
   b. Upholds the dignity of team members and maintains effective interpersonal relationship with them.
   c. Appreciates and nurtures professional role of team members.
   d. Cooperates with other health professional to meet the needs of the individuals, families and communities.
4. **Valuing human being**
   a. Takes appropriate action to protect individuals from harmful unethical practice.
   b. Considers relevant facts while taking conscience decisions in the best interest of individuals.
   c. Encourages and supports individuals in their right to speak for themselves on issues affecting their health and welfare.
   d. Respects and supports choices made by individuals.
5. **Management**
   a. Ensures appropriate allocation and utilization of available resources.
   b. Participates in supervision and education of students and other formal care providers.

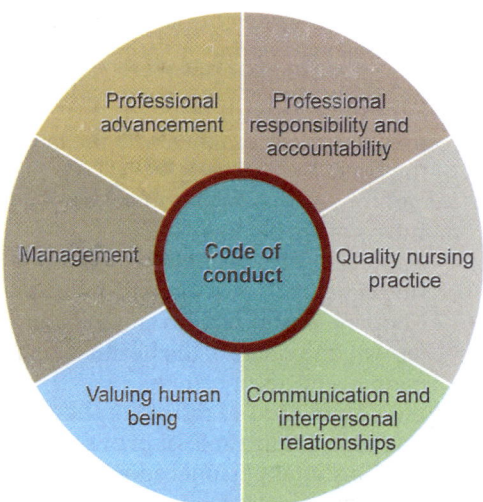

Fig. 3.4: Code of professional conduct for nurses.

c. Uses judgment in relation to individual competence while accepting and delegating responsibility.
d. Facilitates conductive work culture in order to achieve institutional objectives.
e. Communicates effectively following appropriate channels of communication.
f. Participates in performance appraisal.
g. Participates in evaluation of nursing services.
h. Participates in policy decisions, following the principle of equity and accessibility of services.
i. Works with individuals to identify their needs and sensitizes policy makers and funding agencies for resource allocation.

6. **Professional advancement**
   a. Ensures the protection of the human rights while pursuing the advancement of knowledge.
   b. Contributes to the development of nursing practice.
   c. Participates in determining and implementing quality care.
   d. Takes responsibility for updating own knowledge and competencies.
   e. Contributes to the core of professional knowledge by conducting and participating in research.

Need for Nursing Ethics

a. Help the students/nurses to practice ethically.
b. Helps the nurse to identify the ethical issues at her work place.
c. Protect patients right and dignity.
d. Provides care with possible risk to the nurses health.
e. Understand staffing patterns that may limit the patient's access to nursing care.
f. Helps in ethical reasoning.
g. Helps the nurse to respond to ethical conflicts.
h. Helps to differentiate right/wrong behavior.
i. Guide for professional behavior.

j. Help teachers plan education.
k. Prevent below standard practice.
l. Protection against complaints of professional misconduct.

CODE OF ETHICS FOR FORENSIC NURSES

- When faced with ethical choices, forensic nurses should use recognized ethical frameworks for decision making. The guiding principles of ethical decision making are autonomy, justice, beneficence, and nonmaleficence.
- Forensic nurses should consult and collaborate with appropriate ethical resources.
- The ANA and the IAFN Code of Ethics as applied to forensic nursing is given in **Table 3.2**.
   a. **Responsibility to the public:** Forensic nurse has a professional responsibility for health and welfare of the public. Forensic nurses acknowledge the value and dignity of all human beings and strive to create a world where violence is not accepted.
   b. **Fidelity to patients:** Forensic nurses should serve patients faithfully and with honesty. They should respect confidentiality and advice patients

Table 3.2: Code of ethics for forensic nurses.

ANA code of ethics	IAFN code of ethics
1. Respect of human dignity	1. Responsibility to the public and the environment
2. Commitment to patients	2. Fidelity to clients
3. Protecting patient rights	3. Obligation to science
4. Accountability	4. Care of profession
5. Professional growth	
6. Improving healthcare environments	
7. Advancing the profession	
8. Promoting efforts to meet health needs	
9. Participating in the profession's goals	

about the limits of confidentiality as determined by their practice setting. For example, the forensic nurse is required/duty bound to inform the police about the incidence of sexual assault even if the patient refuses for the same. In contrast to usual nursing role, the forensic nurse must remain neutral, objective and detached.
   c. **Obligation to science:** Forensic nurses should seek to advance nursing and forensic science, understand the limits of their knowledge, and respect the truth. Forensic nurses should incorporate evidence-based knowledge in practice decisions.
   d. **Dedication to colleagues:** Forensic nurses should work honestly and competently, fulfill obligations, and safeguard proprietary information. Forensic nurses should treat colleagues with respect, share ideas honestly, and give credit for their contributions.

Forensic Nursing Skills

The following skills can help a forensic nurse in better management of the patient:
1. **Advocacy:** Patient advocacy is about sharing, expressing and highlighting the rights of a patient. It is speaking on behalf of patients and promote the best interests of the patients.
2. **Attention to detail:** Attention to detail can help ensure forensic nurses do not miss anything important. Identifying evidence, sample collection and photography—all require training, focus and high attention to detail.
3. **Communication:** Written and oral communication skills can help forensic nurses write reports, communicate with patients and relay important information to patients, police, patients' families and the court.
4. **Empathy:** Empathy and compassion are very useful. As the patients are most often victims of violence, forensic nurses who can comfort and assure patients in vulnerable states are often more successful at providing proper patient care and earning patient trust and cooperation.
5. **Coping:** Forensic cases can often be traumatic for both the victim and the forensic nurse. Having healthy coping skills can help stay separate from cases and continue providing quality care to the patients.

Professional Secrecy

The healthcare professional has the moral duty to keep the information about the illness of the patient secret or confidential. If the patient is major (≥18 years), the facts relating to the nature of illness *must not be disclosed to anyone else without his consent:*
   i. To parents or relatives even though they may be paying the doctor's fees. In case of minor or insane person, guardians or parents should be informed.
   ii. When requested by a public or statutory body, *except* under notifiable clauses.
   iii. Regarding the husband to his wife and vice versa.
   iv. In divorce and nullity cases.
   v. In the case of domestic servant is examined at the request of the master.
   vi. Person in police custody as an undertrial prisoner.

Punishment

a. Criminal action under **Sec. 499 IPC** (defamation—imprisonment for 2 years and/or fine under **Sec. 500 IPC**).
b. Civil action for damages.
c. Disciplinary action by SNC/INC.

Privileged Communication

It is the disclosure of confidential information by the healthcare professional to the concerned public authority due to his legal, moral and social duty to protect the interest of the community.
- It is an exception to professional secrecy.
- Healthcare professionals have a moral duty to protect the interests of the community. So here, privileged communication plays an important role.

Some examples of privileged communication are:

1. Court of law	In court of law, a nurse cannot claim professional secrecy concerning the facts about illness of her patient
2. Civic benefit	In case drivers are suffering from epilepsy, alcoholism, drug addiction, color blindness, the healthcare professional should advise him to change the employment because of the dangers of his present occupation both to himself and to the public. If the patient refuses, he/she can disclose this information to the concerned authority
3. Venereal disease	If the person is suffering from syphilis or HIV infection and is going to marry, it is the duty of the healthcare professional to advise him not to marry till he is cured. If patient refuses, he/she can disclose the details of the disease to the other party
4. Suspected crime/assault	Healthcare professional is bound to report it to the Magistrate/police officer **(Sec. 39 CrPC)**. It is mandatory to report any sexual abuse in children (≤18 years) **[POCSO Act, 2012]**. • *If he/she intentionally omits to inform the police, then imprisonment up to 6 months with/without fine **(Sec. 202 IPC)**.*
5. Notifiable clauses	It is the duty of the healthcare professional to notify births, deaths, still births, infectious diseases, epidemic and food poisoning to public health authorities.
6. In patient's interest	Healthcare professional may disclose patient's condition to his relatives in case person is suffering from certain symptoms like suicidal tendencies, so that he can be treated properly

Professional Misconduct

Definition: Professional misconduct refers to a nurse's failure to meet the expected professional and ethical standards and legislation.

- Acts that constitute a breach or abuse of nurse-patient relationships are considered as professional misconduct.
- It includes poor ethical competence and neglect of professional guidelines, breaching nurse-patient confidentiality, crossing nurse-patient professional boundaries and threatening patient safety.
- Acts of professional misconduct may result in an investigation by the college/institute/hospital, followed by disciplinary proceedings. This may lead to suspension or cancellation of nurse's registration.
- Some examples of professional misconduct are given in **Box 3.1**.

Procedure of Disciplinary Action (Flowchart 3.1)

State Nursing Councils (SNCs) are empowered with the duty to administer and enforce the Council's rules and regulations. This duty is based on the SNC's overall duty to protect the public from unsafe and/or incompetent nurse practitioners.

Box 3.1: Examples of professional misconduct.

1. Failure to follow nursing practice
2. Substance abuse
3. Sexual misconduct (such as engaging in sexual relationships with patients)
4. Boundary violations (such as soliciting or accepting monetary or valuable gifts)
5. Abuse of patients (either physically or verbally)
6. Procuring certificate/license by fraud or misrepresentation
7. Positive criminal background checks

SECTION I: Introduction to Forensic Nursing and Indian Laws

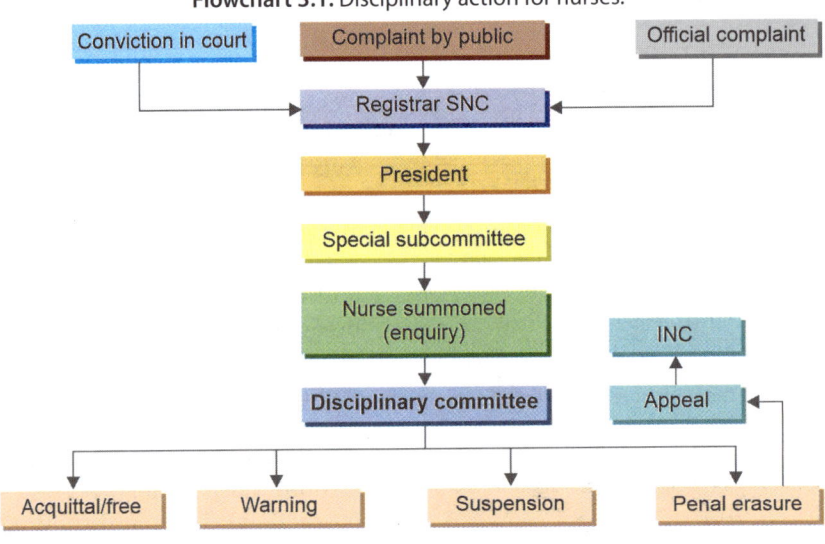

Flowchart 3.1: Disciplinary action for nurses.

Filing a complaint
A patient, family member, employer or member of the public may file a complaint against the nurse with the SNC for any criminal conviction or violation of the State Council regulations, unethical behavior, or behavior that endangers a patient.

Enquiry
Upon receipt of any complaint, the SNC would hold an enquiry and give opportunity to the nurse, patient and witnesses to be heard; asking for a written response and review documentation and other evidence.

Council proceedings and actions
After the enquiry, the SNC may decide to close the case if the complaint is found to be frivolous with acquittal of the nurse. If the nurse is found to be guilty, the Council may punish her as deemed necessary (warning/suspension of license/removal of the name from the nursing register—altogether or for a specified period).

Reporting to INC
The SNC must report the results of any nursing disciplinary action to INC.

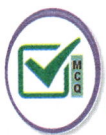

MULTIPLE CHOICE QUESTIONS

1. Who is considered as founder of forensic nursing?
   A. Virginia Lynch
   B. Ann Burgess
   C. Anita Hufft
   D. Nancy Martin

   Explanation: Virginia Lynch, a forensic clinical nurse is recognized as founder and mother of forensic nursing as a formal discipline in the US and across the world.

2. All the activities are included in the forensic nurse's role, *except*:
   A. Documentation of injuries
   B. Providing expert testimony
   C. Collecting evidence
   D. Obtaining a master's degree

   Explanation: The forensic nurse documents and collects evidence and provides expert testimony. Forensic nurses activities do not include obtaining master's degree. However, the ANA designates that a master's degree is required to be considered a specialist.

3. **All are responsibilities of sexual assault nurse examiner (SANE), *except*:**
   A. Conduct detailed physical examination
   B. Identify a victim's future medical needs and associated costs
   C. Providing expert testimony in court of law
   D. Collect forensic evidence

   Explanation: A SANE nurse is responsible for history taking, forensic examination, collection and preservation of evidence and providing expert testimony in court of law. A legal nurse consultant identifies a victim's future medical needs and associated costs.

4. **A patient is brought into the ED by family members who reported a fall, shares that the injury a result of physical abuse. The patient tells the forensic nurse that this is to be kept confidential because of her right. The forensic nurse informs the patient that:**
   A. The patients has the right but it is intended to protect the patient.
   B. The abuser needs to be stopped before any serious harm is caused to her.
   C. The report will not mention the patient's admission that abuse has occurred.
   D. Forensic nurse is required by law to report all incidents of abuse.

   Explanation: Forensic nurse is bound to report any crime or abuse to the Magistrate/police officer. Under Sec. 39 CrPC, every person who is aware of the commission of any offense to give information and aid the Magistrate or police officer by giving such information.

5. **Nursing ethics is defined by:**
   A. Moral principles and values
   B. Written rules
   C. Policy and procedures
   D. Standards of care

   Explanation: Nursing ethics is the applied discipline that addresses the moral principles of nursing practice. Ethics for nurses provides ethical guidance in relation to nurses' roles, duties, responsibilities, behaviors, professional judgement, etc.

6. **Use of code of ethics in nursing profession includes:**
   A. It guides professional behavior
   B. It prevents a nurse from practicing below the standard
   C. It can be used to protect a nurse who is falsely accused of doing something wrong
   D. All the above

   Explanation: Following a code of ethics helps to prevent below standard practice, guide for professional behavior, and serve as a defense in case of alleged unethical behavior.

7. **The duty to provide service for the good of the patient is enunciated in the ethical principle of:**
   A. Beneficence   B. Maleficence
   C. Non-maleficence   D. Autonomy

   Explanation: The principle of beneficence is the obligation of medical provider to act for the benefit of the patient. The principle calls for not just avoiding harm, but also to benefit patients and to promote their welfare.

8. **An example of professional misconduct is:**
   A. Touching a patient without consent
   B. Leaving an unstable patient unattended in the bathroom
   C. Yelling at a patient
   D. Speaking badly of a patient in the cafeteria

   Explanation: Abuse of patients (either physically or verbally) will constitute professional misconduct.

9. **Which of the following is an ethical principle that guides nursing practice?**
   A. Autonomy
   B. Virtue
   C. Care
   D. Utilitarianism

   Explanation: Autonomy is an ethical principle which means respecting patient's choices and self-determination. Utilitarianism (judiciousness), virtue, and care are not ethical principles, but ethical frameworks that help nurses analyze and resolve ethical dilemmas.

10. **A nurse is caring for a patient who is refusing treatment for his condition. The patient's family is pressuring the nurse to persuade the patient to accept treatment. What should the nurse do?**

A. Respect the patient's autonomy and allow him to refuse treatment.
B. Persuade the patient to accept treatment to satisfy the family's wishes.
C. Seek a court order to force the patient to accept treatment.
D. Consult with another nurse to determine the best course of action.

Explanation: The nurse has an ethical obligation to respect the patient's autonomy and right to make decisions about their own care. Persuading the patient to accept treatment against their will would violate their autonomy and could lead to a breach of trust between the patient and healthcare providers.

ANSWER KEY

| 1. A | 2. D | 3. B | 4. D | 5. A | 6. D | 7. A | 8. C | 9. A | 10. A |

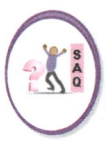

SHORT ANSWER QUESTIONS

1. Write briefly about the function of Indian Nursing Council.
2. Write a note on National Nursing and Midwifery Commission.
3. Why there is a need for nursing ethics?
4. What ethical principles are to be followed by nurses in dealing with the patients?
5. Write briefly about the nursing skills essential for forensic nurses.
6. Discuss in brief professional misconduct with examples.
7. What are privileged communications? Give some examples.
8. Write a note on professional secrecy.

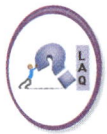

LONG ANSWER QUESTIONS

1. Write briefly about the history of development of forensic nursing.
2. Define forensic nursing. Discuss the various areas of practice and subspecialties related to forensic nursing.
3. Discuss the role and responsibilities of forensic nurse.
4. Discuss the composition and function of Indian Nursing Council.
5. Define nursing ethics. Discuss the code of ethics for nurses.
6. Discuss the code of professional conduct for nurses.
7. Discuss the ethical principles that are required to be followed by forensic nurses.

Answers to Case Study

A1. The death is informed to the police because it is due to trauma i.e., the gunshot wound. The manner of death could be homicide, suicide or accident.
A2. The clothing that is removed must be sent with the body to the forensic pathologist for examination. It should not be rolled/crumpled up, but folded with any defects facing upward. All clothing should be placed in paper bags, signed and handed over to the police.

CHAPTER 4

Comprehensive Forensic Nursing Care of Victim and Family

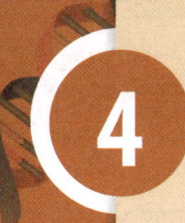

"Every trauma patient should be considered a forensic patient until proven otherwise."
— **Jamie Ferrell**
(Forensic Nurse Examiner)

LEARNING OBJECTIVES

At the end of this topic, the student should be able to:
1. Identify members of forensic team and outline their roles.
2. Describe the role of forensic nurse as member of forensic team.
3. Provide comprehensive forensic nursing care of victim and family vis-a-vis:
   - Physical aspects
   - Psychosocial aspects
   - Cultural and spiritual aspects
   - Legal aspects
4. Assist forensic team in care beyond scope of her practice
5. Deal with admission and discharge/referral/death of victim of violence
6. Understand and explain the role and responsibilities of nurse as a witness

CASE STUDY

You are a forensic nurse and posted in the ER. At night, a 26-year-old female Ms NJ was brought in unconscious by ambulance after her husband Mr X called 108. He stated that Ms NJ was not feeling well for the past few days and fell down the steps accidentally at home. There were swelling and bruising over face, lips, nose, broken front teeth with bruising over right forearm, hands and fingers. Imaging studies showed fracture of right ulna (as shown in **figure**) with acute subdural hemorrhage.

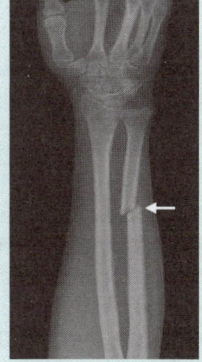

Q1. As a forensic nurse, do you think the patient's injuries correlates with Mr X's description of events?
Q2. What documentation will be most important from the perspective of the forensic nurse?
Q3. What is the nature of injury?*

*Discuss the questions with your teacher/facilitator.

FORENSIC TEAM MEMBERS AND THEIR ROLES IN CRIME SCENE

- **Forensic team:** The forensic analysts deployed on a given case.
- **Forensic analyst:** Person responsible for performing certain specialized forensic work on a case.
- **Crime scene:** Any location that may be associated with a committed crime and forensic evidence may be gathered, such as building, vehicles etc.
- **Crime scene investigation:** A process that aims at recording the scene as it is first encountered, and recognizing and collecting all physical evidence potentially relevant to the solution of the case.

There are certain personnel who are invariably necessary in almost any crime scene investigation; namely:
1. Team leader
2. Photographer and photographic log recorder
3. Sketch preparer
4. Evidence recorder/evidence recovery personnel
5. Specialists

Team Leader

- Assume control—ensure safety of personnel and security at scene. Ensure that the personnel use appropriate protective equipment and follow standard recommendations to protect them from any health hazard which might be presented by blood or any other biological body fluids.
- Conduct initial walk-through for purposes of making a preliminary survey, evaluating potential evidence, and preparing a narrative description.
- Determine search patterns and make appropriate assignments for team members.
- Coordinate with other law enforcement agencies and make sure a cooperative spirit is maintained.
- Ensure that sufficient supplies and equipment are available for personnel.
- Control access to the crime scene and designate an individual to log everyone into the scene.
- Release the crime scene after a final survey and inventory of the evidence has been done.

Photographer

An expert photographer may be needed to best capture images or video at the scene. Low-light, infrared, or aerial photography require skills.
- Photograph entire area before it is entered.
- Photograph victims, crowd, and vehicles.
- Photograph entire scene with overall, medium and close-up coverage, using measuring scale when appropriate.
- Photograph major evidence items before they are moved; coordinate this effort with sketch preparer, evidence recorder, and evidence recovery personnel.
- Photograph all latent fingerprints and other impression evidence before lifting and casting are accomplished.
- Prepare photographic log and photographic sketch.

Sketch Preparer

- Diagram immediate area of scene and orient diagram with sketch (now-a-days apps are available which have made the job easier).
- Describe major items of evidence on sketch.
- Designate and label areas to be searched and advise team leader and all other search members of organization for designated areas.
- Obtain appropriate assistance for taking measurements and double check measurements.

Evidence Recorder

- Have the evidence photographed before collection.
- Describe evidence and its location on appropriate bag or envelope.
- Sign and date evidence container/maintain chain of custody.
- Appropriately collect and package evidence to maximize evidence integrity.
- Maintain evidence log.
- Use appropriate protective equipment (gloves) and methods when dealing with potentially infective evidence (such as blood).

Specialists

The following are some examples of specialty assistance to be considered:

1. **Forensic pathologist:** Depending on the jurisdiction in various countries, either a medical examiner/coroner/forensic medicine specialist is concerned with the examination of the deceased. The medical examiner will determine the cause and manner of death. Medical examiners and their staff (often called "death investigators") carry out investigations at the scene of death, identify the deceased, and may identify and collect evidence.
2. **Forensic nurse:** Forensic nurses provides specialized care for both victims and perpetrators of violence. They care for the physical, psychological, and social trauma that occurs in patients who have been assaulted or abused. Forensic nurses also acquire skills in injury identification, evaluation of the nature and scope of injuries, documentation of the patient's incident, and the collection and proper storage of biological and physical evidence.
3. **Forensic anthropologists** are specialists in physical anthropology, the study of human biological function and variation, particularly skeletal system. The anthropologist's ability to understand the forms and variations of the human skeleton in individuals and populations complements the forensic pathologists' emphasis on soft tissue and body systems.
4. **Forensic entomologist** uses insects to gather information about a crime scene. An analysis of the insects and their life stages can yield information about the time of death.
5. **Forensic odontologist** identifies a person based on the recognition of features present in each person's dental structures; it is particularly useful when identification by the use of friction ridge skin (necessary for fingerprint) is not possible, as in burn victims or airplane crashes. They are also called upon to preserve and perform comparison of bite marks.
6. **Latent fingerprint expert** is skilled in fingerprint collection and comparison.
7. **Bomb technician** is responsible for the deactivation and/or removal of suspected explosive, incendiary devices, explosive chemicals, etc. and investigates post blast scenes and suspected arson crime scenes.
8. **Bloodstain pattern analysts** seek to answer questions about the manner and sequence of events of a crime by examining the bloodstains left behind.
9. **Ballistic expert** is responsible for collecting and analyzing ballistics-related evidence, which includes firearms and ammunition to determine their source.

Several studies have highlighted the benefits of the presence of forensic nurses in forensic team, namely empathy, support, and strengthening the sense of control and empowerment of most patients by forensic nurses.

We will discuss the role of forensic nurse in common settings.

Forensic Nurse as Member of Death Investigation Team (Crime Scene)

- Forensic nurses possesses essential knowledge of anatomy, physiology, pharmacology, growth and development, physical examination and medical history interviewing techniques.
- Additional training and experience in forensic medicine make the nurse ideal candidate for the role of a death investigator.
- The forensic nurse conducts a more thorough investigation—analyzes the scene and examines bodies to determine the time of death and collect any clues that might explain the cause of death.
  1. Nurse death investigators offer a holistic assessment of the death scene.
  2. Being of medical background, she can confirm the death of the victim from presence of clinical signs (pulse, breathing and heartbeat) of life. If otherwise, she should call an ambulance immediately, simultaneously doing whatever she can to save the life of the person. Dying declaration may be recorded, if death is eminent.

3. She can judiciously select biological evidence to be collected in order to achieve maximum utility of their analytical reports. Irrational collection of evidence overburdening police and FSL staff can be avoided. Any materials or evidence which are likely to be lost during transportation of body to the mortuary can be collected (loose fibers or hair). Perineal or vaginal swabbing in sexual assault cases, nail scrapings, swabbing of hands in firearm cases, loose ligature material, etc., can be preserved which may otherwise be overlooked by the crime scene team.
4. Appling her nursing knowledge, she may identify prescription medicines or illicit drugs at a scene and can distinguish overdose from natural death.
5. Sometimes, manner of death may be difficult to determine. For example, autoerotic asphyxia deaths may appear as suicidal in nature. In this, sexual pleasure is obtained by pressure on carotid vessels causing cerebral ischemia which may lead to hallucinations of an erotic nature in some men. But in some cases, *death occurs accidentally* which a skilled forensic nurse may determine from scene (presence of padding under the noose, nakedness of the victim, feminine attire and exposed genitalia), interview with friends and family can lead to a clear picture of the deceased person's intentions at the time of death.
6. Provides a link between pathologists and lay investigative staff.
7. Questions are formulated based on a medical knowledge base.
8. Interacts with and educates family members.
9. Aid families and survivors in terms of the grieving process.
10. Educates the community regarding death investigation and forensic issues.

Forensic Nurse as Member of Autopsy Team

1. Forensic nurse is an ideal complement to forensic pathologists and investigative staff.
2. Collaborate with organ/tissue procurement agencies.
3. *Helps in conducting postmortem:* Nurses have the educational background to understand exactly what the cause and manner of death, and what happens to the body after death occurs. They are also well educated in physiology to accurately distinguish between the cause and the physiologic mechanism of death.
   - Helps in thorough physical examination, document pathological findings.
   - Description via diagrams and dictation.
4. Oversee medical record aspect of the medico-legal examination—reviews the medical, surgical and social history of the deceased. The relevant information is provided to the forensic pathologist to determine the cause and manner of death.
5. Contact family members in order to provide information on cause and manner of death.
6. Discuss medical and familial implications of cause of death, if applicable.
7. Provide education regarding the medico-legal death investigation.

Forensic Nurse as Member of Sexual Assault Investigation Team

- When a person is violated, someone has violated their trust. Nurses, the most trusted health professionals, are the ones who are up close and personal with patients who are frightened, hurt or ashamed. The nurse who is knowledgeable about forensic procedures can establish and maintain trust with the patient and collect important evidence that otherwise might be lost.
- Forensic nurses provide "empowering care" in which all survivors are treated with dignity and respect regardless of circumstances, accepting her as a person, believing the history of assault, assisting her in restoring control over her life and making her own choices and respecting decisions.

1. Forensic nurse willingly conducts examination of sexual assault/child abuse
2. Specialty training in providing survivor centric services
3. Comprehensive and compassionate care
4. Provide community awareness:
    ♦ Where to come
    ♦ How will she be treated
5. Encourage reporting of sexual assaults
6. Fact based documentation
7. Encourage successful apprehension and prosecution of guilty offenders
8. Forensic issue:
    ♦ Evidence collection
    ♦ Chain of custody
    ♦ Courtroom testimony
    ♦ Aid in identifying false reporting/allegations

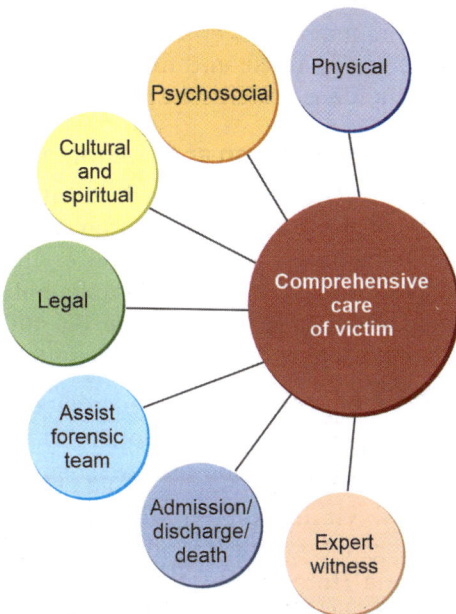

Flowchart 4.1: Comprehensive care of victim.

- The survivors of rape may have to wait for long hours to receive medical services. In order to collect samples, they are not allowed to drink, eat, or use the toilet. It has been found that the waiting time may take up to 12 hours until medico-legal examination is done. This time would decrease to less than 60 minutes with the presence of a forensic nurse.
- In addition, the examinations of rape survivors are hurriedly done and ED doctors usually dislike/reluctant doing it. This situation is worsened by unprofessional conduct when the victims are blamed for being raped. The presence of forensic nurses in examination team may lead to more acceptance of treatment, more often reporting to the police, more likely to consent to evidence collection and shorter stays in hospital.

COMPREHENSIVE CARE OF VICTIM AND FAMILY (FLOWCHART 4.1)

- **Trauma** is an exposure to actual or threatened death, serious injury or violence. Trauma/assault has lasting effects on victim's physical health, psychological, social and spiritual well-being.
- Forensic nurse may be the first person to engage the victim when seeking medical care for any injuries that may have been sustained due to trauma/assault or when neglect has occurred.
- The forensic nurse should provide the required medical treatment and psychological support [compassionate, holistic care (treating the whole person)]. Next, she would assist the victim in their medico-legal proceedings by collecting evidence and ensuring good quality documentation for use in criminal proceedings.
    - The forensic nurse documents the medical history of the victim while considering the potential for comorbidities in their existing health history and the type of abuse that has occurred.
    - Forensic nurses help victims navigate the emotions that come with trauma early on by providing a safe and comfortable environment and asking victims for permission to provide care. Their goal is to work with a possible victim and make sure the proper medical but also forensic tasks are accomplished.
    - While the many types of trauma may elicit different responses in different people, forensic nurses can identify the behaviors generally associated with

PTSD to determine how to address the issue.
- She may discover suspicious/subtle signs of abuse and neglect, and ask questions to assess the patient.

Physical Examination and Treatment

The first and foremost duty of the healthcare professional is to address acute problems and provide treatment for the same. Everything else is secondary. Information to be police should be sent as soon as possible, but under no circumstances, the treatment should be delayed.

History

Brief history of the incident should be taken from the victim/accompanying person regarding time, manner (accidental/suicidal/homicidal/intentional), weapon/means caused and place of event of injury/poisoning, and the time sequence of symptoms/incapacitation developed etc. (when/where/why/what/who) This will help the healthcare provider in proceeding with the examination.
- Due to stigma associated with sexual or domestic violence, many victims remain silent.

Informed Consent

- Permission should be sought before touching.
- The forensic nurse provides information about the process of an examination to allow the victim to make an informed decision about consenting to the medico-legal examination.
- She/he should explain to the victim in simple and understandable language all medical terms, the rationale for history taking, explain the various procedures, and details of how they will be performed.
- The consent form should be signed by the survivor if she is ≥12 years of age, and the guardian/parent if she is <12 years.
- A female patient, even if she is not a medico-legal case, should not be examined without the presence of a female relative of the patient or a female hospital attendant (if the examiner is male).
- Medico-legal report (MLR) should not be written in the presence of a police officer, patient's relatives or any other interested party.
- Whenever a victim of trauma/assault is brought to the ER, it the duty of the healthcare provider to send information to the police station/post of the area.
- Consent of the patient/injured/guardian is not needed for labelling a case as "MLC" and for further police information.

Particulars of Injuries

- Once consent is obtained, the examiner conducts the medico-legal examination and the collection of biological evidence. The examiner documents the findings by use of a written report (MLR) and photographs.
- The person should be examined in a systematic way from front to back, as well as from head to toe. All injuries observed, even insignificant should be noted for potential use as evidence in a later court case, where the examiner may be called as a witness to testify to the injuries.

The following particulars of injury must be recorded:
a. **Type of injury** like abrasion, bruise, wounds (lacerated, incised, stab, firearm etc.), fracture dislocation, bite mark, deformity, swelling, tenderness or burns etc.
b. **Size:** Exact dimensions (in centimeters using a ruler) of each injury should be noted down in respect of its length, breadth and depth, wherever possible.
c. **Shape:** Whether circular, oval, spindle, triangular, elliptical, crescentic etc., margins/edges of wounds (use magnifiers/hands lens wherever necessary), regular or irregular having bruise on its vicinity should be noted.
d. **Location of wound** with reference to some anatomical landmark, e.g., midline, bony structure or umbilicus should be noted.
e. **Direction of the wound** i.e., horizontal, vertical or oblique should be noted with regard to anatomical position of the body.

f. Foreign matter like grease, dirt, mud, paint, glass, bullets, wads, clothes, hair etc. should be noted and must be preserved for further analysis.
g. **Duration of injuries:** Time elapsed between infliction of injuries and examination can be determined from the color changes of abrasion and bruise, and healing process.

Psychosocial Aspects

- Psychosocial support involves the culturally sensitive provision of psychological and social care.
- Forensic nurses play a unique role in supporting patients. By initiating dialogue with patients, she/he can begin to understand how patients view themselves as individuals, what is important to them, and how their relationship with others may affect their decisions and their ability to live with those decisions during their treatment and beyond.
- Good communication and assessment skills are essential to building a rapport with patients and can help the nurse develop a clinical relationship with the patient and their family.

> **Communication skills for caring of victims**
> - **Effective communication**
>   a. Forensic nurse needs effective and good communication skills to make the victim regain the strengths which was lost due to the trauma.
>   b. The use of clear and concise language in a timely and accurate way is essential to avoid misunderstanding and confusion.
>   c. A forensic nurse with poor communication skills can re-victimize and traumatize the victim.
> - **Active listening techniques**
>   a. The forensic nurse should try to understand the victim's perspective, which includes both verbal and nonverbal signs.
>   b. Effective communication involves active listening techniques, such as making eye contact, rephrasing, asking follow-up questions, good presence of mind, and absence of interruptions.
>   c. If interrupted while the victim is narrating, such as taking a call in the mobile, may send a wrong message that the examiner is uncaring and uninterested.
>
> Contd....

> Contd....
> - **Open-ended and closed-ended questions**
>   a. Open-ended questions will allow the forensic nurse to gather maximum qualitative information from the victim.
>   b. Close-ended "yes or no questions" are short with virtually no description; should be asked only when necessary.

- The provision of good psychosocial care has been shown to be beneficial for patients by reducing both psychological distress and physical symptoms.
- It is important that the forensic nurse should be sensitive to the victim, since she/he has experienced a traumatic episode and may not be able to provide all the details. An environment of trust should be created so that the victim is able to speak out.
- Forensic nurse should:
  - Ensure consultation is conducted in safe, private and comfortable conditions.
  - Ensure confidentiality, while informing the victims of limits of confidentiality.
  - They should be nonjudgmental and supportive and validate what the victim is saying.
  - Provide practical care and support that responds to her/his concerns but does not intrude.
  - Ask about the history of trauma/violence, listening carefully, but not pressuring her/him to talk.
  - Help her/him access information about resources, including legal.
  - Provide or mobilize social support.

Cultural and Spiritual Aspects

- Sociocultural factors such as race, ethnic background, religious beliefs, beliefs about health and illness, sexuality, mental and physical disability status, and traditions also impacts the thoughts, affect and behavior of the forensic nurse, as well as her patients. The forensic nurse should rather maintain neutrality while dealing with the victims.
- Sociocultural theory states that human cognition and learning are social and cultural phenomena. They are applicable

to forensic nursing because language and cultural issues with patients can present barriers to receiving healthcare and can lead to disparities and inequalities in health outcomes and quality of care.
- The spiritual and religious needs of a patient should be given due consideration.

Legal Aspects

- The forensic nurse should mark on the top of first page of the file of the patient the letters "MLC" or put the stamp "Medico-legal case".
- An injury report is a form of medico-legal report (MLR) giving the details of the condition of a patient, solicited for legal purposes.
- This report is prepared wherever requested/consented, brought in the emergency by the police or those coming of their own for medico-legal examination or any other case in which foul play is suspected.
- Currently, a casualty medical officer or any other medical officer is called upon to examine the injured person. Forensic nurses can complement and help in this regard, and in future may be able to do it independently.

> **Medico-legal case (MLC):** A case of injury or complaint where the healthcare provider after history taking and clinical examination considers that investigations by police is required to ascertain circumstances and fix responsibility for the case.
> **Medico-legal report (MLR):** A document that describes the examination findings and opinion of a doctor prepared for the purpose of litigation.
> *Some examples of medico-legal cases are:*
> 1. Cases of injuries by any means—physical (assault/violence) or firearms.
> 2. Cases of suspected/evident sexual assault (both the accused and the victim).
> 3. Cases of burns, scalds, chemical and electrical injuries.
> 4. Suspected or evident homicides or suicides, including attempted.
> 5. Accidents—road traffic, fall from height, railway, factory, construction site or any other unnatural accident cases.
> 6. Cases of suspected or evident criminal abortion.
> 7. Cases of unconsciousness where its cause is not natural or unclear.
> 8. Cases of suspected or evident poisoning including snake bite poisoning or intoxication (alcohol).
> 9. Cases of drug overdose and drug abuse.

- A complete list of the injuries or conditions complained of by the patient along with a body diagram (*body chart*) to describe the exact anatomic location of a person's injuries should be present. Diagrams are visual supplements to written assessment findings.
- Color photographs of injuries are recommended. Photographs should be taken from different angles with a wide-angle lens. Close-ups should be taken both with and without a scale (such as a ruler) in the picture to show the size of the focal point.
- **Nature and duration of injuries:** Against each injury, it should be noted whether it is simple or grievous (as per **Sec. 320 IPC**). Injured person must be kept 'under observation', if nature of particular injury cannot be made out at the time of examination, e.g., head injury or abdominal injury. Opinion regarding duration of injuries (time of infliction) is based on the state of healing of the injuries as was recorded in the column of examination of the injuries.
- **Weapon used to inflict the injury:** In many cases, examination of the wound and clothing (presence of cuts, tears or burns) give fairly definite information about the kind of weapon. With stab and incised wound, there is not much difficulty.

> *As per **Sec. 320 IPC**, the following kinds of hurt are designated as "grievous":*
> 1. Emasculation.
> 2. Permanent privation of the sight of either eye (permanent loss of eye-sight).
> 3. Permanent privation of the hearing of either ear (permanent loss of hearing).
> 4. Privation of any member or joint (permanent loss of any body part, like ears, fingers, etc.).
> 5. Destruction or permanent impairing of the powers of any member or joint.
> 6. Permanent disfiguration of the head or face.
> 7. Fracture or dislocation of a bone or tooth.
> 8. Any hurt which endangers life or which causes the sufferer to be during the space of 20 days in severe bodily pain, or unable to follow his ordinary pursuits.

- The MLR should be handed over to the police immediately after the examination. If any injury is kept under observation, the

same may be recorded as such and result thereof communicated to the police at the earliest.
- Details of all samples and specimens should appear in the report to establish the chain of custody. Failure to collect, destruction or loss of such an exhibit is punishable under **Sec. 201 IPC**.
- The report should be impartial and unbiased, comprehensible and easy to read. Further, it should be clear about the opinion regarding the nature, cause and duration of injury.

Assist Forensic Team in Care beyond Scope of her Practice

- Forensic nurses can help in photographic documentation of the injuries when a forensic pathologist is documenting the injuries in the medico-legal report.
- She/he has a unique position in emergency care to attend to family members and provide support.
  - The inclusion of family members may be difficult or too great a risk if the perpetrator is within the family or has close connections to other family members.
  - However, in cases when there is no risk for the victim, involvement of family members in care may strengthen the family and alleviate suffering and emotional distress.
- In addition to providing care, forensic nurses work together with multidisciplinary team members and consultants and medical professionals and the police.
- She/he may provide referrals for follow-up care, written discharge instructions, community resources, and facilitation of a safe place post discharge. This occurs if the victim is not admitted for further evaluation and treatment of injuries or if the return to the residence or facility is unsafe for the victim.
- Crime victims face a higher risk of PTSD, depression, suicide, and medical complications than other patients; forensic nurses can improve both legal outcomes and quality of life for these patients.

Admission and Discharge/ Referral/ Death of Victim of Violence

Admission and Discharge

- No MLC should be discharged or leave against medical advice (LAMA) without information to the police. Whenever a MLC is admitted or discharged, the same should be intimated to the police at the earliest.
- If the patient is not serious and can take care of himself, he may be discharged on his own request, after taking in writing that he has been explained the possible outcome of such a discharge. Police have to be informed before the said patient leaves the hospital.
- While discharging or referring the patient, care should be taken to see that he receives the discharge card/referral letter, complete with the summary of admission, the treatment given in the hospital and the instructions to the patient to be followed after discharge. Failure to do so renders the healthcare provider liable for "negligence" and "deficiency of service".
- Sometimes, the patient, registered as a "MLC", may abscond from the hospital. Police have to be immediately informed, the moment such an instance comes to the notice of the nurse.

Referral Cases

If patient is serious and proper arrangements are not available, then he/she should be referred to higher centre for treatment with full details clearly stating that MLR could not be prepared due to seriousness of the patient.

Death of a Person Admitted as MLC

- Whenever a patient of MLC dies, inform the police immediately and a note mentioning the same is recorded on the file of the deceased.
- The body should be shifted with dignity to the mortuary for preservation. Clear instructions should be given to the

mortuary staff, not to hand over the body to the relatives till the legal formalities are completed and the police releases the body to the lawful heirs.
- Dead bodies should be shifted to mortuary with proper body identification tag. The tag should include details of case, name, age, sex, address, CR No., ward, etc.
- The name of the ward attendant or any other employee/police staff transporting the dead body shall be recorded in the mortuary register/file/OPD register.
- Complete chain of custody of the dead body shall be maintained at all times, till the body is finally handed over to the police.
- Medico-legal postmortem examination is done to determine the cause of death.
- Death certificate is not issued, even if the patient was admitted.

Patient is MLC but not Admitted

- If a patient of MLC is not admitted, entry shall be made in the OPD register. MLR will be prepared by the doctor on duty in ER.
- A copy of the MLR should be given to the patient only on request or if the same is required for the purpose of further treatment at any other hospital.

> - Cases which are admitted as *non-MLC* but in which the healthcare provider suspects foul play should be immediately brought to the notice of the police in writing so that they may take necessary action in the matter.
> - In the event of death of such a case, a written report should be sent to the police so that a medico-legal postmortem could be arranged. The body of such a case should be sent to the mortuary and not be handed over to the relatives.

Responsibilities of Nurse as a Witness

A witness is a person who gives sworn testimony (evidence) in a court of law as regards facts and/or inferences that can be drawn from these.

Types (Diff. 4.1)

1. **Common/Ordinary/Percipient Witness**
- Gives evidence about the facts observed/perceived by him **(Sec. 118 IEA)**.

Diff. 4.1: Common and Expert Witness.

Features	Common witness	Expert witness
Definition	Gives evidence about the facts observed or perceived by him (Sec. 118 IEA)	Person especially skilled in foreign law, science or art (Sec. 45 IEA)
Volunteering a statement	Not allowed	Can volunteer
Drawing inference from observations	Not allowed	Can draw
Responsibility	Less	Highly responsible
Punishment on false evidence	Less punishment	Severely punished
Conduct money	Cannot claim	Can claim
Examples	Any person	Forensic nurse, doctor, chemical examiner, fingerprint expert

- This is when a nurse in the course of practice is in possession of facts, direct observations and/or personal knowledge of the case at trial.
- The nurse can testify to physical findings such as lab results, photographs or anatomical drawings, observations of behaviors, specimen collection procedures, instruments used to examine the patients etc.

2. **Expert/Skilled Witness**
- A person whose professional training and experience in technical or scientific subject can provide the court with an assessment, opinion or inference from the facts observed by him or noticed by others, which is not considered known to the layperson, e.g., handwriting or fingerprint expert, forensic nurse, doctor, chemical examiner, etc.
- An expert nurse witness can testify in case of professional negligence or in cases

where there is a disciplinary hearing against another nurse since they can give professional opinion on the actions of others.

Hostile Witness

- A person who willfully or with motive (bribe/intimidation) conceals part of the truth or gives completely false evidence in a court.
- Any of the above two witnesses can be declared hostile witness.

Forensic Nurse as Expert Witness

- A nurse expert witness acquires specific expertise and competencies in acting as an expert witness.
- The forensic nurse who serves as an expert witness is held to higher standards of relevant education and experience than the nurse testifying about the care provided to a specific medico-legal case. An expert nurse may be called by the defense to evaluate the procedures or counteract the testimony of a common nurse witness.
- Forensic nurse should prepare herself well in time with the case documents and review the notes before reaching the court. Efforts must be made to discuss with the public prosecutor and ask him about the role that she needs to play. This would help her to be well prepared and respond to questions asked in the court.
- Forensic nurses' testimony should covey impartiality; their role represents search for the truth, not a "win" for the victim (or defendant). They are required to be objective witnesses of the facts and the science base, contributing information to the judges and court so that the most informed deposition can be made.
- Assertive patient advocacy is appropriate in the hospital setting, but not in the court of law. Forensic nurses should never testify that they believe the victim is telling the truth about being assaulted or whether victim consented to sexual intercourse—that is for the judge to decide.
- As an expert witness, forensic nurse testifies as to her opinion about some element of the case. Only when the facts of the matter have been determined by the court, a decision can be based on the relevant law.

Following are some of the do's and dont's in the witness box **(Fig. 4.1)**:
- Take all records and relevant reports that may have to be quoted in the box.
- Be well dressed and modest. Switch off your mobile or set in vibration mode.
- Do not discuss the case with anyone in the court except the lawyer by whom you were asked to testify.
- Stand up straight, be relaxed, calm and not be frightened or nervous.
- Address the Judge by his proper title such as 'Sir' or 'Your honor'.
- Never attempt to memorize. You can refresh your memory from copies of reports.
- Speak slowly, distinctly and audibly so that the typist can record your evidence.
- Use simple language, avoiding technical terms to the best of your ability.
- Be polite, pleasant and courteous to the lawyer. Do not underestimate the medical knowledge of the lawyers.
- Do not evade a question or "guess" an answer. Say "I don't know" if it is so, for no one can be expected to know everything.
- Do not lose your temper. An angry witness is often a poor witness.
- Retain independence of your mind. A biased expert is a useless expert.
- Listen carefully to the questions. Do not hesitate to ask the questions to be repeated, if you do not understand it. Consider your response before speaking.
- If you believe the question is unfair, look at your lawyer before answering. If he fails to object, turn to the Judge and ask whether you should answer the question.
- Watch for double questions. The answer to each part of the question may be different.
- When asked to comment upon the competence of a colleague, avoid any insulting remarks.
- Say 'In my opinion....', do not use phrase such as 'I think...' or 'I imagine...' Be prepared to give reasons for your opinion, if asked.
- Do not be drawn outside your particular field of competence.
- Do not volunteer any information beyond that is asked for in the question, unless clarification is needed.

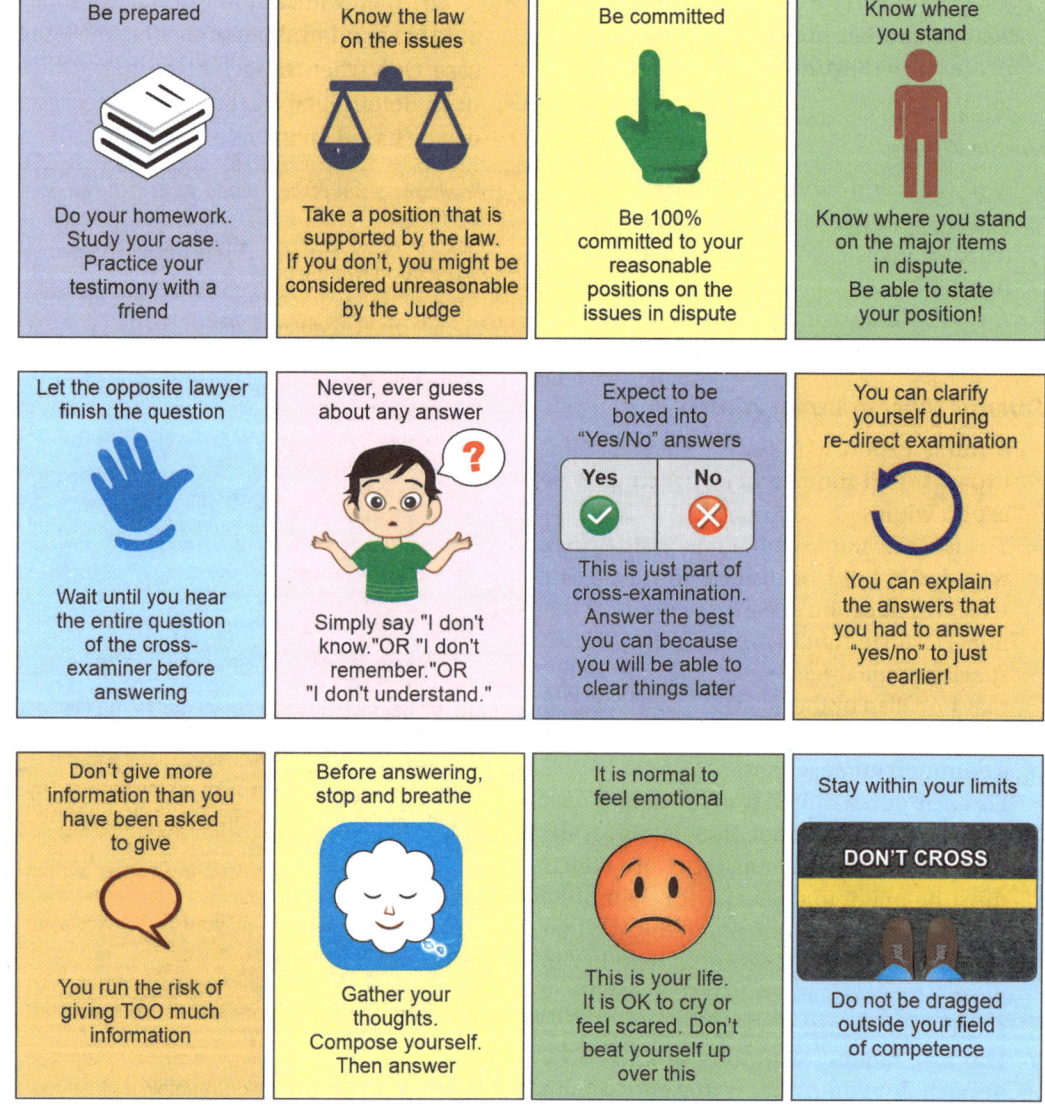

Fig. 4.1: Testimony: Do's and don'ts.

CHAPTER 4: Comprehensive Forensic Nursing Care of Victim and Family

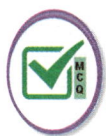

MULTIPLE CHOICE QUESTIONS

1. Following are members of forensic team, *except*:
   A. Team leader
   B. Photographer
   C. Evidence recorder
   D. Police constable

   Explanation: Police constable can be a member of first responder team to a crime scene as he may receive the information of a crime. The first responders include emergency medical services personnel, firefighters, and police officers. They are usually not a member of the investigating forensic team.

2. All are examples of cases where the emergency forensic nurse should be involved, *except*:
   A. Victim of road traffic accident
   B. School student reporting rape
   C. Elderly person with signs of abuse
   D. Patient who has sued for negligence

   Explanation: The forensic nurse may address victims of road traffic accidents, rape or abuse (all are MLCs) but need not attend a patient who sued for negligence in the emergency department. It is not her current concern but may encounter as legal nurse consultant later in legal proceedings.

3. A 27-year-old female patient presented with history of domestic violence. There was a fracture of left central incisor teeth and some bruises around mouth. The injury is:
   A. Simple injury
   B. Grievous injury
   C. Dangerous injury
   D. Culpable homicide

   Explanation: Fracture or dislocation of a bone or tooth is considered as grievous hurt as per Sec. 320 IPC.

4. A 30-year-old male was admitted in the emergency with alleged history of being stabbed by his neighbor. The forensic nurse is required to inform the police under:
   A. Sec. 174 CrPC
   B. Sec. 39 CrPC
   C. Sec. 193 IPC
   D. Sec. 176 CrPC

   Explanation: Under Sec. 39 CrPC, every person who is aware of the commission of any offense is required to give information and aid the magistrate or police officer by giving such information. Sec. 174 CrPC and Sec. 176 CrPC is for police and magistrate inquest respectively. Sec. 193 IPC is for punishment for false evidence.

5. Consent for medico-legal examination can be given by a person who is:
   A. Above 10 years of age
   B. Above 12 years of age
   C. Above 16 years of age
   D. Above 18 years of age

   Explanation: The consent for medico-legal examination can be signed by the victim/survivor if he/she is ≥12 years of age, and the guardian/parent if she is <12 years.

6. **All of the following are true of written consent:**
   A. It must be taken prior to the examination
   B. It must include the evidence to be collected
   C. It must include the forensic nurse's interpretation of the events that took place
   D. It must include the taking of photographs during the examination

   Explanation: Written informed consent should be obtained before the examination, collection of specimens, release of information to authorities, and taking of photographs. There is no requirement for nurse's interpretation of the events that took place.

7. Which of the following examples is NOT a good example of the forensic nurse's documentation?
   A. Measuring the wound in centimeters
   B. Using photographs instead of written documentation
   C. Documenting statements exactly as the victim stated them
   D. Marking a wound on a body diagram

   Explanation: Forensic documentation includes a written component, a diagrammatic component, and a photographic component. Using photographs instead of written documentation is not the correct way for documentation.

8. **In case of a death of a medico-legal case, the dead body is handed over to:**
   A. Next of kin/relatives
   B. Police
   C. Municipal corporation
   D. Ambulance personnel

   Explanation: In MLCs, the body will not be handed over to the NOK/relatives. The police is informed and the body is handed over to them. The police will, after the medico-legal formalities, hand over the body to the NOK/relatives.

9. **The term "expert witness" is defined under:**
   A. Sec. 131 IEA
   B. Sec. 131 CrPC
   C. Sec. 45 CrPC
   D. Sec. 45 IEA

   Explanation: Sec. 45 IEA refers to 'opinions of experts': "When the court has to form an opinion upon a point of foreign law, or of science, or art, or as to identity of handwriting, or finger impressions, the opinion of persons especially skilled in such foreign law, science or art or handwriting or finger impressions, are relevant facts. Such persons are called experts."

10. **All are considered as expert witnesses, *except*:**
    A. Forensic nurse
    B. Ward nurse
    C. Chemical examiner
    D. Forensic pathologist

    Explanation: The ward nurse can testify as a common witness to physical findings such as lab results, photographs or anatomical drawings, observations of behaviors, specimen collection procedures, etc., but cannot draw an opinion on any technical matters.

ANSWER KEY

| 1. D | 2. D | 3. B | 4. B | 5. B | 6. C | 7. B | 8. B | 9. D | 10. B |

SHORT ANSWER QUESTIONS

1. Discuss in brief the role of forensic nurse in death investigation team.
2. Discuss in brief the role of forensic nurse in sexual assault investigation team.
3. What all are noted while describing the injuries in a victim of assault?
4. What is a medico-legal case? Give some examples.
5. Discuss in brief the psychosocial aspects of care of assault victim.
6. Write a note on communication skills required for forensic nurses.
7. What are the legal issues related to assault victim?
8. Write a note on grievous hurt.
9. What are the various types of witnesses? Describe briefly.
10. Write a note on "forensic nurse as expert witness".

LONG ANSWER QUESTIONS

1. Discuss the role and responsibilities of members of forensic team.
2. Discuss how forensic nurse can help in providing comprehensive care of victim of assault.
3. Discuss the role of forensic nurse in admission, discharge, death and referral of medico-legal case.
4. Discuss the do's and don'ts while testifying in the court of law.

CHAPTER 5

Comprehensive Forensic Nursing Care of Survivor of Sexual Assault

> "In order to escape accountability for his crimes, the perpetrator does everything in his power to promote forgetting. If secrecy fails, the perpetrator attacks the credibility of his victim. If he cannot silence her absolutely, he tries to make sure no one listens."
> — **Judith Lewis Herman (Psychiatrist, Researcher, Teacher, and Author)**

LEARNING OBJECTIVES

At the end of this topic, the student should be able to:
1. Provide comprehensive forensic nursing care of survivor of sexual assault vis-a-vis:
   - Physical aspects
   - Psychosocial aspects
   - Cultural and spiritual aspects
   - Legal aspects
2. Understand the responsibilities of nurse as a witness

CASE STUDY

A 19-year-old college student Ms CK comes to the ER. She informs that two nights back she woke up in the lobby of her building with her clothes backwards, and she was not wearing any underwear. The last thing she remembers is drinking and dancing at a party in another resident's room.

Q1. What should the forensic nurse do?
Q2. Do you consider it as a case of sexual violence?
Q3. Should the nurse send police information regarding this incident?*

*Discuss the questions with your teacher/facilitator.

INTRODUCTION

- **Sexual assault** is known to cause physical, psychological, social and economic consequences which can endanger the well-being of survivors and their families.
- The presence of trained forensic nurses provides survivors of sexual assault with medical, psychological, and legal services at hospital and community level.
- Fear of police investigation procedures, threat from perpetrators, shame related to the sexual assault, lack of support from the community, fear that nobody will believe them and lack of information about negative health consequences may lead survivors to hide such incidents.

Health Consequences of Sexual Assault

Survivors of sexual assault may present to hospital with varying signs and symptoms. Some may not reveal a history of sexual assault, but the following signs and symptoms should prompt one to suspect the possibility **(Table 5.1)**.

Table 5.1: Physical and psychological consequences of sexual assault.

Physical health consequences	Psychological effects	
	Short term	Long term
Severe abdominal pain	Fear and shock	Depression and anxiety
Burning micturition/UTI	Powerlessness	Feelings of vulnerability
Dyspareunia	Denial	Nightmares
Sexual dysfunction	Worthlessness	Emotional distress
Menstrual disorders	Apathy	Impaired sense of self
Unwanted pregnancy	Intense self-disgust	Loss of self-esteem
Unsafe abortion	Numbing	Self-blame
Miscarriage of an existing fetus	Withdrawal	Mistrust
Sexually transmitted infections (HIV/AIDS)	Physical and emotional pain	Post-traumatic stress disorder
Pelvic inflammatory disease		Suicidal ideation
Infertility		Avoidance
Mutilated genitalia		Substance abuse
		Rape trauma syndrome

COMPREHENSIVE CARE OF SEXUAL ASSAULT SURVIVOR

- **Survivor:** The term 'survivor' is preferably used instead of 'victim' since it recognizes that the person is capable of taking decisions despite being victimized, humiliated and traumatized due to the assault.
- **Victim:** It is a person in need of compassion, care, validation and support, and is not fully capable of comprehending situation at hand because of the victimhood faced.

Although in the text, we have used victim or survivor liberally, it is recommended to use the terminology "the patient who experienced sexual assault" or "the patient who is a victim/survivor of sexual assault" during documentation as the word "victim/survivor" indicates that the healthcare provider is confirming that the patient has been raped or sexually assaulted (advocacy), in the same sense we cannot refer to the perpetrator as the "perp". They are both patients. They are not a victim or a perpetrator until they go to court and are found innocent or guilty by the judge. It is part of being neutral in our role as healthcare providers.

The guidelines describe in detail the stepwise approach to be used for a comprehensive response to the sexual violence survivor **(Flowchart 5.1)**:

i. Initial resuscitation/first aid.
ii. Establish a rapport with the survivor and take informed consent.
iii. Detailed history taking.
iv. Medical examination—general physical and local.
v. Age estimation (physical/dental/radiological)—if required.
vi. Documentation.
vii. Treatment of injuries.
viii. Evidence collection.
ix. Packing, sealing and handing over the collected evidence to the police.
x. Testing/prophylaxis for sexually transmitted disease, HIV, hepatitis B and pregnancy.
xi. Psychological support and counseling.

The purpose is:

- Establish a uniform method of examination and evidence collection by following the protocols using the sexual assault forensic evidence (SAFE) kit.
- Search for physical signs that will corroborate the history given by the victim.
- Search for, collect and preserve all trace evidence for laboratory examination.
- Treat the victim for injuries, to prevent/treat sexually transmitted infections (STIs) or pregnancy, and to prevent or alleviate psychological damage.
- Maintain a clear and full-proof chain of custody of medical evidence collected.
- Refer to appropriate agencies for further assistance (e.g., legal support services, shelter services, etc.).

This will help in forming an opinion on:

i. Whether a sexual act has been attempted or completed?
ii. Whether such a sexual act is recent?
iii. Whether any harm has been caused to the survivor's body?
iv. The age of the survivor needs to be verified in the case of adolescent girls/boys.
v. Whether alcohol or drugs have been administered to the survivor?

CHAPTER 5: Comprehensive Forensic Nursing Care of Survivor of Sexual Assault

Flowchart 5.1: Examination protocol of patient who is a survivor of sexual assault.

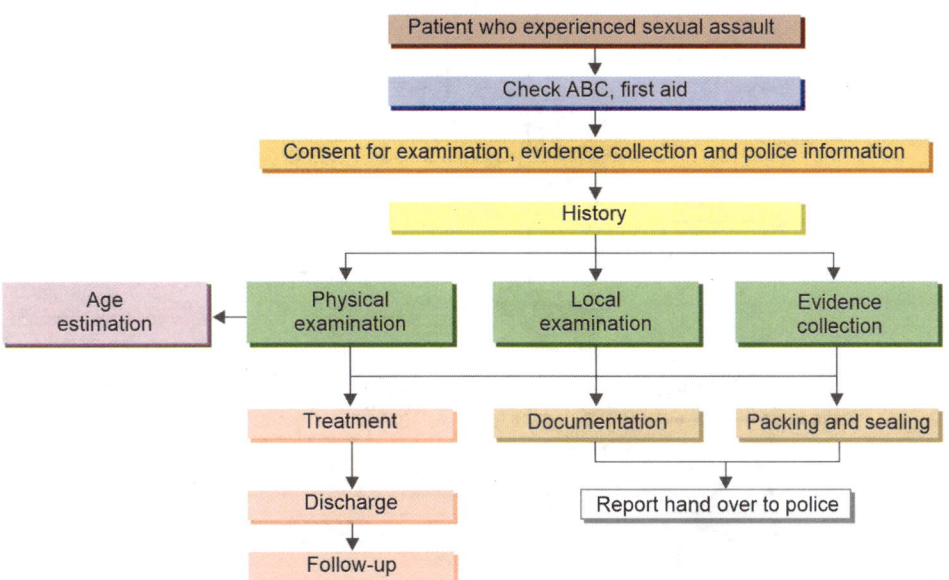

Sexual Assault Forensic Evidence (SAFE) Kit

- It is a set of items used by medical personnel for gathering and preserving physical evidence following an allegation of sexual assault **(Table 5.2 and Figs. 5.1 and 5.2)**.
- It is used to maintain uniform method of examination and evidence collection. It is also called "rape kit" or "physical evidence recovery kit (PERK)".

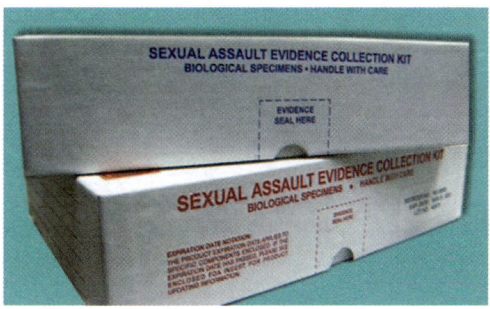

Fig. 5.1: SAFE kit.

Table 5.2: Sexual assault forensic evidence kit.	
Detailed instructions for the examiner	Large sheet of paper for patient to undress
Forms for documentation	Paper bags for clothing collection
Catchment paper	Disposable gloves
Nail cutter, comb, scissor	Sterile/distilled water
Glass slides	Urine sample container
Unwaxed dental floss	Sealing wax, labels
Nail scrapper for fingernail scrapings	Tubes/vacutainers (EDTA, plain, NaF)
Sterile swabs	Syringes and needles
Envelopes or boxes for individual evidence samples	Clean clothing and shower/hygiene items (for the survivor's use after examination)

Examination Guidelines (Fig. 5.3)

1. Guidelines and protocols of medico-legal care for survivors/victims of sexual violence by Ministry of Health and Family Welfare advocates a structured format for documentation which needs to be followed in case of rape/sexual assault examination.
2. Under **Sec. 164-A CrPC** (medical examination of the victim of rape), the examination should be conducted without delay by a registered medical practitioner (RMP) employed in a Government hospital or any other RMP with the consent of the survivor or person competent to give consent on her behalf, and she should be sent to the RMP

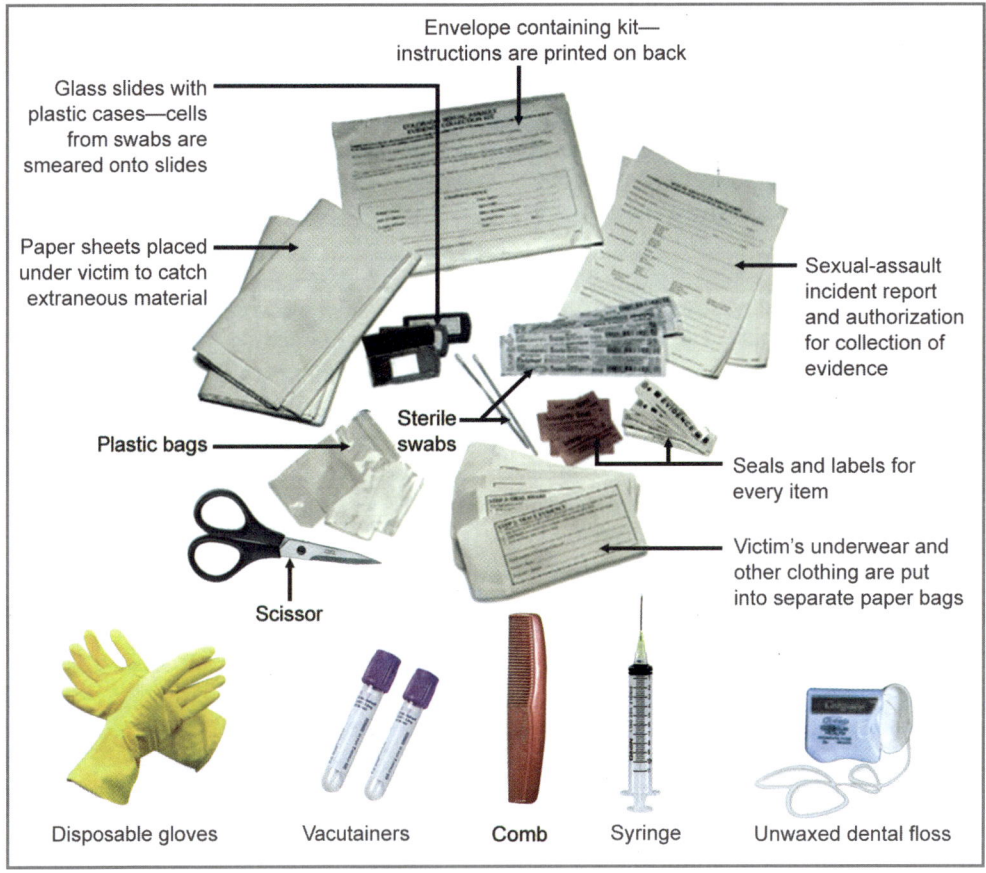

Fig. 5.2: Contents of SAFE kit.

within 24 hours from the time of receiving the information by the police relating to the commission of such offense.
3. The healthcare provider should prepare a detailed report and describe the material taken from the female for DNA profiling.
4. Even if there is informed refusal for medico-legal examination, medical treatment should not be denied.
5. In case of refusal for police intimation, the healthcare provider is duty bound to inform the police.
6. Per-vaginal examination, commonly referred to as *"two-finger test"* to check the hymen and to determine the laxity and rugosity of vaginal muscles, **must not be conducted for establishing rape/sexual violence.**

Examination Procedure
i. A requisition for examination of the survivor should come from an authorized person, either from the magistrate or incharge of a police station. If she has approached the healthcare provider by herself to get a medical examination, the provider is bound to conduct her medico-legal examination without any delay. A police requisition is not required for this. Information is sent to the police for recording her statement and lodging of complaint.
ii. Police officers, regardless of their sex, should never be in the examining room.
iii. If possible, the survivor is examined by or under the supervision of a female healthcare provider. If a board of examiners

CHAPTER 5: Comprehensive Forensic Nursing Care of Survivor of Sexual Assault

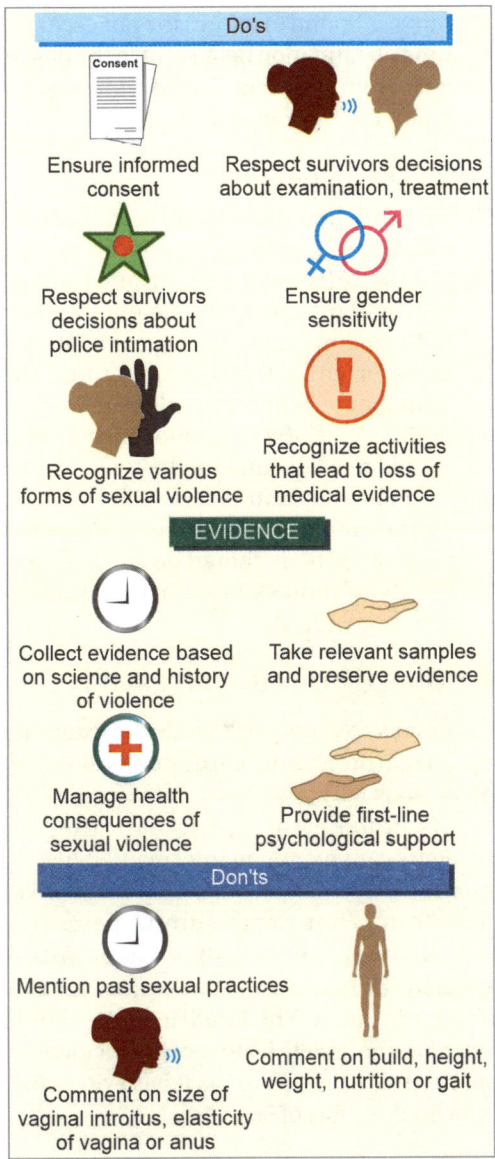

Fig. 5.3: Guidelines for rape survivor examination.

is examining her, at least one must be a female. Otherwise, a female attendant should be there, if she is examined by a male healthcare provider. If the survivor requests, her relative may be present while the examination is done.
- At many places, getting a doctor for medico-legal examination of rape survivor may be difficult. In such scenarios, a forensic nurse can be very useful to conduct examination and handle such cases (if amendment is made in CrPC). Otherwise, she can complement the examining healthcare provider.

iv. The examination should be carried out without delay. Minor degrees of injury may fade rapidly, and swelling and tenderness of vulva may disappear in a few hours. Chances of detection of spermatozoa from the genital tract diminish with delay.

v. Statements of the survivor and others accompanying her are recorded separately. This is particularly important in cases of children wherein she may be accompanied by the abuser. In such situations, a female person appointed by the head of the hospital may be present during the examination.

vi. Since abuse by near and dear ones are common, it is important not to let the history be dictated by the person accompanying the survivor. History must be sought independently, directly from the survivor.

INFORMED CONSENT

i. The forensic nurse should explain to the survivor in simple and understandable language the rationale for history taking and details of various procedures/stages of examination, and how they will be performed **(Box 5.1)**.

ii. Only in life-threatening situation, the healthcare provider may initiate treatment without consent **(Sec. 92 IPC)**.

iii. In case of persons with mental disability, their informed consent is taken from their parents or legal guardians and the patient need to provide assent* after providing the necessary information and adequate time. Assistance of a friend/colleague/caregiver can be taken in forming the decision.

iv. Consent should be obtained before the examination, collection of specimens,

---

*Assent is an agreement of someone not able to give legal consent to participate in the activity.

> **Box 5.1:** Informed consent for examination of survivor of sexual assault.
>
> - The medico-legal examination may involve an examination of the mouth, breasts, vulva, vagina, anus and rectum depending on the particular circumstances.
> - The fact that genital examination may be uncomfortable but is necessary for legal purposes should be explained to the survivor.
> - The survivor should be informed about the need to carry out additional procedures, such as X-rays which may require her to visit others departments.
> - Forensic evidence may be collected which may include removing and isolating clothing, scalp hair, foreign substances from the body, saliva, pubic hair, samples from the vulva, vagina, anus, rectum, mouth and collecting a blood sample.
> - She has the right to refuse either a medico-legal examination or collection of evidence or both, but that refusal will not be used to deny treatment. The court or the police have no power to compel a woman for medico-legal examination against her will **[Sec. 164-A (7) CrPC]**. She has a right for partial examination— she may also decide on whether she wants to undergo a physical examination and/or genital examination and allow collection of bodily evidence.
> - The hospital/examining healthcare provider is required/duty bound to inform the police about the incidence. However, if she does not wish to participate in the police investigation, she has the right to refuse to file FIR and it would not result in denial of medical examination and treatment.
> - Any evidence obtained may be used in court, and that she will then be exposed to publicity and cross-examination.

release of information to authorities and taking of photographs. The form should be signed by the survivor, a witness and the examining healthcare provider. Any major 'disinterested', person may be considered a witness.

v. The survivor may refuse to give consent for any part of examination, particularly genital examination. In this case, the forensic nurse should explain the importance of examination and evidence collection for legal purposes; however, the refusal should be respected and documented. Even if there is informed refusal for police intimation, the forensic nurse is bound to inform the police. At the time of intimation being sent to the police, a clear note stating '*informed refusal for police intimation*' should be made.

Particulars of the Survivor

i. Name of the survivor, age, marital status, residence, occupation and social status.
ii. Date, time (commencement and completion) and place of examination. Date and time are important, because the interval between the alleged incident and the examination is important. If there was any undue delay, the reason for such a delay should to be documented.
iii. Two identification marks such as moles, scars or tattoos, preferably on the exposed parts of the body should be documented. Left thumb impression is to be taken in the space provided.

THE MEDICO-LEGAL INTERVIEW

The details of history will guide the examination, treatment and evidence collection **(Flowchart 5.2)**.

It is noted as to who is narrating the incident—survivor or an informant. If history is narrated by a person other than the survivor herself, his/her name should be noted. Especially, if the identity of assailants is revealed, it is better to have a countersignature of the informant. The forensic nurse should record the complete history of the incident, in the survivor's own words as it has evidentiary value in the court of law.

History of Chief Complaints

- It should include date, time and place of alleged offense, description of the assailant(s) and number of persons, relationship to assailant (stranger, acquaintance, internet connection), use of threats or restraints, exact relative positions of the partners, details of struggle or resistance, calls for help, sensation as to penetration and emission (whether emission was within the vagina or outside), any condom used during the act, and

CHAPTER 5: Comprehensive Forensic Nursing Care of Survivor of Sexual Assault

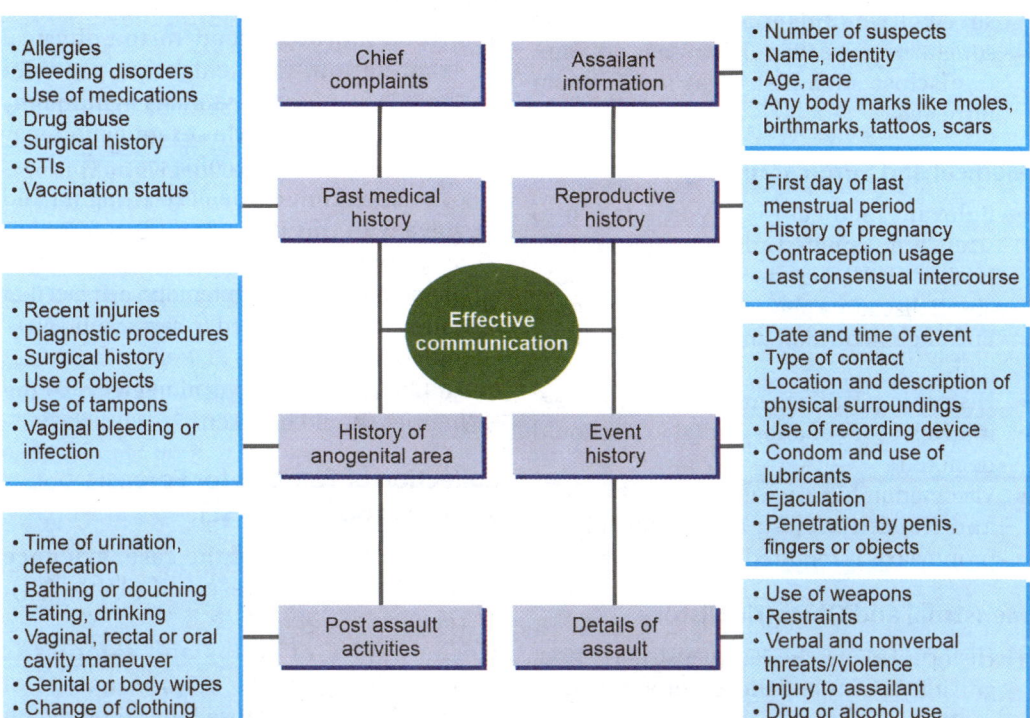

Flowchart 5.2: History.

any bleeding or pain during or after the incident.
- Other nongenital acts, such as kissing, touching, licking, and biting, and where on the body.
  - Information about emission of semen outside the orifices should be elicited as swabs taken from such sites can have evidentiary value.
  - Information regarding use of condom during the assault is relevant because in such cases, vaginal swabs and smears would be negative for sperm/semen.
  - Information regarding attempted or completed penetration by penis/finger/object in vagina/anus/mouth should be recorded.
- Whether any drug or alcohol was taken (it may help establish lack of consent)?

Physical Violence
- Use of any physical violence is recorded with description of the type of violence and its location on the body (e.g., beating on the legs, biting cheeks, pulling hair, hitting, choking, or kicking the abdomen).
- History of injury inflicted by the survivor on the assailant's body is noted so that it can be matched eventually with the findings of the assailant's examination.
- Whether consciousness was lost at any time during the attack?

Post-assault Activities
Details of the events after the alleged assault, such as douching or bathing, cleaning or changing clothes, using tampon or sanitary napkin, urination or defecation, eating or drinking, and use of toothpaste, mouthwash, enemas or drugs.

Sexual History
- Date and time of the last consensual intercourse (because sperm from this encounter may still be present in the vaginal canal and cervix and confuse the issue).

- While seeking such history, explain to the survivor why this information is being sought, because the survivor may not want to disclose such history as it may seem intrusive.

Medical and Surgical History

- Relevant medical history in relation to sexually transmitted infections (gonorrhea, HIV or HBV) can be elicited by asking about discharge per urethra, warts, ulcers, burning micturition and lower abdominal pain.
- History in relation to treatment of fissures/injuries/scars of ano-genital area should be noted.
- Vaccination history with regard to tetanus and hepatitis B, so as to ascertain if prophylaxis is required.

Menstrual and Obstetric History

- History of menarche, last menstrual period, gravidity, parity and the method of contraception.
- If the survivor is menstruating at the time of examination, then a second examination is required at a later date in order to record the injuries clearly. Some amount of evidence is lost because of menstruation.

PHYSICAL EXAMINATION (TABLE 5.3)

- After a thorough head-to-toe physical examination, the healthcare provider should examine the genitalia in lithotomy position (**Fig. 5.4**). This examination may involve the use of a colposcope (process of examination of the cervix, vagina and vulva with this instrument is referred to as colposcopy). Old injuries related to previous consensual intercourse or fact that a person is 'habituated to sex' should NOT be recorded.
- Full body photographs along with all the injuries should be taken.

Collection of Samples for Forensic Science Laboratory (FSL)

- After assessment of the case, evidence is collected and preserved (**Table 5.4**). *(details in Chapter 6)*
- The nature of swabs and samples is determined by the history, nature of assault, and time lapse between incident and examination, and if she has bathed/washed herself since the assault.
- The likelihood of finding evidence after 72 hours (3 days) is greatly reduced; however, it is better to collect evidence

Table 5.3: Examination protocol and brief findings in sexual assault cases.

Physical examination	Local (genital) examination

1. **General**
  – Pulse
  – Temperature
  – Respiratory rate
  – Blood pressure
  – Mental status
2. **Clothes of victim**
  – Should stand over a clean sheet of paper and then remove all her clothes by herself
  – Clothes are packed in paper bag and sent to FSL
	Genital examination
	1. Vulva—assessed for tears, swelling, abrasions, or discharge
	2. Hymen
	  – Laceration of hymen occurs with the first intercourse
	  – Tears at posterolateral position (most common), edema
	3. Fourchette often tears during first intercourse
	4. Vagina
	  – Bruises seen on anterior vaginal wall (lower 1/3) and posterior wall (upper 1/3)
	  – Look for vaginal discharge
	5. Cervix—presence of abrasions (away from external os)

Contd....

CHAPTER 5: Comprehensive Forensic Nursing Care of Survivor of Sexual Assault

Contd....

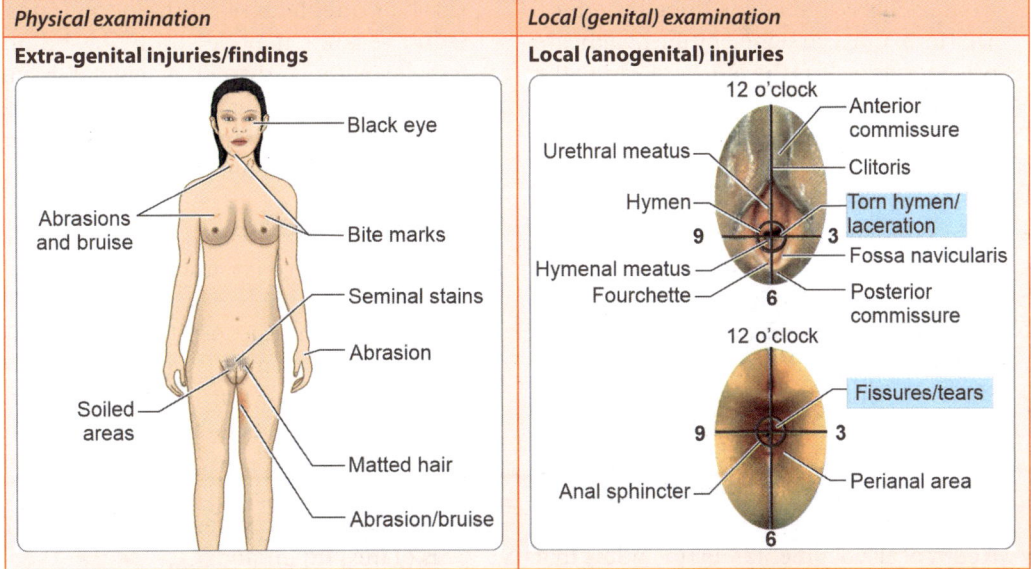

Physical examination	Local (genital) examination
Extra-genital injuries/findings	**Local (anogenital) injuries**

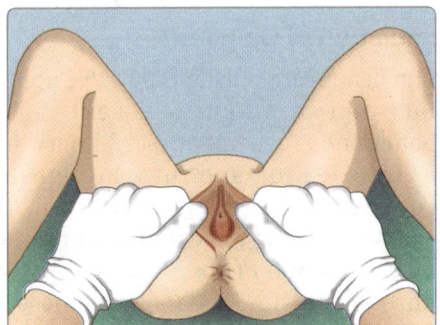

Fig. 5.4: Lithotomy position.

up to 96 hours in case the survivor may be unsure of the number of hours lapsed since the assault.
- Evidence on the outside of the body and on materials, such as clothing can be collected even after 96 hours.
- The collected samples for evidence are preserved in the hospital till such a time that police are able to complete their paperwork for dispatch to FSL.
- Vaginal swabs and blood samples need to be refrigerated if not sent immediately for testing.
- While handing over the samples, a requisition letter addressed to the FSL,

Table 5.4: Evidences to be preserved.

Samples preserved	Remarks
Clothes	• Worn at the time of incident • Foreign material collection, that falls off patient's when undressing • Collect sheets on the exam table and/or from the ambulance as evidence may be present in the debris
Swabs	• Soiled areas, bite marks • Mouth, pharynx, vagina, anus (depending upon history) • Buccal swab (for DNA)
Hair	• Loose hairs on the body/scalp (combings) • Pubic hair (for comparison) • Matted pubic hair
Fingernail clippings	Tissue sample, blood of the accused
Blood	• ABO blood grouping • Alcohol/drugs • HIV/Hepatitis B
Scrapping	• Dried blood stain • Dried seminal stain
Saliva	Secretor grouping

stating what all samples are being sent and what each sample needs to be tested for. This form must be signed by the healthcare provider, as well as the officer to whom the evidence is handed over. A chain of custody must be maintained.

Post-examination

- After completion of examination, she is allowed to wash-up using the toiletries provided by the hospital, change clothing, use mouthwash, and urinate or defecate, if needed.
- Survivors should receive all services free of cost. This includes OPD/inpatient registration, laboratory and radiology investigations, urine pregnancy test and medicines.
- A copy of all documentation (including that pertaining to medico-legal examination and treatment) must be provided to her free of cost.

OPINION

- The *provisional opinion* must, in brief, mention relevant aspects of the history of sexual violence, clinical findings and samples which are sent for analysis to FSL.
- The *final opinion* of whether sexual intercourse has taken place or not is based on a consideration of:
  - Signs of struggle and injuries.
  - Presence of blood and/or seminal stains on clothes and body.
  - Presence of seminal matter in the vagina.
  - Transmission of venereal disease.
  - FSL reports.

Absence of Injuries

- Sometimes, there may be absence of injuries on the survivor which has to be interpreted based on medical knowledge and details of the episode provided by survivor.
- Lack of injuries have to be based on the time lapse between the incident and reporting to hospitals, information pertaining to luring the child or adult survivor, or factors such as fear, shock and surprise, intoxication or other circumstances that rendered the survivor unable to resist the perpetrator. Other reasons may be simply based on female anatomy—hymen or vaginal tissue can stretch without any visible injury and vaginal mucosal barrier is resistant to abrasion from friction, etc.

Negative FSL Findings

Absence of negative laboratory results may be due to:
 i. Delay in reaching a hospital for examination and treatment.
 ii. Activities, such as urination, washing, bathing, changing clothes, menstruation can lead to loss of evidence after the assault.
 iii. Use of condom or vasectomy/diseases of vas of the perpetrator.
 iv. No ejaculation of semen by the perpetrator.

Formulation of Opinion

- The healthcare provider may give opinion that there are signs of recent vaginal penetration, general physical injury and/or intoxication and that the signs are consistent with the history given. The examiner must ensure that comments on past sexual history, status of vaginal introitus must not be made as these are unscientific and the courts too have determined them as biased.
- The healthcare provider may need to clarify in the court that normal examination findings neither refute nor confirm forceful sexual intercourse.
- Health professionals must not entertain questions from the police such as "whether rape has occurred", "whether the person is capable of having sexual intercourse or habituated to sexual intercourse". He/she should never make a diagnosis of "rape" because it is a legal term determined by the judiciary.
- The provider should explain the nature of medico-legal evidence, its limitations, as well as the role of examiner as expert witnesses.

ROLE OF FORENSIC NURSE EXAMINER

Establishing trust and offering support are the cornerstones of the medico-legal history taking and documentation process in any sexual assault interview. Moreover, survivor of sexual assault deals with the assault differently. The forensic nurse can play a vital role in mitigating some of the concerns of the survivor.

PSYCHOSOCIAL CARE

Establishing Rapport with the Survivor

a. A forensic nurse should believe when a patient says that sexual assault has happened. Never say or do anything to suggest disbelieve regarding the incident.
b. Do not pass judgmental remarks or comments that might appear unsympathetic.
c. Appreciate the survivor's courage in reaching the hospital as she has to overcome several barriers.
d. Convey important messages, such as she is not responsible for precipitating the act of rape by any of her actions or inactions like wearing of certain clothes or being drunk.
e. Explain to the survivor that rape is a crime and not an act of lust or for sexual pleasure.
f. Emphasize that this is not a loss of honor, modesty or chastity but a violation of her rights.

This would enable the survivor to discard feelings of self-blame.

Addressing Survivor's Emotional Wellbeing

- Recognize that survivors may present varied emotions.
- Encourage the survivor to express her feelings.
- Encourage survivors to seek crisis counseling.
- Assess for suicidal ideation.
- Make a safety assessment and safety plan.
- Involve family and friends in the healing process of survivor.

Creating an Enabling Atmosphere and Establishing Trust

- Speak to survivor in a private room/space.
- Recognize the dilemma faced by survivors in reporting violence.
- Do not label nonreporting to police as false case.
- Assure the survivor that her treatment will not be compromised.
- Ensure confidentiality and explain to the survivor that she must reveal the entire history without fear.
- Inform survivor of available resources, referrals, legal rights so that she can take an informed decision.

Role of Family, Friends and Community

- Recovery from sexual violence is dependent on the extent of support received from family, friends and community. The forensic nurse is best suited to engage with family and discuss ways of promoting survivors' well-being.
- It must be discussed with all care givers that survivor should not be held responsible for the assault.

In Situations of Child Sexual Abuse

- Parents may experience anger, confusion, and guilt. Some may also blame themselves for not having taken adequate care of or paid attention to the child.
- Reiterate that it is the perpetrator who misused their position.

Dealing with Adolescents Survivors

- Communicate that she was not at fault; encourage her to share feelings, fears and concerns. For an adolescent, acceptance by family and peers becomes a critical aspect in healing.
- Parents and friends should encourage survivor to seek counseling and crisis intervention support as adolescence is an age of turbulence and the survivor may not be comfortable talking about several issues with parents such as "contraception",

"healthy sexual relationships", fears of contracting infections such as STI/HIV, anxiety about how they are perceived by others in the school/college.
- Parents/guardians should exercise caution and not become over protective and restrictive in their approach. This could occur due to fear of recurrence of the assault and fear for survivor's safety. These concerns need to be discussed openly with the survivor and her parents and encourage them to make informed decisions.

Perpetrator of Sexual Abuse is Parent/Guardian

- Survivors under 18 years are likely to be accompanied by parents/guardians. If a healthcare provider finds out that the perpetrator is the guardian, it is critical to involve social worker/counsellor to discuss safety of the child.
- As per the POCSO Act, the social worker would have to speak with the child to assess whom the child trusts and can be called to the hospital. The social worker would also have to contact the police if the child is in need of protection and care.

CULTURAL AND SPIRITUAL ASPECTS

Specific steps when dealing with a survivor from marginalized groups such as children, persons with disability, LGBTQIA+ (lesbian, gay, bisexual, transsexual, queer, intersex and allies) persons, sex workers or persons from minority community, may be required.
- **LGBTQIA+:** There should be no judgment on the person's sexual orientation in general or as a cause of the assault. The survivor should be given a choice as to whether she/he wants to be examined by a female or male healthcare provider. Confidentiality of their sexual orientation should be maintained. The inadvertent discovery during history or examination that a person is transgender/intersex should not be treated with ridicule, surprise or shock.
- **Sex worker:** The Supreme Court has acknowledged that a woman who is a sex worker has the right to decide with whom she will have sex, and so any non-consensual intercourse with her would therefore amount to rape. Only information of the current episode of violence that the survivor is reporting must be documented.
- **Caste and religion:** One should not pass any explicit or implicit comments about the person's caste or religion while medically treating them, except if relevant to the nature of injuries or for treatment purposes.

LEGAL ASPECTS

A forensic nurse should know the legal provisions under which the offense of rape has been described. Rape is defined under **Sec. 375 IPC as:**

A man is said to commit rape, if there's:
 i. Penetration of penis into vagina, anus, urethra or mouth.
 ii. Insert any object or body part into vagina, urethra or anus.
 iii. Applies mouth to vagina, urethra or anus.
 iv. Manipulates any part of victim's body to cause penetration into vagina, anus or urethra.

If any of the above act is done:
1. Against her will
2. Without her consent
3. With her consent, if consent is obtained/given due to
   - Fear of death or hurt
   - Impersonation or fraud
   - Mental illness or intoxication
4. With or without consent, when she is <18 year of rape—is considered as **statutory rape.**
5. When she is unable to communicate her consent (such as an unconscious patient).

Exceptions

- Any medical intervention shall not constitute rape.
- Sexual intercourse by a man with his wife >15 years of age is not rape.

Supreme Court has held that sexual intercourse by a man with his minor wife (15–18 years) is *rape*. The man can be prosecuted if she registers a complaint within 1 year of the offense.

- **Custodial rape:** Rape of a woman by a person in position of authority, e.g., police officer, jail warden or hospital staff.
- **Gang rape:** Rape of a woman by >1 person.
- **Statutory rape:** Sexual intercourse with a girl under the age of consent (<18 years).

PUNISHMENT OF RAPE

Punishment for rape is given as per **Sec. 376 IPC**:

IPC	Offense (rape)	Punishment
376(1)	Rape committed on a girl ≥18 years	≥10 years to life imprisonment and fine
376(2)	Rape under special circumstances 1. Custodial rape 2. Rape of pregnant female 3. Rape during communal violence 4. Rape by armed forces 5. Rape on same female repeatedly	≥10 years to life imprisonment (remainder of natural life) and fine
376(3)	Rape of a girl <16 years	≥20 years to life imprisonment (remainder of natural life) and fine
376 A	Rape causes persistent vegetative state/death of the victim	≥20 years to life imprisonment (remainder of natural life) or death
376 D	Gang rape	≥20 years to life imprisonment (remainder of natural life) and fine

Consent

- A woman of ≥18 years *(age of consent)* can give valid consent for sexual intercourse.
- Consent must be free and voluntary, in sound mind, not intoxicated and obtained prior to the act.

Absence of Consent

- Evidence of resistance (tearing of clothes or infliction of injuries on body and genitalia) from a woman unwilling to yield to sexual intercourse may be seen.
- Absence of signs of struggle or injuries does not mean the victim has consented to sexual activity. As per law, resistance was not offered does not mean the person has consented.

What Constitutes Rape?

- As per the current law, even slight penetration to the vagina, anus, mouth or urethra by penis or any other object constitutes the offense of rape. Applying mouth/finger to vagina, anus or urethra will also constitute rape.
- Rape can be committed even when there is inability to produce an erection or ejaculation.

Medico-legal Aspects

1. Ordinarily, the burden to prove unwillingness and absence of consent lies with the prosecution. *But in rape case, under **Sec. 376 IPC**, it lies with the accused to prove that she consented for intercourse.*
2. Consent is required for intercourse with a prostitute.
3. *Medical proof of intercourse is not legal proof of rape.* Rape is not a medical diagnosis, but a legal definition.
4. **By a man:** *No age limit* under which a boy is considered incapable of committing rape. In a charge of rape brought against a boy,

the court is guided by **Secs. 82 and 83 IPC and Juvenile Justice Act, 2017** in awarding punishment. Likewise, there is no upper limit.
- **Of a woman:** Only a man can rape a woman (*except in France* where a woman can also be charged for rape on a man).

> **Legal sections related to rape**
> - **Treatment and information to police:** Hospitals should immediately provide first-aid or medical treatment free of cost, to the survivor of rape/acid attack, and immediately inform the police **(Sec. 357-C CrPC)**.
>   - *Denial of treatment:* Imprisonment up to 1 year with/without fine. Offense is noncognizable and bailable **(Sec. 166-B IPC)**.
> - **Punishment of revealing the identity of rape victim:** Punished with imprisonment for up to 2 years and fine **(Sec. 228-A IPC)**.
> - **Presumption of consent:** When sexual intercourse is established, and if the woman states that she did not consent, the court shall presume that she did not consent **(Sec. 114 IEA)**.
> - **Cross-examination in rape trial:** Not permissible to put questions in cross-examination of victim about her general immoral character or describe her as loose character **(Sec. 146 IEA)**.
> - **Courts in which rape offenses to be tried:** Should be tried by a court presided over by a woman (in-camera) **[Sec. 26 (a) CrPC]**.
> - **In-camera:** Proceedings are heard in a Judge's private chamber or in a courtroom which has been cleared of all spectators.
> - **Recording of statement of survivor:** Recorded and video-graphed by a woman police officer and get the statement recorded by a judicial magistrate **(Sec. 154 CrPC)**.

EXPERT WITNESS

Forensic nurse may appear in the trial court as "fact witness" or as "expert witness".
- The forensic nurse may meet the public prosecutor to discuss the procedures and the type of questions that will be asked by the public prosecutor. The information provided during testimony should be concise, objective and factual. There is an expectation that the nurse should be unbiased.
- Opinions and interpretations are provided by the forensic nurse when appearing as "expert witness" but should be qualified to do so. The requirement for expert witness is more stringent.

SUMMARY

Basic Elements of Health Response
The basic health response to a survivor of sexual violence involves:

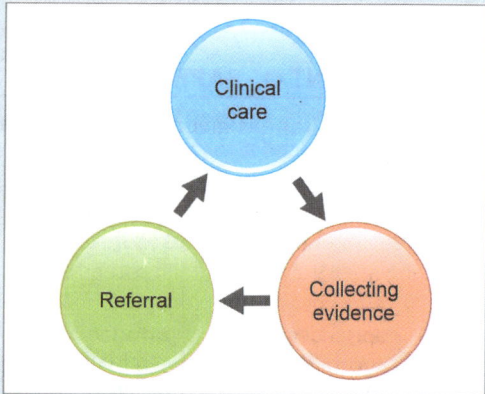

Clinical care
- Taking a detailed history of the incident
- Performing and documenting a thorough physical examination
- Providing treatment for injuries
- Evaluating the patient for STIs and providing preventive care
- Evaluating for risk of pregnancy and pregnancy prevention
- Providing supportive counseling and psychosocial support
- Following-up through subsequent visits

Collecting Evidence
- Collecting evidence to support a criminal investigation, as appropriate to the context
- May include collection of forensic material (from the survivor's body and/or clothing), photographs of injures, etc.
- In some cases, the evidence may be kept for a period of time, in case the survivor decides to pursue legal action at a later date.

IMPORTANT! The healthcare provider's response to sexual violence does not include the determination of whether rape has occurred. The role of the healthcare provider is to indicate all examination findings objectively and accurately and to provide treatment.

CHAPTER 5: Comprehensive Forensic Nursing Care of Survivor of Sexual Assault

Referral
Good quality, compassionate care means providing:
- Referrals for additional assistance and services
- Information on possible additional services that survivors might want:
  – Psychosocial support
  – Security
  – Legal aid
  – Livelihood programs

Service providers should provide information about what services are available and where/how the survivor can access them. However, a survivor should never be pressured into seeking additional services. It is up to the individual survivor to decide to take the referral.

MULTIPLE CHOICE QUESTIONS

1. **Disclosure of name of rape victim punishable under:**
   A. Sec. 304A IPC
   B. Sec. 354 IPC
   C. Sec. 376 IPC
   D. Sec. 228-A

   Explanation: Punishment of revealing the identity of rape victim is imprisonment for up to 2 years and fine under Sec. 228-A IPC. Sec. 304A IPC is causing death by negligence, Sec. 354 IPC is assault or criminal force to woman with intent to outrage her modesty and Sec. 376 IPC is punishment for rape.

2. **When providing care to an assault female victim, the forensic nurse will initially:**
   A. Notify the police that an assault has occurred
   B. Assess the individual for any resulting physical trauma
   C. Bag all clothing to preserve any relevant evidence
   D. Determine whether the victim has been sexually assaulted as well

   Explanation: Initial medical care for acute problems needs immediate attention before the medico-legal examination and evidence collection. Information to be police should be sent, as soon as possible but the treatment should not be delayed.

3. **A 13-year-old girl was brought by parents to hospital for treatment with alleged history of rape committed by their tenant. They refused any medico-legal examination to be conducted by doctor. What should the healthcare examiner do?**
   a. Inform police
   b. Start medical examination
   c. Record refusal of consent for medico-legal examination
   d. Take vaginal sample
   e. Start treatment for STD and pregnancy
   A. a, b, c, e are true
   B. a, c, d, e are true
   C. b, c, d are true
   D. b, c, e are true

   Explanation: Even if there is informed refusal, the examiner is required/duty bound to inform the police about the sexual assault. She may not wish to participate in the police investigation, but medical examination and treatment is to be provided. Medico-legal examination and evidence collection is not done. At the time of intimation being sent to the police, a clear note stating 'informed refusal for police intimation' should be made.

4. **All are true of examination of an 11-year-old rape victim, *except*:**
   A. Consent for examination should be taken from her
   B. Male doctor with a female attendant can do the examination
   C. Per-vaginal examination should not be done
   D. Police information should be sent

   Explanation: The consent form should be signed by the survivor if she is ≥12 years of age, and the guardian/parent if she is <12 years. Per-vaginal examination can be done only in adult women when medically indicated and not recommended in children. Even, per speculum examination is not a must in the case of children/young girls when there is no history of penetration and no visible injuries.

5. Helpful strategies in the examination by forensic nurse of sexually assaulted clients include:
    A. Being made to feel safe
    B. Controlling client's response
    C. Maximizing trauma
    D. Rushing the client through examination

    Explanation: Providing safety and physical and emotional support is cornerstone of forensic nurse response to sexual assault. The environment where history is taken should be safe, private and comfortable.

6. While interviewing a survivor of sexual assault, the forensic nurse should be:
    A. Compassionate
    B. Pitiful
    C. Judgmental
    D. Indifferent

    Explanation: Engaging using a compassionate nonintrusive manner is essential to elicit the history. The forensic nurse should not be pitiful, judgmental or indifferent.

7. Which of the following is NOT one of the components of forensic documentation?
    A. Photography
    B. Written documentation
    C. Diagrammatic documentation
    D. Scanning with a Wood's lamp

    Explanation: Forensic documentation includes a written component, a diagrammatic component, and a photographic component. Examination using a Wood's lamp is used to detect semen or foreign debris on the skin—not a component of documentation but useful for evidence collection.

8. Which statement by the victim might compromise the evidence to be collected?
    A. I took a shower immediately after the men raped me
    B. I tried fighting them off as best I could
    C. I came to the emergency room as fast as I could
    D. I grabbed a bunch of hair from one of the men

    Explanation: The police usually advise the survivor not to change clothes or have a bath—to prevent the loss of physical evidence and to ensure that medical attention is not delayed.

9. Which of the following areas sustains the most injury during a sexual assault involving penile penetration only?
    A. Cervix
    B. Vaginal walls
    C. Perineum
    D. Fourchette

    Explanation: Laceration of hymen and fourchette occurs with the penile penetration. Tears in the deeper part of vagina and cervix are not likely to occur during sexual intercourse but are often caused by sexual perverts using instruments.

10. All are true regarding trace evidence and biological evidence material collection to be carried out, *except*:
    A. Less than 72 hours after the alleged assault
    B. With consent
    C. Using colposcopy
    D. After police reporting

    Explanation: Examinations conducted after 72 hours have lower rates of finding trace and biological evidence. It should be collected with consent and colposcopy is helpful to detect and collect evidences. But the examiner should not wait for police reporting to collect the evidences.

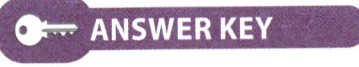
ANSWER KEY

| 1. D | 2. B | 3. A | 4. A | 5. A | 6. A | 7. D | 8. A | 9. D | 10. D |

CHAPTER 5: Comprehensive Forensic Nursing Care of Survivor of Sexual Assault

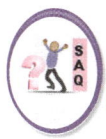

SHORT ANSWER QUESTIONS

1. What are the common health consequences of sexual assault?
2. Write a note on SAFE kit.
3. Write briefly on Sec. 164-A CrPC.
4. Define rape as per Sec. 375 IPC.
5. What constitutes rape as per Indian law?
6. Write a note on punishment for rape as described in under Sec 376 IPC.
7. Discuss briefly the cultural and spiritual aspects while dealing with survivors of sexual assault.
8. Discuss in brief the role of forensic nurse as a witness in rape trial.

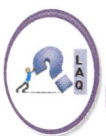

LONG ANSWER QUESTIONS

1. Discuss the examination protocol of survivor of sexual assault.
2. Discuss the components of informed consent taken from survivor of sexual assault.
3. Discuss the components of medico-legal history taking in relation to survivor of sexual assault.
4. What are the common physical and local findings seen in survivor of sexual assault.
5. Discuss the role of forensic nurse in comprehensive care of survivor of sexual assault.
6. Discuss the psychosocial care provided by the forensic nurse for survivor of sexual assault.

CHAPTER 6

Collection and Preservation of Evidence

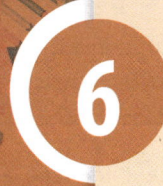

"Physical evidence cannot be intimidated. It does not forget. It sits there and waits to be detected, preserved, evaluated, and explained."

— **Herbert Leon MacDonell**
(Inventor of the MAGNA Brush fingerprint device, and expert in blood splatter analysis)

LEARNING OBJECTIVES

At the end of this topic, the student should be able to:
1. Define and discuss forensic evidence.
2. Explain the role of forensic nurses in collection and preservation of evidence.
3. Describe the documentation of biological and other evidence related to criminal/traumatic event.
4. Discuss forwarding of biological samples for forensic examination.

CASE STUDY

You are a forensic nurse posted in the emergency room (ER). Ms SM, a 22-year-old female presents with alleged history of stabbing by her ex-boyfriend because of jealousy and frustration (as shown in **figure**). She is bleeding profusely and her clothes are soaked in blood. She is to be taken to the emergency OT shortly.

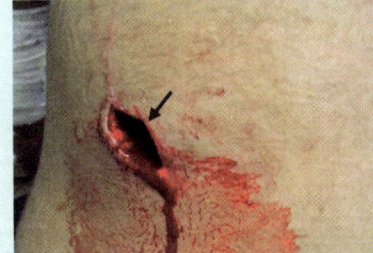

Q1. What can the forensic nurse do to help in this case?
Q2. What evidence can be collected that may be used in the court case?
Q3. What documentation will be most important from the perspective of the nurse?*

*Discuss the questions with your teacher/facilitator.

INTRODUCTION

- **Forensic evidence:** Any item or information legally submitted and accepted by a court to prove or disprove a claim (determine the truth of any matter under investigation).
- The collection, preservation, and analysis of the evidence from the crime scenes and victim's/perpetrator's body are often critical in determining a suspected person's guilt or innocence.
- In addition to providing comprehensive health care, forensic nurse also has the legal, ethical, and professional responsibility of identifying, collecting, storing, documenting and maintaining the chain of custody of evidence which contributes to the effectiveness of the care provided to the victims and to justice.

- Forensic evidence collection is a systematic process that follows legal requirements and guidelines. Forensic nurse should:
  a. Ensure that proper documentation is made prior to handling evidence.
  b. Maintain the chain of custody by whom the evidence was handled.
  c. Apply appropriate analysis and preservation methods.
  d. Uphold legal and ethical standards.
  e. Preserve evidence properly so that it is usable in the future.

The advent of DNA testing has revolutionized forensic analysis of biological evidence and greatly affected criminal proceedings. The following sections comprise an overview of forensic evidence collection.

TYPES OF EVIDENCE

There are various types of evidence which can be produced before the court:

1. **Oral evidence:** All statement which the court permits or requires to be made before it by witnesses, in relation to matter of fact under inquiry. It must be direct.
   - **Direct evidence** will prove the point in fact without interpretation of circumstances. An ED nurse may be called as a witness regarding what happened while caring for a patient and any documentation related to the case.
2. **Documentary evidence:** All documents including electronic records produced for the inspection of the court.
   - *Primary evidence:* Documents itself produced for the inspection of the court, e.g., clinical notes, injury documentation, photographs showing the injuries, etc. It is considered to be the *best evidence*.
   - *Secondary evidence* is allowed by the court in the absence of the primary evidence, e.g., certified copies.
3. **Real evidence (or physical evidence)** consists of material items involved in a case, objects and things the court can physically hold and inspect.

Table 6.1: Real evidence.

Physical evidence	Biological evidence
- Clothing - Tool markings - Fingerprints - Bullet and shell casings, gun - Gunpowder particles - Fibers - Shoe and tire impressions - Creams, lotions, toothpaste - Electronic devices - Glass fragments, paint chips, soil	- Blood and seminal stains - Teeth and bite marks - Insects - Plants and plant materials, wood chips - Saliva, vomitus, urine, feces - Tissue and organs - Hair - Skeletal remains, bones or bone fragments

   - Some consider physical evidence as *nonliving inorganic matter* (any material, condition, solid, liquid, or gas), whereas biological evidence as *living organic matter* **(Table 6.1)**.
   - Physical evidence is admitted because it tends to prove or disprove an issue of fact in a trial.
4. **Indirect/Circumstantial evidence** relies on an inference to connect it to a conclusion of fact.
5. **Hearsay evidence** is the statement of a witness not based on his personal knowledge but on what he heard from others.

Purpose of Evidence Collection

Physical evidence establishes a link between victim and perpetrator **(Box 6.1)**.

Box 6.1: Reasons/purpose for evidence collection and preservation.

a. Proves that a crime has been committed
b. Helps establish a modus operandi of a crime
c. Confirm or refute an alibi or statement
d. Identify weapon(s) of injury
e. Connect the presence of a suspect(s) in relation to a crime
f. Acquits the innocent
g. Substantiates the testimony of the victim
h. Identification of biological markers specific to a particular individual (e.g., DNA)
i. Identification of ingested substances, such as drugs, poisons, or any other substance
j. More reliable than an expert witness

PRINCIPLE OF EXCHANGE

- The principle governing evidence collection was put forth by Edmond Locard, a 20th century French criminologist. Locard's theory is the basis for linking victims, perpetrators and crime scenes.
- Locard's **principle of exchange** states that "When two objects come into contact with each other, there is always some transfer of material from one to the other". It means that *every contact leaves a trace, i.e.*, during a criminal act, the perpetrator brings something into the scene and takes away something from the scene. For example, footprints, fingerprints, hair, fibers, broken glass, tool marks, or DNA from skin, blood, semen or other body fluids etc., **(Fig. 6.1)**.
- Once this transfer is detected and the substance classified and/or individualized, the forensic specialist will have a clue as to what may have occurred at the scene.
- The forensic scientist's job is to uncover and reconstruct how the evidence fits into the investigation of a crime.

CONSENT

- Written, informed consent from persons more than 12 years should be obtained prior to evidentiary examination or else from parents/guardian if he/she is <12 years.
- This consent should inform the patient what evidence will be collected (including photography, if planned).
- Consent forms should address confidentiality issues.

GUIDELINES FOR COLLECTING AND PRESERVING EVIDENCE

- The essential requirements for evidence collection and preservation are shown in **Fig. 6.2**.

> **Forensic uses of "Vacutainers":**
> a. **Yellow top Vacutainers (contain acid citrate and dextrose solution):** Useful for conventional serological testing and DNA testing.
> b. **Purple top Vacutainers (contain EDTA):** Useful for DNA testing; may inhibit certain conventional serological tests.
> c. **Red top Vacutainers (no additives):** Useful for conventional serological tests; less useful for DNA testing; can be used for pregnancy and HIV testing.
> d. **Grey top Vacutainers (contain sodium fluoride and sometimes EDTA):** Useful for toxicological testing; not suitable for conventional serological analysis and may not be suitable for DNA analysis.

- Physical evidence with the greatest potential value is often present on the victim's/perpetrator's body.
- Whenever forensic nurses are required to collect items for forensic evaluation, it is important to prevent contamination and loss.

Following are do's and don'ts in evidence collection and preservation:

a. Wear clean nonpowdered gloves while handling evidence to reduce cross contamination.
b. Wear masks, shoe cover and head cover, and hair should be tied back—to prevent contamination.
c. Trace evidence is particularly at risk for contamination and loss—should be handled as little as possible.
d. Treat all biological samples as infective material.
e. Avoid talking, sneezing, and coughing over evidence.
f. Be careful to open evidence bags and collection containers without touching the inside.
g. Dry stains are obtained with wet swabs and wet stains are obtained with dry swabs.
h. Paper bags/envelopes are used for packing. Plastic bags are avoided as they gather moisture and degrade evidence.

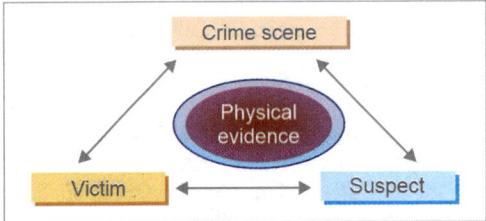

Fig. 6.1: Locard's principle of exchange.

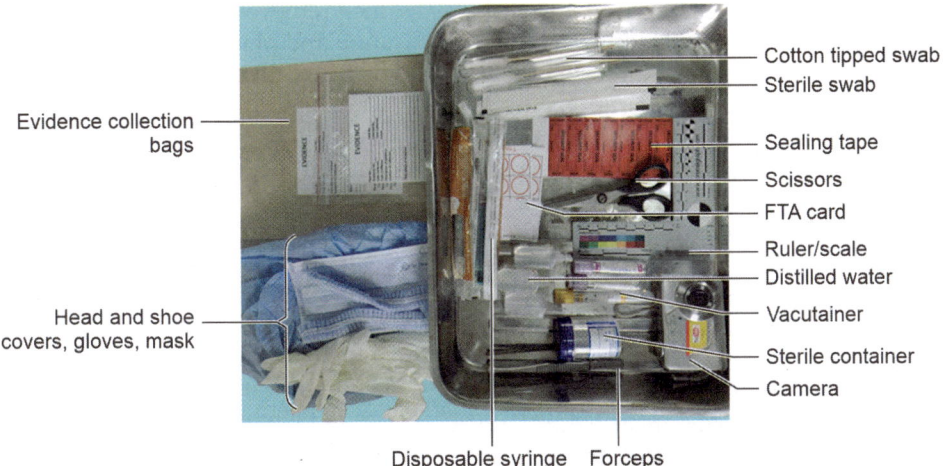

Fig. 6.2: Essential requirements for evidence collection and preservation.

i. The articles (swabs, clothes, smears) must be air dried before packaging them. Drying of swabs is absolutely mandatory as there may be decomposition/degradation of evidence. Do not dry stained material by heating or placing the article in bright sunlight.
j. Use containers of appropriate size for the specimen and use one container per item of evidence to minimize cross contamination.
k. Following collection, every paper bag should be labeled and sealed.
l. Seal it tightly and seal each evidence bag with breakaway tape or wax seal.
m. Store evidence in secure locker or area until it is handed over to the police.

Observation and Recognition of Evidence

- Before collecting, recognition of something as physical evidence is a major objective in crime scenes and hospital settings. Evidence recognition and recovery requires experience and extensive training.
- Typically, the recognition of physical evidence starts by observing the scene/victim/perpetrator.
- Based on initial observations and taking into consideration the context of the case, possible scenarios, the nature of the incident, a search strategy is formulated. This includes searching with the naked eye and magnifiers, and also using light sources.
- Once the evidence is recognized, appropriate recovery methods (e.g., cotton swabs) and adequate packaging (e.g., collection bags/boxes, containers for sharp objects) are used.
- Priorities in evidence recovery might have to be decided to avoid unnecessary loss or degradation of evidence.
- Selecting what is relevant evidence is a challenge of the recognition and recovery phase. It requires a good understanding of what can be done on the various types of physical evidence in a FSL, as well as the information that can be obtained. However, it might be preferable to recover more evidence, and select at a later stage of the investigation.

COLLECTION AND PRESERVATION OF EVIDENCE

Collection Techniques

- The techniques for collecting trace evidences are picking, lifting, scraping, vacuum sweeping, combing, and clipping.
  - The swabbing collection technique should be used for the recovery of biological evidence in a dried or liquid state.

- Several tools can be used for the collection of trace evidence (e.g., blunt end forceps, tweezers, adhesive tape lifts, spatulas, nail clippers, etc.).
- The collected evidence should be immediately packed and secured to avoid sample loss.
a. **Picking:** Trace evidence may be separated from an item by using clean forceps.
b. **Lifting:** An adhesive tape is repeatedly and firmly patted or rolled over the item causing loosely adhering trace evidence to stick to the tape. The collected tapes are then placed on a transparent backing (e.g., clear plastic sheeting, glass slides, and clear plastic/glass petri dishes).
c. **Scraping:** A clean spatula is used to remove the trace evidence from an item onto a collection surface, such as clean paper.
d. **Vacuum sweeping:** A small vacuum cleaner equipped with a filter trap is used to recover trace evidence from an item or area.
e. **Combing:** A clean comb is used to recover trace evidence from the hair of an individual. The combing device and collected debris from the hair should be packed together.
f. **Clipping:** Trace evidence can be recovered from fingernails by nail clipping. Fingernails may be clipped with clippers and packed in clean paper/glass tube.

Collection procedures for some of the most common types of physical/biological evidence are as follows:

1. Clothing

- **In sexual assault**
  - If the patient is wearing the clothes they had during the assault, all items are preserved. If the patient is not wearing the same clothes—clothing put on later by the patient, such as underwear, may still contain bodily fluids other than the patient's.
  - The examiner sets two layers of clean papers/sheets on the floor. The patient then removes one item of clothing at a time and places it in a separate paper bag (to prevent cross-contamination) while standing over the sheet placed on the floor.
  - The top sheet captures the loose debris that may fall from the clothing, which is folded inwards, and secured in a paper evidence bag separately. Debris may include leaves, grass, or loose hair that may not be the patient's.
- **In gunshot injury**
  - Garments with suspected gunshot holes are to be handled carefully to prevent the loss of gunshot residues and its distribution around the hole/defect (**Fig. 6.3A**).
  - Clean polythene/paper may be kept under and above the suspected hole.
- Each piece of clothing must be dried thoroughly, if wet or damp. All stains or tears to the clothing must be documented and marked (**Figs. 6.3B and C**). Use protective paper to prevent stains from touching.
- If possible, the patient's clothes should remain intact. However, if the clothes need to be cut, it is done without cutting through any stains, tears, holes, or other defects in the fabric.

2. Footwear

- Footwear should be packaged separately from the clothing, and each shoe packed individually.
- Soil or other trace materials may collect within the grooves and ridges of the soles of shoes and may be linked to a source at a scene or from a vehicle.

3. Bed/Trolley Sheets

Some patients may have also been brought in by ambulance on a bed sheet; this too can be collected for evidence as it may contain debris that fell off the patient and may be valuable in establishing where the crime occurred.

Biological Stains or Deposits

Since DNA analysis is important for many inquiries involving biological evidence, the forensic nurse must ensure that the biological evidence is not subjected to alteration, degradation or deterioration during collection, storage or laboratory analysis.

Control Swabs

Control swabs may be used as a standard. These swabs are moistened with sterile water and used for the entire evidence collection process.

4. DNA

- The application of DNA technology revolutionized the field of forensic science. DNA analysis is applied in both criminal and civil cases.
- Commonly collected is blood or buccal sample. Hair sample is also useful.
  a. **Blood (most common sample):** 5 mL of venous blood is collected in a purple stoppered vacutainer (EDTA tube) and mixed thoroughly without shaking. Sample can be preserved at 2–8°C (not frozen).

  Blood and buccal smear samples can be stored on Whatman FTA® cards at room temperature with subsequent amplification by PCR.

  Advantages of FTA
  i. Simple collection
  ii. Convenient room temperature storage and transport
  iii. Safe handling and easy shipping

  Format
  - Blood sample collection kit
  - Buccal sample collection kit

Blood collection using Whatman FTA blood collection kit
1. Place the contents of the kit out on a clean dry table.
2. Wear gloves and unfold protective flap of FTA to expose the printed circle.
3. Use alcohol swab to clean the finger properly.
4. Firmly hold the end of the lancet on the part of the finger that was cleaned and press the trigger to prick the finger.

Contd....

Contd....

5. Press the finger to deposit a drop in the printed circle without touching the card **(Fig. 6.4)**.
6. Do not over-saturate, as DNA cannot be recovered from FTA card that is saturated with too much blood.
7. Allow the card to dry for 1–2 hours at room temperature. Close the protective cover of the FTA card and insert the card with desiccant packet into the Multi-barrier pouch.
8. Insert the Multi-barrier pouch in the envelope provided.

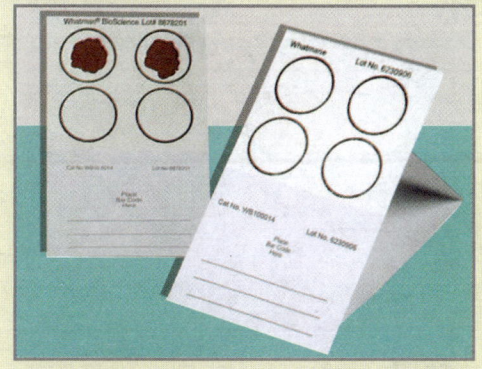

Fig. 6.4: FTA card with blood sample.

b. **Buccal epithelial cells (buccal swabs)** are considered a convenient alternative for collecting genetic material, as they are relatively easy to collect, inexpensive and noninvasive.

Buccal cell collection using Whatman FTA Buccal collection kit (Figs. 6.5A and B)
1. Place the indicating FTA card and other components on a clean dry surface.
2. Remove one sterile foam tipped applicator.
3. Holding the plastic handle of the applicator, place the foam applicator in the mouth.
4. Soak up as much saliva as possible by running the foam applicator on the inside cheek for 30 seconds. Repeat the process with the opposite side of the applicator.
5. Carefully lift the paper cover of the indicating FTA card to expose the pink sample area.
6. Apply pressure; rock the foam applicator from side to side three times.
7. Run the applicator over and repeat the other side within the same circle.
8. The sample area will turn white indicating the transfer of sample.

Contd....

Contd....

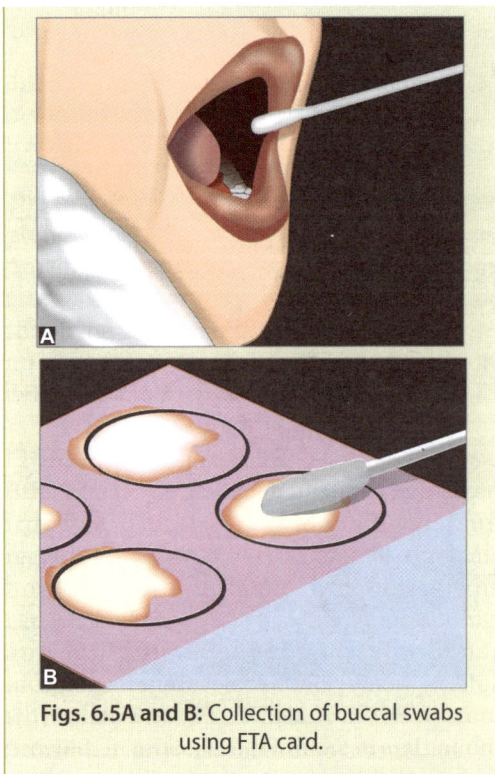

Figs. 6.5A and B: Collection of buccal swabs using FTA card.

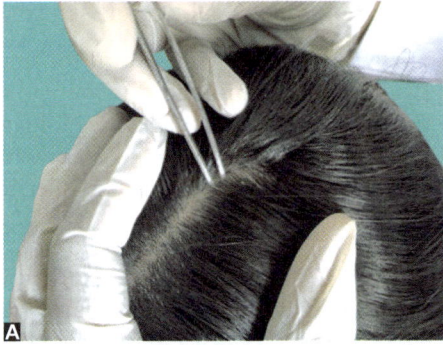

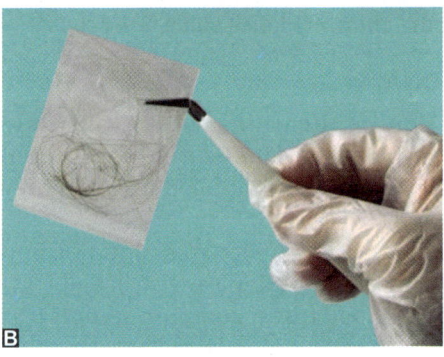

Figs. 6.6A and B: (A) Plucking the hair from roots. (B) Collected hair sample.

c. **Hair follicles with roots (plucked hair)**, about 10–20, from the head is used as a reference standard **(Figs. 6.6A and B)**. The root of the hair contains nuclear DNA, and the shaft contains mitochondrial DNA.

5. Blood

Blood sample are collected for grouping and also helps in comparing and matching bloodstains at the scene of crime.
- Venous blood is collected with a sterile syringe and needle and transferred to 3 sterile vials/vacutainers for the following purposes: plain vial/vacutainer—blood grouping and drug estimation; sodium fluoride—alcohol estimation; EDTA—DNA analysis **(Figs. 6.7A and B)**.
- Collect blood before administration of crystalloids, medications or blood products.
- Soap and water are used to clean the site to be venipunctured for blood alcohol sampling.

6. Oral Swabs

- If there was an oral assault, oral swab is collected for detection of semen and spermatozoa. The likelihood of evidence beyond 24 hours is low.
- Prior to swabbing, there should be an assessment of the mouth for any injuries.
- Swabs are taken from the posterior parts of the buccal cavity, behind the last molars or area beneath the tongue where the chances of finding any evidence are highest and rotate the swabs during collection **(Fig. 6.8)**.
- A mouth rinse can be collected (before she eats or drinks anything) for any evidence of semen, if the survivor reports oral sex in the last 48 hours. She can rinse her mouth with sterile water into a sterile container and then sealed and labelled.

7. Fingernail Scrapings

- In case of struggle, the accused and the survivor may have scratched each other,

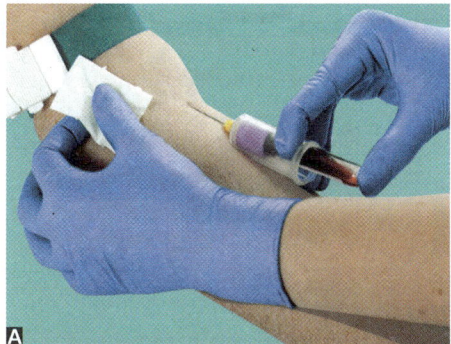

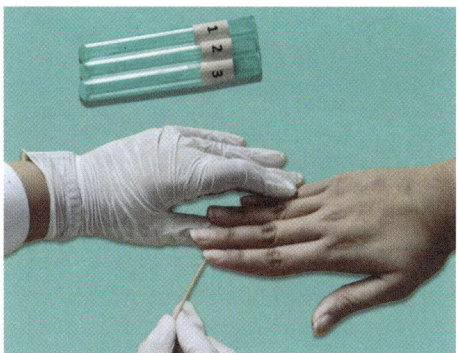

Fig. 6.9: Fingernail scraping.

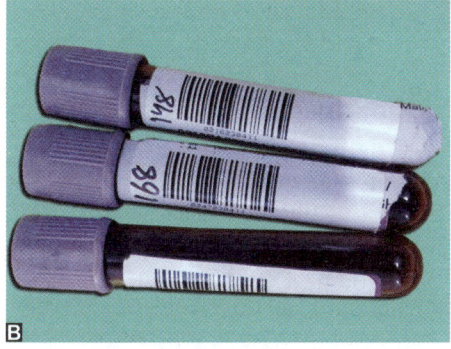

Figs. 6.7A and B: (A) Drawing of blood sample. (B) Blood sample in EDTA vacutainers.

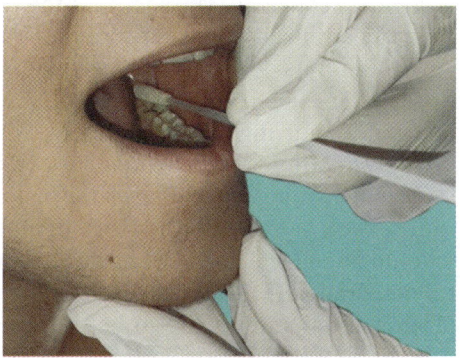

Fig. 6.8: Oral swab collection.

of paper and then collect the contents, as well as the scraper for evidence collection **(Fig. 6.9)**.
- Alternatively, nails can be clipped close and collected in an envelope.
- Skin obtained may provide material for DNA typing and the assailant identification.

8. Hair

- Hair and fiber evidence are among the most common forms of trace evidence encountered in crime investigations.
- Detection of scalp hair and pubic hair of the accused on the survivor's body (and vice-versa) has evidentiary value.
- **Scalp hair:** Obtaining head hair samples include a small comb and piece of paper; the hair is combed over the paper so that any loose hair or debris falls onto the paper. The comb and paper are collected for analysis.
- **Pubic hair:** Matted pubic hair should be cut and placed in an envelope. The forensic nurse should gently comb the hair to collect any foreign material or hair that may identify the assailant **(Figs. 6.10A and B)**. The comb and specimens obtained are placed in a clean paper towel, then in an envelope. Next, 10–20 pubic hairs plucked or cut, and are placed in a separate envelope or container as "controls" **(Fig. 6.10C)**.
- Alternatively, all hair may be collected in a catchment paper which is then folded and sealed.

and epithelial cells of one may be present under the nails of the other that can be used for DNA detection. It may contain skin cells or blood of the perpetrator transferred during the attack.
- Nail clippings and scrapings are taken from both hands and packed separately.
- Using a nail scraper/cuticle stick, scrape nail debris from each hand over a piece

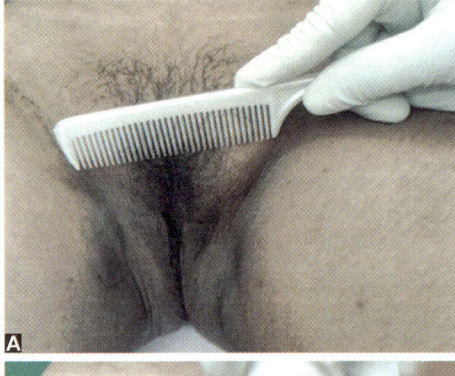
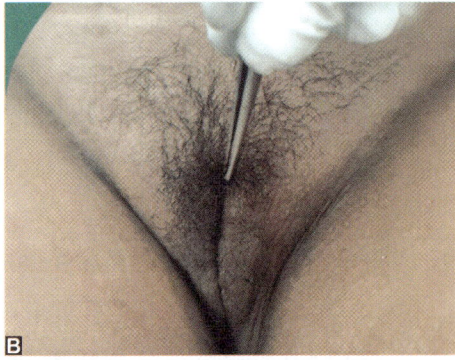
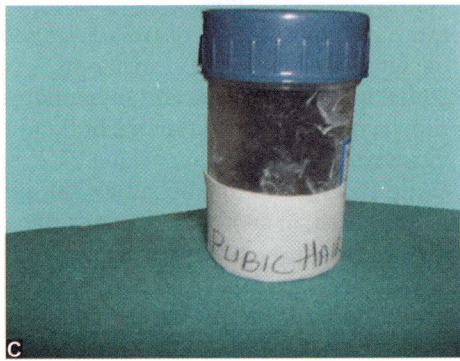
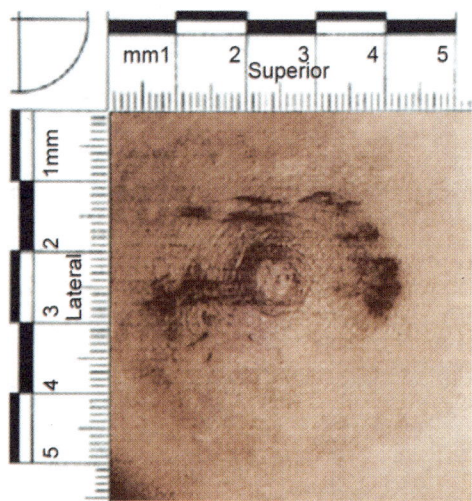

Fig. 6.11: Bite marks on breast of the victim of sexual assault.

(Courtesy: Nitul Jain, Eklavya Dental College and Hospital Kotputli, Rajasthan)

Figs. 6.10A to C: Collection and preservation of pubic hair: (A) Combing; (B) Plucking; and (C) Control sample.

9. Bite Marks

- Bite marks need to be swabbed and measured **(Fig. 6.11)**.
- Use moistened swabs on the area where the teeth and lips of the assailant would have pressed on the patient's skin (best place to obtain evidence).
- A *double swab technique* is recommended for collection of evidence from bite marks—use of moist swab followed immediately by a dry swab.

10. Genital and Anal Swabs

If a woman reports within 72 hours (3 days) of the assault, all swabs based on the nature of assault are collected. The spermatozoa can be identified till 72 hours after assault. If she reports after 3 days, swabs for spermatozoa are useless. In such cases, swabs should only be sent for identifying semen.

- Two swabs are taken from the vulva, vagina and anal opening depending on the history and examination. Swabs from orifices should be collected only if there is a history of penetration **(Fig. 6.12A)**.
- Two vaginal smears are to be prepared on the glass slides provided, air-dried in the shade and sent for seminal fluid/spermatozoa examination **(Fig. 6.12B)**.
- Often lubricants are used in penetration with finger or object, so swabs must be taken for detection of lubricant.
- Vaginal washing is collected using a syringe and a small rubber catheter. Two milliliter of normal saline is instilled into the posterior fornix of vagina and fluid is aspirated. Fluid filled syringe is sent to FSL for motile sperms after putting a knot over the rubber

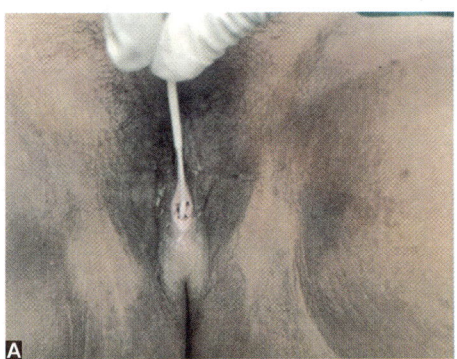

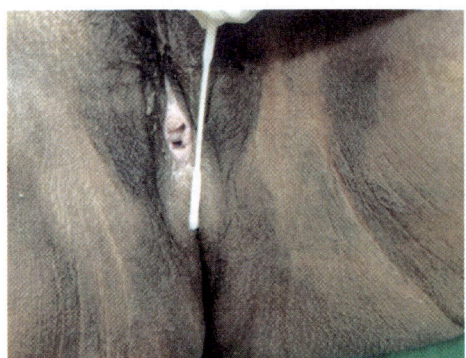

Fig. 6.13: Perineal swab.

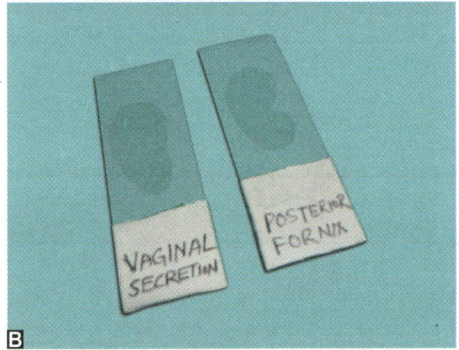

Figs. 6.12A and B: (A) Vaginal swab; (B) Vaginal smears.

catheter. Spermatozoa are best recovered from the posterior fornix.
- Any foreign bodies found within the vagina (including tampon) should be collected, air dried and preserved.

11. Perineal Swab
- Swabbing the perineal area is required if there was a rectal or vaginal assault since it may contain the perpetrator DNA (such as sperm or penile epithelial cells).
- The area should first be inspected for any injuries and swabbed with moistened swabs **(Fig. 6.13)**.
- If there was a rectal assault, then swabs should be taken within 24 hours.
- When taking an anorectal swab, swab the area for the smear slides and then repeat the procedure with the second set of swabs.

12. Penile Swabs
- Penile swabs are taken from the accused, minor or any nonconsensual victim.

- Using moistened swabs, swab the glans, shaft, and base of the penis with a rotating motion to ensure uniform sampling.

13. Additional Swabs
- Swab any area when there is an indication based on the history or suspicion of bodily fluid transfer, such as licking, kissing or biting for trace evidence. Swabs are taken from bloodstains, foreign material, seminal stains and other stains on the skin/body surfaces.
- An alternative light source may be used. Any area that fluoresces under the florescent light should be swabbed with moistened swabs.
- It is best to have the patient undress, and then turn off the lights and examine the patient's body to see if any areas indicate the need for a swab. Dried seminal stains on the skin appear as pale-yellow glistening areas, and will fluoresce under a Wood's lamp (long wave UV source of light).
- Particular attention should be paid to the thighs, buttocks and genitalia when viewing the skin for possible seminal stains.

14. Firearms, Bullets, and Projectiles (Box 6.2)
- Firearms and projectiles may contain various types of physical evidence, such as fibers, hair, blood and tissue. In the case of bullets, they also may contain primary markings that allow for comparison to known firearms.

Box 6.2: Collection of firearm evidence.

1. Clothes with trace evidence
2. Wound dressings
3. Victim's hair, fibers and blood
4. Gunpowder and other evidence on the hands
5. Unspent ammunition and empty cartridges
6. Gun used in the crime

- Clothing, bullets and wound dressings are important for detection of gunshot residue (GSR)* which can identify a link between the firearm, suspect and the victim.
- Swab the hands of suspect (preferably upper left hand, palm of left hand, upper right hand and palm of right hand) using 5% HNO_3 (or use sticky tape) and one control sample should be taken for GSR. Wrap the suspect's hands in a paper bag for GSR, if swabbing is not done.
- **Firearms** should never be packaged in a paper envelope. They should be handled as little as possible and only while wearing gloves (to preserve biological material, fingerprints and other evidence). Ideally, firearms should be placed in a clean cardboard box and kept secure.
- **Bullet:** All bullets and recognizable parts of bullets in the victim must be recovered from the body and preserved with correct labeling of each bullet to the corresponding wound and placed in a separate envelope. It should be removed with fingers or with a rubber tipped forceps **(Fig. 6.14A)**. The recovered bullet should be dried and not washed, since washing removes the powder residue.
- **Pellets:** In a shotgun injury, few pellets and all wadding should be recovered to determine the shot size, bore and type of ammunition.
- **Preservation and packing:** Fired cartridge cases, bullets, pellets, slugs and wads are wrapped in sterile cotton or gauze padding and packed in cardboard box or plastic container and sealed, after drying **(Fig. 6.14B)**.

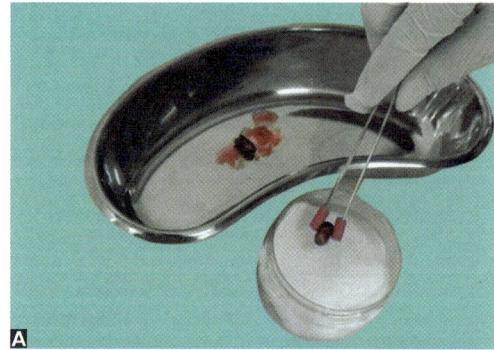

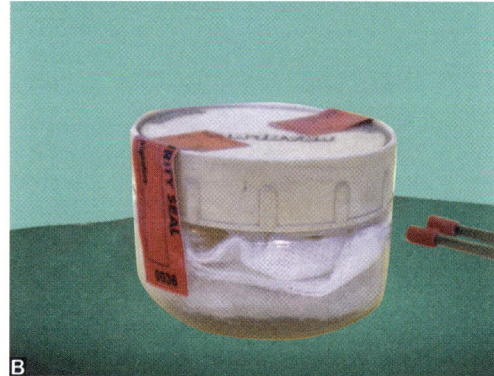

Figs. 6.14A and B: (A) Bullet is handled with rubber coated forceps; and (B) Preservation of bullet.

15. Sharp Objects

- Sharp objects, such as knife, syringe with needle, razor blades, or glass fragments should be packed in rigid, puncture-resistant, and leak-proof containers so as to prevent injury to others and preserve trace evidence on the item.
- The knife may be tied into cardboard holders or placed into specially designed sharps containers with air vents **(Figs. 6.15A and B)** and secured in cardboard boxes of the appropriate size.

Cases Pertaining to Toxicology

Chemicals and Drugs

In cases of suspected poisoning, use of controlled substances or effects from prescription medications, the collection of appropriate

---

* GSR contains trace amounts of primer and burnt and unburnt gunpowder when firearm is discharged which gets deposited on clothing, hands or face of the shooter. This GSR is highly perishable and transient.

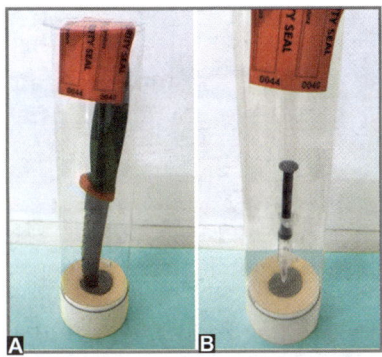

Figs. 6.15A and B: Preservation and packaging of (A) Knife; and (B) Syringe with needle.

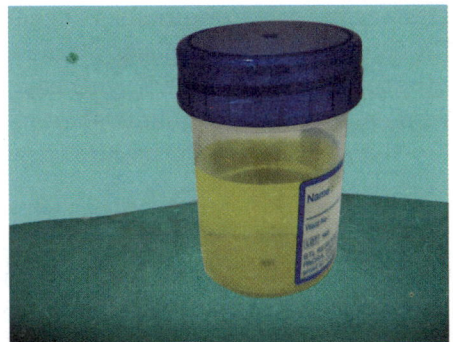

Fig. 6.16: Urine sample.

evidence and documentation is important for treatment of the patient who presents at the hospital.

The evidences commonly encountered in toxicological cases are **(Table 6.2)**:
i. Vomitus of the patient
ii. Container of the poison
iii. Tumbler, cup or similar utensil used to consume/administer the poison
iv. Bottles of water, cold drinks or liquor etc.
v. Clothes suspected to have poison/vomit stain
vi. Empty injection vial/ampoules, hypodermic syringes and needle etc.
vii. Gastric lavage
viii. Blood and urine sample

Table 6.2: Sample preservation for toxicological analysis.

Sample	Quantity	Preservative
Whole blood	10 mL	Lithium heparin or EDTA tube; fluoride/oxalate, if alcohol is suspected
Urine	20–50 mL	No preservative; sodium fluoride is added, if alcohol is suspected
Gastric contents	25–50 mL	No preservative
Scalp hair	About 100–200	No preservative
Exhaled air	As required	No preservative
Scene residues	As appropriate	No preservative

16. Urine

- Urine sample is collected to test for drugs and alcohol levels **(Fig. 6.16)**. The time limit for toxicology testing is about 96 hours since the time of the assault or the time during which substances were believed to be ingested.
- For estimation of alcohol levels, full quantity of urine passed must be collected. It is collected in a large clean, sterilized, screw capped bottle.
- If drug/alcohol is found in the blood/urine, the validity of consent is called into question. There may not be any physical or genital injuries, since this may have affected the survivor's ability to offer resistance.
- Urine samples should be stored in a locked refrigerator.

17. Vomitus and Stomach Contents

- Vomitus is placed either in a clean glass jar or a plastic tub with a tight-fitting lid. There is no need to add any preservatives.
- Gastric lavage *(stomach washing)* is most useful within 1 hour after ingestion of any poison (can be done till 4-6 hours after ingestion). The fluid is taken out initially after gastric lavage is preserved for chemical analysis **(Fig. 6.17)**.

Motor Vehicle Accidents

Clothing should be inspected for evidence of tire tread marks, glass pieces, dirt, vegetations, foreign bodies or paint transfer, and should be

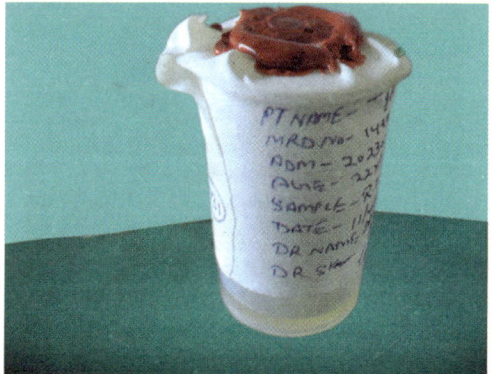

Fig. 6.17: Ryle's tube aspirate.

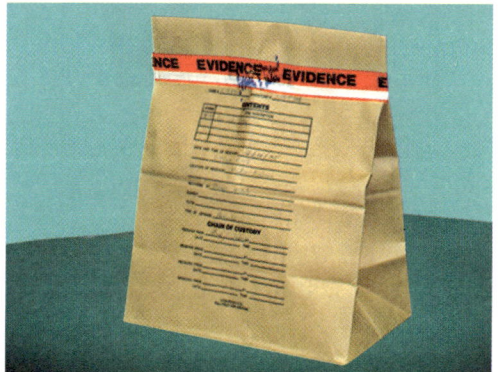

Fig. 6.18: Evidences packed in a single paper bag, sealed and the chain of custody mentioned over it.

preserved as described earlier. This may help in reconstruction of the events.

Burns

In case of burns, clothes and hair of the victim should be preserved/sealed separately in a similar fashion by the examiner.

LABELLING OF EVIDENCE

- Label it correctly and clearly with black pen (permanent marker) with the case number/MLR number, type of specimen, (e.g., blood/urine/vaginal swab/anal swab etc.), site of collection, name, age and sex of the patient, date and time of collection, and examiner's name and signature.
- Each bag is then placed in a larger bag, properly labeled with the patient's identifying information, MLR/Case No., examiner's name and signature, date and time **(Fig. 6.18)**.
- Write across the edge of the tape onto the paper in several places to ensure it cannot be removed and replaced.

CHAIN OF CUSTODY

- The chain of custody of evidence is a written record of every individual who has had physical possession of the evidence. Every time the evidence is opened from its collection container and the evidence seal is broken or moved, there must be a log of that activity.
- Maintaining proper chain of evidence is as important as collecting proper evidence.
- Without complete documentation (along with signatures) of chain of custody from the individual who collected the evidence to the courtroom, the evidence will be inadmissible.
- In collecting and processing evidence, the fewer people who handle that evidence, the better. There is less chance of contamination and a shorter chain of custody for court admissibility.
- The chain of custody:
  a. Begins with the first person who has contact with the piece of evidence.
  b. Ensures that items have been under constant surveillance, have remained in a secure area, and have not been tampered with during handling or transfer, except for analysis by authorized laboratory personnel.
- The forensic nurse must maintain control of evidence during examination, while the evidence dries, and until the evidence is in container/bag and sealed. If the police is unable to pick up the evidence, it can be stored in a locked storage area.
- To maintain the chain of custody, all evidence should be locked up with limited access until it is handed over to the police.
- Documentation of evidence transfer should be noted in medical notes and on the chain

of custody form. Documentation should include:
a. Type of evidence being transferred (evidence kit, photographs, clothing, copies of the medical chart, etc.).
b. Number of bags of evidence being transferred.
c. Time and date of the transfer.
d. Name and signature of the person releasing the evidence.
e. Name and badge number of the police officer collecting the evidence.

The original chain of custody form accompanies the evidence.

DOCUMENTATION OF EVIDENCE

- If physical evidence, such as body fluid, stains or trace evidence is identified at a scene or during the examination of a patient, that evidence should be thoroughly documented prior to collection. Documentation is an integral part of the recovery process, including the precise location of the evidence before recovery.
- Body diagrams, notes, photographs and video recording are important methods of documentation and are considered as evidence in legal proceedings. Each method has advantages and disadvantages—should be employed as seems appropriate to the situation.
- As with other aspects of nursing, thorough and extensive notes are the foundation of good evidence documentation **(Box 6.3)**. These notes can also provide the examiner with important information after evidence collection. Notes also provide the link to other evidence documentation methods and key documents, such as chain of custody.

Box 6.3: Documentation of firearm injury.

- Record the patients' statements accurately.
- Record the patient's appearance (condition), behavior, attitudes and concerns.
- Record location, size and appearance of injuries and take photographs.
- Document the presence of tattooing, soot, abrasion collar.
- Record the location of the projectile(s) recovered.
- Record firearm collection.
- Identify the container in which the projectile is preserved with the patient's data.
- Report incident to the police.

- Photographs of the injuries should also be taken at the time of examination. Whenever photographs are taken, an appropriate scale should be included to document the size and appearance of those injury patterns. Afterward, photographs should be taken without a scale.

FORWARDING OF BIOLOGICAL SAMPLES

The forwarding letter signed with stamp by the competent authority should be addressed to the Director, Forensic Science Laboratory. It should include:
1. Details of all the exhibits sent indicating the impression of the seal.
2. Nature of examination required on each exhibit.
3. Copy of medico-legal report, if any.
4. Copy of postmortem report in cases of death.
5. Copy of all medical treatments given before death, if hospitalized.
6. Sample seal.
7. Chain of custody form.

MULTIPLE CHOICE QUESTIONS

1. Evidence which is sensitive to absolute temperature or fluctuations of temperature?
   A. Physical evidence
   B. Latent print evidence
   C. Biological evidence
   D. Trace evidence

   Explanation: Some evidence, particularly biological evidence, may be sensitive to absolute temperature or fluctuations in temperature. Temperature in the extremes can cause problems with evidence either being "cooked" or "frozen". Blood when exposed to the sun would be decomposed or contaminated by bacteria to a point where further analysis would be impossible or inconclusive.

2. Which of the following refers to proper collection and preservation of evidence?
   A. Storage and packing
   B. Bag it Tag it
   C. Evidence analysis and storage
   D. Acquiring proper storage of evidence

   Explanation: Used in the field of forensic science, "bag it" refers to putting evidence in a sealed bag or container, and "tag it" refers to the tag or label attached describing the contents and context of their retrieval.

3. Best method to identify a person is by:
   A. Scars   B. Blood groups
   C. Fingerprints   D. DNA analysis

   Explanation: Fingerprinting is a very useful method in the identification of a person. A fingerprint is unique to an individual and is permanent. However, the best method is DNA fingerprinting. One of the most common DNA fingerprinting procedures is restriction fragment length polymorphism) (RFLP).

4. Which of the following types of fluids are useful for DNA collection?
   A. Blood   B. Saliva
   C. Semen   D. All of the above

   Explanation: Semen, blood and saliva are useful for DNA collection.

5. Assertion (A) Wet blood stains on cloth should be preserved after drying under room heater.
   Reason (R): Drying under heater causes disintegration of blood stains.

   A. Both (A) and (R) are correct.
   B. Both (A) and (R) are incorrect.
   C. (A) is correct, but (R) is incorrect.
   D. (A) is incorrect, but (R) is correct.

   Explanation: Wet stains must be air dried before packaging them; else there may be decomposition/degradation of evidence. But it should not be dried by heating or placing the article in bright sunlight as it gets denatured.

6. The following steps are followed to avoid contamination/denaturation of DNA evidence:
   A. Touch the area where one believes DNA may exist
   B. Wear gloves
   C. Avoid coughing, sneezing or talking over evidence
   D. Air dry evidence before packing

   Explanation: Avoid touching the area where you believe DNA may exist. Single hair, perspiration and/or saliva deposited mistakenly by an investigator can cost valuable time and create the potential for excluding a suspect, as well as confuse the interpretations of the physical evidence.

7. Collection of evidence from bite marks is particularly useful in
   A. Identifying motive
   B. Creating a firm legal case
   C. Determining the timeframe of assault
   D. Identification of the perpetrator through DNA-tested saliva

   Explanation: Bite marks may be seen in assaults, homicides, and child abuse. The presence of bite marks is useful for guiding saliva collection, which can be used to connect the victim to the suspect thru DNA analysis.

8. When documenting gunshot wounds, forensic nurses should:
   A. Identify the caliber of bullet
   B. Identify entrance or exit wounds
   C. Remove gunshot powder residue with a clean, damp cotton swab
   D. Remove bullets or fragments with rubber-coated forceps and handle as little as possible.

Explanation: Bullets when removed from victims, they should be extracted with rubber-coated forceps and handled as little as possible. When documenting gunshot wounds, they need not identify entrance or exit wounds or determine the caliber of the bullet.

9. An appropriate container for the collection and preservation of dried blood in clothing is:
   A. Plastic container
   B. Glass jar
   C. Paper bag
   D. Plastic bag

   Explanation: Container should be cardboard box, envelope or a paper bag. Never pack in plastic container. The packaging of biological evidence in plastic or airtight containers must always be avoided, because the accumulation of residual moisture could contribute to the growth of DNA-destroying bacteria and fungi.

10. Why is it important for the forensic nurse to maintain a proper chain of custody?
    A. It will exonerate the perpetrator
    B. It will assist in gathering enough data for conviction
    C. Evidence will convict the assailant
    D. It will be accepted as evidence and can be used in the court of law

    Explanation: The chain of custody is important to maintain the authenticity of the collected evidence and make it admissible to court for legal proceedings.

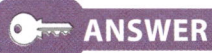

ANSWER KEY

| 1. C | 2. B | 3. D | 4. D | 5. D | 6. A | 7. D | 8. D | 9. C | 10. D |

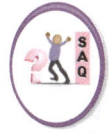

SHORT ANSWER QUESTIONS

1. Write a short note on principle of exchange.
2. Discuss briefly the various types of evidences.
3. What are the essential requirements for collection and preservation of evidence?
4. What is the purpose behind evidence collection?
5. Describe in brief how firearm evidences are collected.
6. Write a note as to how fingernail scraping is collected and preserved.
7. Write a note as to how hair evidence is collected and preserved.
8. Describe briefly how clothing evidence is collected and preserved.
9. What is meant by "chain of custody?" Explain.
10. Explain why documentation of evidences is necessary.

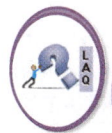

LONG ANSWER QUESTIONS

1. Describe how blood is collected in FTA card.
2. Describe how buccal swab is collected in FTA card.
3. Describe how genital and anal evidences are taken from a victim.
4. Discuss in detail the collection and preservation of biological evidences.

CHAPTER 7

Fundamental Rights and Human Rights Commission

"To deny people their human rights are to challenge their very humanity."
— **Nelson Mandela**
(Anti-apartheid activist and politician)

LEARNING OBJECTIVES

At the end of this topic, the student should be able to:
1. Describe fundamental rights and human rights commission
   - Introduction of Indian Constitution
   - Fundamental Rights
     — Rights of victim
     — Rights of accused
   - Human Rights Commission

INDIAN CONSTITUTION

Introduction

- The Constitution of India is a written document drafted by a committee headed by Dr Bhimrao Ambedkar which came into effect on 26 January 1950. It is not the creation of Parliament but of the people of India and is therefore supreme.
- The constitution declares India a sovereign, socialist, secular, and democratic republic, assures its citizens justice, equality and liberty, and endeavors to promote fraternity.
- The Constitution of India is referred to as a "cosmopolitan document" and "the Bag of Borrowing" because it derives several of its features from foreign sources, most notably the UK, Ireland, US, Canada, Australia, South Africa, and the former USSR.

Salient Features

The main features of the Indian Constitution are federalism, parliamentary form of government, separation of powers, fundamental rights, an independent judiciary and secularism **(Fig. 7.1)**.

Federal System

The constitution establishes a federal government system in India. All the expected features of a federal state such as two government levels, division of power, supremacy and rigidity of the constitution, written constitution and bicameralism are present. But, the constitution also contains many features of a unitary form of government such as single citizenship, strong center, single constitution, flexibility of constitution, all-India services, integrated judiciary, appointment of State Governor by the centre, emergency provisions, and so on.

Parliamentary Form of Government

The parliamentary form, borrowed from the British system, is based on the principle of cooperation and coordination between the legislative and executive. It is also called responsible government and cabinet government. According to the constitution,

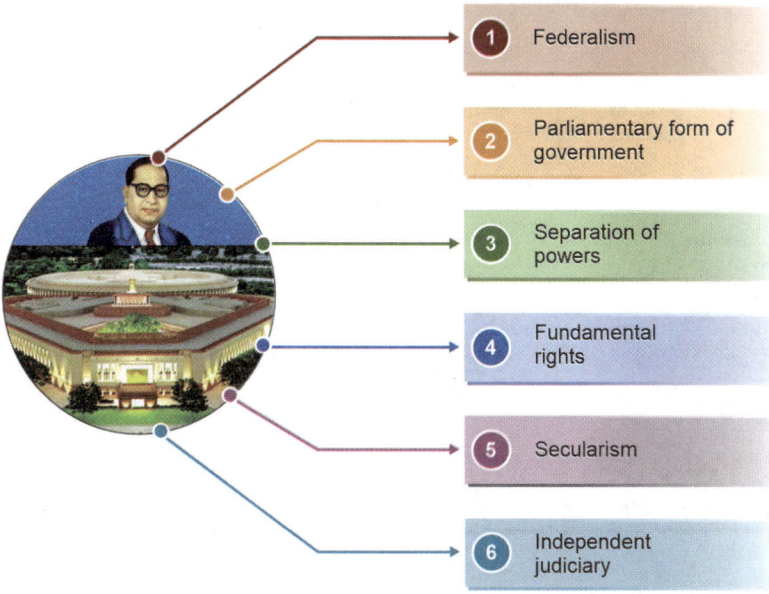

Fig. 7.1: Salient features of our Constitution.

not only the center, the parliamentary form is to be followed even in the States.

System of Governance

Head of State

- The President is the constitutional head of the Union of India, commander-in-chief of the Indian armed forces and head of the government. The "real" executive power is vested with the Prime Minister and the council of ministers (and the President must act on their "aid and advice").
- A similar system is established at the state level. While the Governors are the head of the states, the executive powers are exercised by the Chief Ministers (leader of the state government) and their council of ministers.

Structure

The Indian Parliament comprises two houses:
1. Lok Sabha (House of the people). The political party or coalition of political parties with a majority in the Lok Sabha forms the government. The members of the Lok Sabha are directly elected by the people from their territorial constituencies.
2. Rajya Sabha (Council of States). The members of the Rajya Sabha are indirectly elected from the state assemblies.

Fundamental Rights and Constitution

- Fundamental rights are the basic human rights enshrined in the Constitution of India which are guaranteed to all citizens. They are applied without discrimination on the basis of race, religion, caste, gender, etc.
- India is also a signatory to the Universal Declaration of Human Rights. Most of the rights provided in it have been incorporated as Fundamental Rights in the Constitution of India.
- There were seven fundamental rights in the constitution. Currently, there are only six, as the 'Right to property' was removed as a fundamental right. It is now only a legal right.

The fundamental rights include (Fig. 7.2):
1. **Right to equality:** Right to equality, including equality before law, prohibition of discrimination on grounds of religion, race, caste, gender or place of birth, and equality of opportunity in matters of employment.

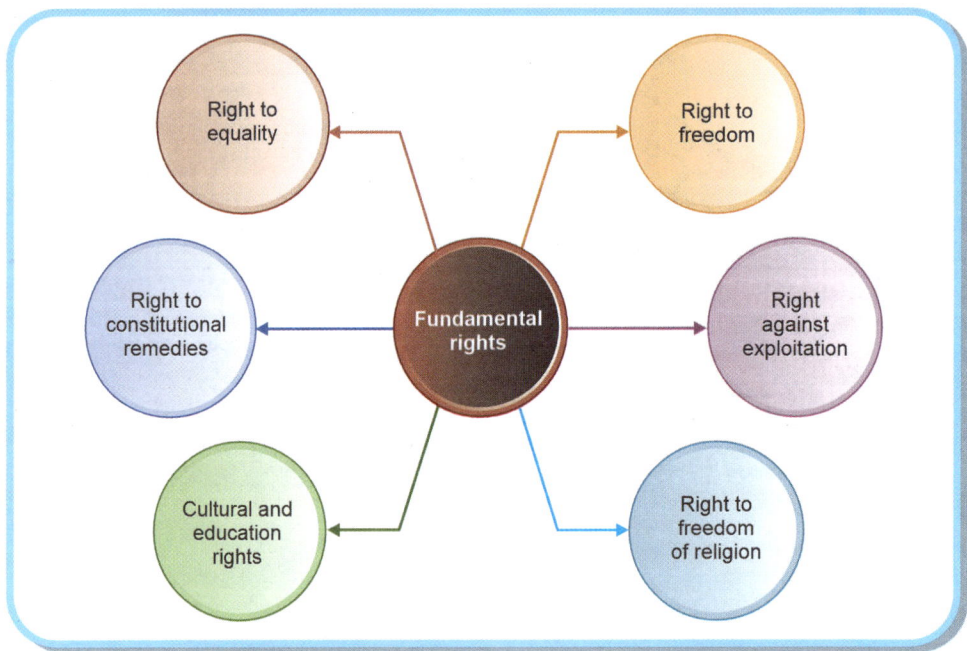

Fig. 7.2: Fundamental rights in India.

2. **Right to freedom:** Right to freedom of speech and expression, assembly, association or union, movement, residence, and right to practice any profession or occupation.
3. **Right against exploitation:** Right against exploitation, prohibiting all forms of forced labor, child labor and traffic in human beings.
4. **Right to freedom of religion:** Right to freedom of conscience, and free profession, practice and propagation of religion.
5. **Cultural and educational rights:** Right of any section of citizens to preserve their culture, language or script, and right of minorities to establish educational institutions and administer education of their choice.
6. **Right to constitutional remedies** for enforcement of fundamental rights.

RIGHTS OF VICTIM

- A "victim" is a person who has suffered harm, either physical or psychological injury, emotional suffering, economic loss or violation of their fundamental rights, through acts or omissions considered to be violative of Indian criminal laws including those laws that prescribe criminal abuse of power.
- In general, a victim's rights can be classified into following classes:
    i. Right to be treated fairly, with self-respect and dignity
    ii. Right to be notified of the events and proceedings in the criminal justice process
    iii. Right to protection during the criminal justice process from threats and injury
    iv. Right to be notified or informed of their various legal rights
    v. Right to speedy proceedings/trail
    vi. Right to be present
    vii. Right to be heard
    viii. Right to compensation
    ix. Rights to privacy
    x. Right to file appeal (under Sec. 372 CrPC)

Provisions for Victims under United Nations Declaration

- Victims should receive the necessary material, medical, psychological and social assistance through governmental, voluntary, community-based and indigenous means.
- Victims should be informed of the availability of health and social services and other relevant assistance and be readily afforded access to them.

Provisions for Victims under Indian Laws

Victim's Rights under Constitution of India

The Indian Constitution includes some provisions for victim's rights, their protection, and respects the idea of victim compensation. Article 14 and Article 21 includes some vital fundamental rights.

- State to offer free legal assistance and guarantee for promoting justice on the grounds of equal opportunity.
- Assures against unfair deprivation of life and liberty by compelling the State to compensate victims of criminal violence.

Victim's Rights under Indian Penal Code (IPC)

- The Criminal Law Amendment Act, 2013 provided for victims and introduced a number of new provisions (sections) for protection of women against acid attacks (Sec. 326A and 326B), sexual harassment (Sec. 345A), voyeurism (Sec. 345C) and stalking (Sec. 345D) and it also widened the scope of definition of rape (Sec. 375) in IPC.
- The two significant remedies of criminal justice system are compensation and restitution which now, have become civil remedies during the modern period.

Victim's Rights under Code of Criminal Procedure (CrPC)

- The victim is represented by the "public prosecutor" who is appointed by the State. The victim can choose an advocate of his choice for assisting the public prosecutor. The code also grants a right to victim to choose his own private lawyer but the authority given to that lawyer is limited.
- **Compensation to victim:** According to Sec. 357(3) CrPC, the court has the right to grant compensation for any loss or injury suffered by the victim, even in cases where fine was not levied upon on the accused.

> **Victim Impact Statement**
> - To empower victims and ensure the protection of their rights, the courts are emphasizing the need to introduce victim impact statements (VIS) in the Indian criminal justice system.
> - A VIS is a written or oral statement given by the victim during the trial.
> - VIS describes the impact of the offense on the victim, including details of the harm suffered by the victim as a result of the offense. These include the physical, financial, psychological, or emotional impact of the crime. It helps judges to assess the real physical, financial, and psychological damage of that crime on the victim and to determine the quantum of punishment accordingly.
> - In a recent case, the Delhi High Court held that filing of the victim impact reports should be made mandatory and courts shall order the accused to pay compensation to the victim especially in cases where fine does not form a part of the sentence. The victim impact report must be processed through the District Legal Services Authorities to verify the impact of the crime victimization on the victims and payment capability of the offender.
> - The Supreme Court highlighted the need of VIS in a recent judgment.
> - The Parliament introduced the Code of Criminal Procedure (Amendment) Bill, 2020, to forward this cause.

RIGHTS OF ACCUSED

Rights of Accused under Constitution of India (Fig. 7.3)

In India, the rights to the accused are given on the lines of *"let hundreds go unpunished, but never punish an innocent person".* Accused is given fair equality at par with other citizen.

- Right to get a fair representation in a criminal procedure is an important aspect of right to equality (Article 14). Article 20 says that "no person shall be convicted of any offense except for violation of a law in

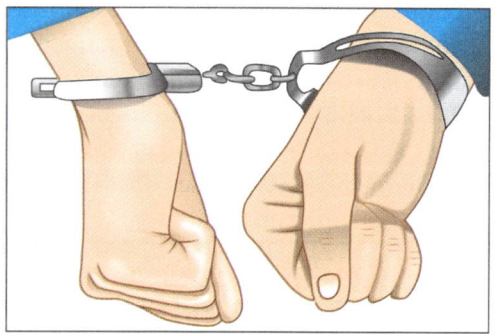

Fig. 7.3: An accused person.

force at the time of the commission of the act charged as an offense."
- Article 22 states that "no person shall be detained in custody without being informed, as soon as may be, of the grounds for such arrest nor shall he be denied the right to consult and to be defended by legal practitioner of his choice."

Under Criminal Law

Presumption of innocence: The essence of criminal trial lies in that "the accused is to be presumed innocent until a charge is proved against him without any reasonable doubt."

The right of accused persons at different stages include:
- Rights of an accused person before his/her trial begins.
- Rights of an accused during a court trial.
- Rights of an accused person after his/her trial is completed.

Pre-Trial Rights of Accused

1. **Right to know about the accusations and charges:** Under the CrPC, the arrested person has the right to know the details of the offense for which he is being arrested and the charges filed against him.
2. **Right to be taken before a Magistrate without delay:** Irrespective of the fact, that whether the arrest was made with or without a warrant, the CrPC provides the accused must be produced before a Judicial Magistrate within 24 hours of arrest.
3. **Right to be examined by a medical practitioner:** Under Sec. 54 CrPC, an arrested person may be examined by a doctor at his request to detect evidence in his favor, a copy of the report is to be furnished by the doctor to the arrested person.
4. **Right to privacy and protection against unlawful searches:** The police officials cannot violate the privacy of the accused on a mere presumption of an offense. The property of an accused cannot be searched by the police without a search warrant.
5. **Right against self-incrimination:** A person cannot be compelled to be a witness against himself as per the constitution.
6. **Right against double jeopardy:** A person cannot be prosecuted and punished for the same offense more than once as per the constitution.
7. **Right against the ex-post facto law:** A person cannot be tried for an offense that was the earlier crime and now is not. This means that the retrospective effect law is not applicable. An act that was not a crime on the day when it was done, cannot be considered as an offense.
8. **Right to have bail:** Any person who is arrested without a warrant and is accused of a bailable offense has to be informed by the police officer that he is entitled to be released on bail on payment of the surety amount.
9. **Right to legal aid:** The accused person can hire a lawyer to defend himself, and in case he is not able to afford a lawyer, the State has to provide free legal aid to him for his representation in court.
10. **Right to expeditious trial:** The accused has the right to fair and speedy trial, which is free of any bias or prejudice.

Rights of the Accused during Trial

1. **Right to be present during a trial:** Sec. 273 CrPC provides that all evidence and statements must be recorded in the presence of the accused or his lawyer.
2. **Right to get copies of documents:** The accused has the right to receive copies of all the documents filed by the prosecutor in relation to the case.
3. **Right to be considered innocent till proven guilty:** The accused has the right to be considered innocent until his guilt is proven in court on the basis of evidence and statements by witnesses.
4. **Right to cross-examination:** The accused has the right to be cross-examined by the prosecutor to prove his innocence.

Post-Trial Rights of the Accused Person

An accused person also has certain rights once his trial is over. These rights of the accused depend upon the outcome of his trial. This means, whether he has been acquitted by the court or has been held guilty and arrested by police.

a. **Rights of the accused, if declared innocent:** When a person is declared innocent and acquitted by the court, the following rights are given to him:
   1. Accused persons have a right to get a copy of the judgment
   2. Right to receive protection from police if there is a threat to his life post-acquittal.

b. **Rights of arrested person**
   1. **Right to appeal:** The arrested person has the right to file an appeal against his conviction in a higher court.
   2. **Right to humane treatment in prison:** The accused has a right to his human rights when in prison and be subjected to humane treatment by the prison authorities.
   3. Right to have family visits in jail.
   4. Right against solitary confinement.

- In Nandini Sathpathy vs PL Dani 1978 SCR (3) 608, it was held that no one can forcibly extract statements from the accused and that the accused has the right to keep silent during the course of interrogation (investigation).
- In DK Basu vs State of WB (1997) 1 SCC 416, the Supreme Court issued some guidelines which were required to be mandatorily followed in all cases of arrest or detention which include, the arresting authority should bear accurate, visible, and clear identification along with their name tags with their designation, the memo be signed by the arrestee and family member, the family or the friend must be told about the arrest of the accused, The arrestee may be permitted to meet his lawyer during interrogation, though not throughout the interrogation.

NATIONAL HUMAN RIGHTS COMMISSION

Introduction

- The National Human Rights Commission (NHRC) established in 1993, is an independent statutory body as per the provisions of the Protection of Human Rights (PHR) Act, 1993.
- Sec. 2(1)(d) of the PHR Act defines human rights as the rights relating to life, liberty, equality and dignity of the individual guaranteed by the constitution or embodied in the international covenants and enforceable by courts in India.
- Composition of NHRC is given in **Flowchart 7.1**.

Functions and Powers

i. Investigate any complaints related to violations of human rights either suo-moto or after receiving a petition.
ii. Interfere in any judicial process that involves any allegation of violation of human rights or negligence in the prevention of such violation by a public servant.
iii. Visit any prison/institute under the control of the state governments to observe the living conditions of inmates,

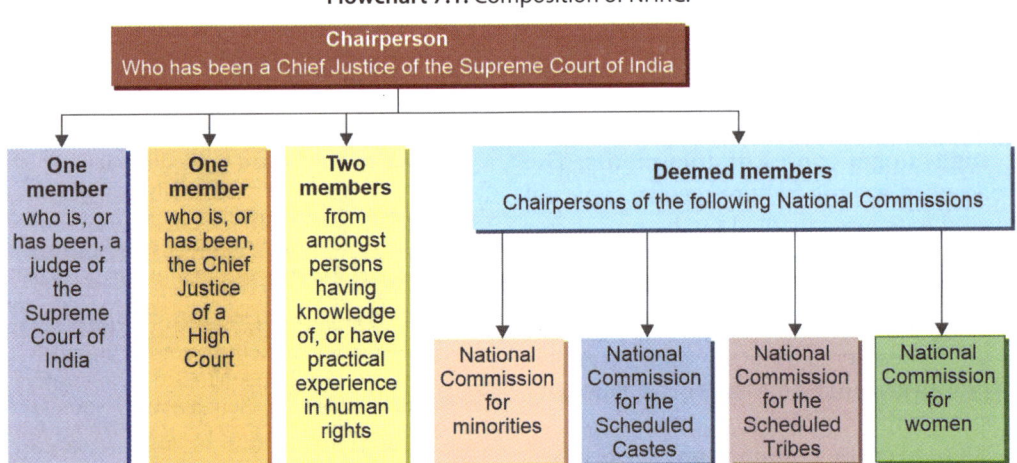

Flowchart 7.1: Composition of NHRC.

and make recommendations based on its observations to the authorities.

iv. Studies treaties and international instruments on human rights and make recommendations for their effective implementation to the government.
v. Review the provisions of the constitution that safeguard human rights and can suggest necessary restorative measures.
vi. Research in the field of human rights.
vii. Recommend suitable steps that can prevent violation of human rights to both central, as well as state governments.

Role

The NHRC is responsible for spreading of human rights awareness amongst the masses and encouraging the efforts of all stake holders in the field of human rights literacy not only at the national level but at international level too.

Major Issues Related to NHRC

NHRC is involved in dealing with the following human rights violations:
a. Custodial torture
b. Child labor
c. Violence and discrimination against women and children
d. Sexual violence and abuse
e. LGBTQIA+ community rights
f. Arbitrary arrest and detention
g. Extrajudicial killings
h. Excessive powers
i. SC/ST, disabled people and other religious minority issues

Limitations of NHRC

1. The recommendations made by the NHRC are not binding.
2. It does not have the power to penalize the authorities that do not implement its orders.
3. Violation of human rights by private parties cannot be considered under its jurisdiction.
4. It has limited jurisdiction over cases related to armed forces.
5. Members may not necessarily be human rights experts.
6. The NHRC does not consider the following cases:
   - Cases older than one year.
   - Cases which are anonymous or vague.
   - Frivolous cases.
   - Cases pertaining to service matters.

Violation of Human Rights and Doctors

- Torture and other human rights abuses have been common throughout history.
- Doctors/nurse may participate in torture either by act of commission (certifying

someone fit for interrogation or intentionally inflicting severe pain or suffering) or by act of omission (falsifying medical certificate or withholding treatment).
- Human Rights Watch has reported on a wide range of abuses against individuals under medical supervision, including the practice of forcible anal and vaginal examination, female genital mutilation and the failure to provide life-saving abortion, palliative care and treatment for drug dependency.
- Ethical guidelines uniformly prohibit healthcare professionals from any form of participation in torture.
- Doctors/forensic nurse have an important role in detecting, documenting and prosecuting those involved in torture.
- Doctors/forensic nurse working in places where systematized abuse is common, such as prisons and interrogation centers are likely to observe and link patterns of injury.
- They may come across sequelae of physical abuse during autopsy.

In India, NHRC has issued guidelines for doctors to deal with cases involving human right violation which emphasizes on right of prisoners regarding prompt medical assistance whenever felt necessary.
- This includes prevention of torture while in custody, and therefore, provisions have been made for mandatory medical examination by doctors every 48 hours during his detention in custody and at the time of his release from the police custody.
- In cases of death in custody, it is mandatory for the DMs and SPs of every district to report to the Secretary General of the Commission about such incidents of death in police or judicial custody within 24 hours of occurrence or having come to know about such incidents.
- Postmortem examination is to be conducted by board/panel of doctors including forensic expert and video recording of examination in such cases is mandatory.

In all these scenarios, forensic nurse can be actively involved and offer immense help to the community.

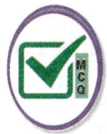

MULTIPLE CHOICE QUESTIONS

1. Which of the following is the ultimate guarantor of fundamental rights in India?
   A. Supreme Court
   B. Parliament
   C. Prime Minister
   D. President of India

   Explanation: Article 32 makes the Supreme Court the defender/guarantor of fundamental rights. Whenever rights of individuals stand breached, they can seek redress from the Supreme Court. It has been given the supreme authority by the Constitution of India to enforce the fundamental rights.

2. Who is the constitutional head of the State governments?
   A. Chief minister of the State
   B. High court judge
   C. Governor
   D. President of the country

   Explanation: The Head of the state governments is the Governor. While the Governor is the nominal executive of the State Government, the person who becomes the Chief Minister is the real executive of the government.

3. How many fundamental rights have been provided by the Constitution of India?
   A. Eight
   B. Seven
   C. Five
   D. Six

   Explanation: The Constitution of India has provided six fundamental rights.

4. Which of the following fundamental right has been deleted from Indian Constitution?
   A. Right to equality
   B. Right to property
   C. Right to speech
   D. Right to freedom

   Explanation: The 44th Amendment in 1978 deleted the right to property from the list of fundamental rights. A new provision, Article 300-A, was added to the constitution, which provided that "no person shall be deprived of his property save by authority of law."

5. India is called a secular country because citizens have the fundamental right to:
   A. Freedom of speech and expression
   B. Freedom to profess the religion of one's choice
   C. Assemble peaceably and without arms
   D. Form associations or unions or co-operative societies

   Explanation: The term "secular" was added to the Preamble of the Indian Constitution by 42nd Amendment in 1976. The Indian Constitution guarantees the freedom of profession, practice, and propagation of religion to all citizens, freedom to manage religious affairs, freedom as to payment of taxes for the promotion of any particular religion.

6. In India, under which of the following legal provisions the crime victim can receive compensation?
   A. Indian Penal Code
   B. Code of Criminal Procedure
   C. Protection of Civil Rights
   D. National Human Rights Commission Act

   Explanation: Compensation can be granted to the victim and families under the schemes enacted under Sec. 357 CrPC.

7. Sec. 162 of the Code of Criminal Procedure, 1973 is for the protection of:
   A. Accused
   B. Witnesses
   C. Police officer
   D. Magistrate

   Explanation: Sec. 162 is aimed at statements recorded by a police officer while investigating into an offense. The object of the section is to protect the accused both against overzealous police officers and untruthful witnesses.

8. The National Human Rights Commission is a:
   A. Constitutional institution
   B. Public sector entity
   C. Department under the central government
   D. Statutory body

   Explanation: NHRC of India is an independent statutory body established in 1993 as per provisions of Protection of Human Rights Act, 1993, later amended in 2006.

9. Who can be appointed as the chairman of the NHRC?
   A. Any sitting judge of the Supreme Court
   B. Any retired Chief Justice of the Supreme Court
   C. Any person appointed by the President
   D. Retired Chief Justice of any High Court

   Explanation: A person who is a retired Chief Justice of the Supreme Court of India can only be appointed as the Chairman of the NHRC.

10. Which of the following is NOT a function of the NHRC?
    A. To interfere in the proceedings related to any human rights violation case pending in the court
    B. To provide economic compensation to any victim of human rights violation
    C. Protecting the human rights of prisoners
    D. Promoting research in the field of human rights

    Explanation: The NHRC does not have the right to penalize the guilty of human rights violation or to provide any financial assistance to the victim.

ANSWER KEY

| 1. A | 2. C | 3. D | 4. B | 5. B | 6. B | 7. A | 8. D | 9. B | 10. B |

CHAPTER 7: Fundamental Rights and Human Rights Commission

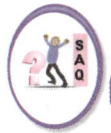

SHORT ANSWER QUESTIONS

1. Write briefly about the salient features of Indian Constitution.
2. What are the fundamental rights given under the constitution?
3. What are the functions of National Human Rights Commission?
4. What are the guidelines issued by National Human Rights Commission for healthcare provider in relation to violation of human rights?

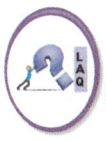

LONG ANSWER QUESTIONS

1. Discuss the rights of victim.
2. Discuss the rights of accused.
3. Discuss briefly the National Human Rights Commission.

CHAPTER 8

Indian Judicial System and Laws

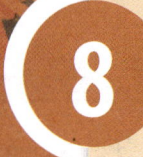

"Justice will not be served until those who are unaffected are outraged as those who are."
— Benjamin Franklin
(Writer, scientist, inventor, statesman, diplomat, and political philosopher)

Learning Objectives

At the end of this topic, the student should be able to:
1. Describe the sources of laws and law-making powers
2. Explain Indian judicial system and laws
   - Overview of Indian Judicial System
     - Apex court
     - High court
     - District court
     - Judicial Magistrate First Class (JMFC)
   - Civil and Criminal case procedures
   - Indian Penal Code (IPC)
   - Criminal Procedure Code (CrPC)
   - Indian Evidence Act (IEA)
3. Discuss the importance of POSCO Act
   - Overview of POSCO Act

SOURCES OF LAWS AND LAW-MAKING POWERS

The main sources of law are the following:
1. **The Constitution of India:** Supreme authority in regard to all matters relating to the executive, legislature and judiciary.
2. **Statutes:** Parliament enacts legislation on a particular subject matter and so do State legislature which prevails in form of law.
3. **Customary law:** In certain aspects, local customs and conventions (usually religious in nature) that are not against any statute or morality are also recognized by law.
4. **Judicial decisions:** Judicial decisions of superior courts like the Supreme Court and High Courts mostly on the points when there is absence of any express law acquires the form of law and has precedential value.

International Sources of Law

- International sources of law (such as a treaty or a convention signed by India) can generally be enforced in India if they have been ratified and incorporated in Indian law, e.g., Geneva Convention.
- In certain cases, customary rules and principles of international law can be applied even without formal ratification in the interests of justice and if the international law in question is not inconsistent with Indian law.
- If there is a conflict between a domestic law and an international law, the domestic law will prevail.

Overview of Indian Judicial System

The Constitution of India divides the Indian judiciary into superior judiciary (the Supreme Court and the High Courts) and the subordinate judiciary (the lower courts under the control of the High Courts) **(Flowchart 8.1)**.
1. **Supreme Court** is the highest judicial tribunal and the highest court of appeal; located in New Delhi. It has the power of supervision over all courts in India. The law

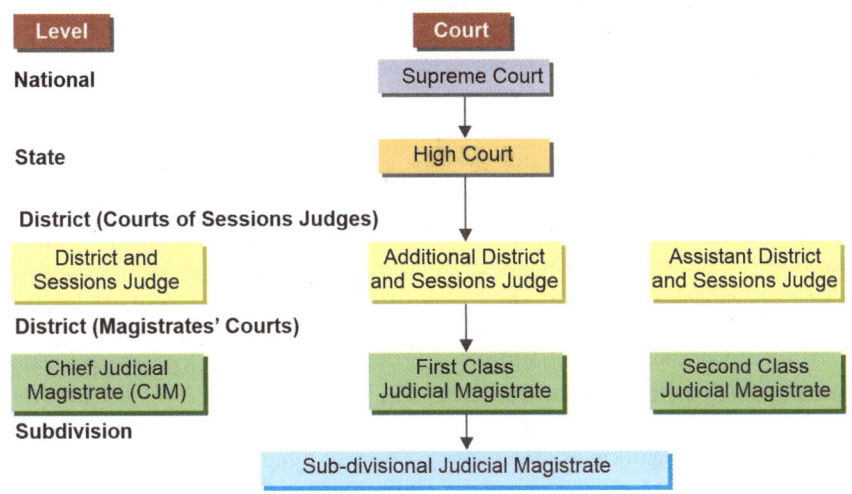

Flowchart 8.1: Indian judicial system (criminal courts).

declared by it is binding on all courts. It is presided by the Chief Justice of India.
2. **High Court** is usually located in the capital of every State (with few exceptions as some High Courts have jurisdiction over multiple States and Union Territories) and is the highest court in the State. There are 25 High Courts in the country. It deals with appeals from lower courts and writ petitions. It may try any offense and pass any sentence authorized by law (Sec. 28 CrPC).
3. **Sessions Court** is usually located at the district headquarters and is also known as *District Session Court* and presided over by a 'District and Sessions Judge'.
   - He is known as a District Judge when he presides over a civil case, and a Sessions Judge when he presides over a criminal case.
   - Appointment of District Judge is done either by the State Government in consultation with the High Court or by way of elevation of Judges from courts subordinate to district courts.
   - It can pass any sentence authorized by law including death sentence which is subject to confirmation by the High Court (Sec. 28 CrPC).
4. **Magistrates' Courts**
   i. Chief Judicial Magistrate
   ii. First Class Judicial Magistrate
   iii. Second Class Judicial Magistrate.

- In metropolitan cities with more than 1 million population, the Chief Judicial Magistrate and First Class Judicial Magistrate are designated as Chief Metropolitan Magistrate and Metropolitan Magistrate respectively.
- The High Court appoints the Judicial Magistrate of First Class to the Chief Judicial Magistrate (Sec. 12 CrPC).
- Powers of Magistrate Court is given in Sec. 29 CrPC. Higher court can enhance the sentence awarded by it.

Powers of Judges and Magistrates are given in **Table 8.1**.

Labor Courts

Labor court is a governmental judiciary body which deals with disputes between an employee and employer (e.g., wrongful termination, unpaid salary, sexual harassment, denied maternity benefit etc.) during the course of employment.

Family Courts

- Family courts were established to hear all cases that relate to familial and domestic relationships, such as marriage, divorce, domestic violence, alimony, child custody, etc.
- In India, the Family Courts Act, 1984 was implemented for the welfare of women.

Table 8.1: Powers of Judge/Magistrate.

Judge/Magistrate	Punishment	Amount of fine
Supreme Court	Imprisonment for any period including death sentence	Any amount
High Court	Same as above	Any amount
District and Session	Same as above (death sentence needs confirmation by High Court)	Any amount
Assistant Session	Imprisonment for up to 10 years	Any amount
Chief Judicial/Chief Metropolitan	Imprisonment for up to 7 years	Any amount
First Class Judicial/Metropolitan	Imprisonment for up to 3 years	Up to ₹ 10,000
Second Class Judicial	Imprisonment for up to 1 year	Up to ₹ 5,000

- **Main purpose:** Try the cases away from the intimidating atmosphere of regular courts and reduce the backlog of cases.

Executive Magistrates

- Executive Magistrates (including DM, SDMs, Tehsildars) are officers of the executive branch.
- State government appoints these Executive Magistrates.
- Judicial Magistrate can handle all cases including criminal cases, whereas Executive Magistrate can handle cases relating to public peace, maintenance of law and order, etc.
- These officers cannot try any accused nor pass verdicts.
- Usually, they are officers of the Revenue Department who are invested with specific powers under both CrPC and IPC.

Juvenile Justice Board

- Under the Juvenile Justice (Care and Protection of Children) Act, 2015, the State Government constitutes the Juvenile Justice Boards for each district.
- The Board consists of a Metropolitan Magistrate/Judicial Magistrate First Class (Principal Magistrate) and two social workers, out of which at least one should be a female.

Functions are:
  i. To adjudicate cases of juvenile offenders (<18 years of age) and monitor institutions for juvenile offenders.
  ii. Ensure that the children's rights are protected in the process of inquiry, arrest and rehabilitation.
  iii. Maintain liaison with the Child Welfare Committee.

Apart from the courts, the Indian judicial system comprises tribunals, commissions and quasi-judicial authorities that derive their authority from specific statutes, e.g., National and State Human Rights Commissions for the protection of human rights, consumer disputes forums at national, state and district level to deal with consumer disputes.

Civil and Criminal Case Procedures (Refer to Diff. 8.1 and Flowchart 8.1)

- The main parties to civil matters are the claimant (plaintiff) and the defendant.
- In criminal matters, the main parties are the State prosecution and the accused.
- The main function of a trial is assessing the available evidence by the court, and weighing and balancing it before pronouncing the verdict.
- A trial usually includes examination-in-chief and cross-examination of witnesses, interrogation of the accused (defendant) and scrutiny of the evidence. Re-examination of witnesses may also be allowed (with the permission of the court).

INDIAN PENAL CODE

- The Indian Penal Code (IPC) is the official criminal code of India intended to cover all aspects of criminal law.

Diff. 8.1: Civil and criminal case.

Features	Civil case	Criminal case
Definition	Dispute between two or more parties in their individual capacities	Prosecution by the State against a person/organization, for committing a public wrong (offense against the State)
Complainant	Sufferer party	Public prosecutor on behalf of the State
Trial by	Civil Court	Criminal Court
Punishment	Pay damages (fine)	Fine, community service, probation, imprisonment, death
Standard of proof	'Preponderance of the evidence'—the winner's side of the story is more probably true than not true	'Beyond a reasonable doubt'—party needs to prove that his version of the facts is highly likely
Examples of cases	Negligence, divorce, custody, consumer disputes, etc.	Assault, robbery, murder, arson, rape, etc.

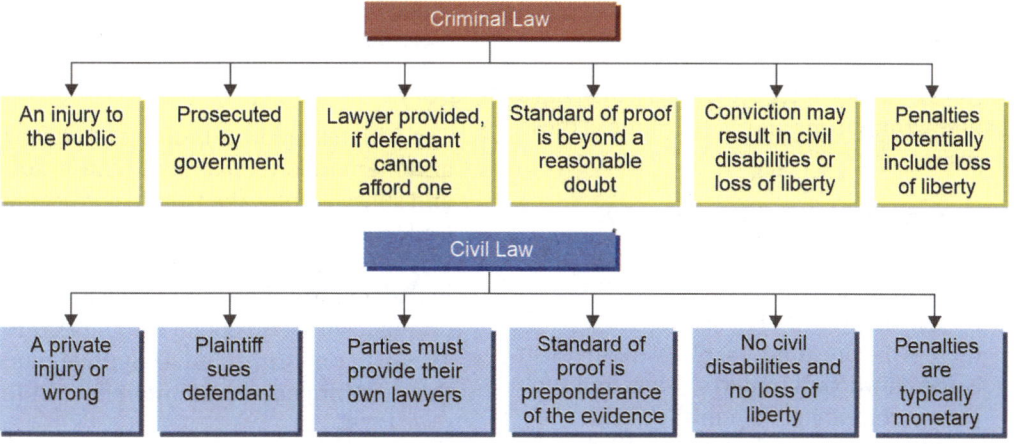

Flowchart 8.1: Criminal and Civil Law.

- It came into force in 1862 in all British Presidencies, although it did not apply to the princely States, which had their own courts and legal systems.
- Before the advent of the British, the penal law prevailing in India, for the most part, was the Mohammedan Law.

Structure of the IPC

The IPC defines specific crimes and provides punishment for them. Some examples are cited below:

a. **Crimes against the human body**
   - These offenses are provided for in Chapter XVI of the Code from Sec. 299, which deals with culpable homicide to Sec. 377, which deals with unnatural offenses.
   - The chapter deals with all kinds of offenses which can be committed against the human body, from the very lowest degree i.e., simple hurt or assault to the gravest ones which include murder, kidnapping and rape.

b. **Crimes against property**
   - These crimes are defined and punished under Chapter XVII from Sec. 378 which defines theft, to Sec. 462 which prescribes punishment for the offense of breaking upon an entrusted property.
   - The offenses dealt under this chapter include theft, extortion, robbery, cheating, forgery etc.

c. **Offenses against the State**
   - These crimes are defined and punished under Chapter VI from Secs. 121 to 130 and are some of the most rigorous penal provisions of the entire code.
   - This includes the offense of waging war against the State under Sec. 121 and sedition under Sec. 124A.
d. **General exceptions**
   - Secs. 76–106 (Chapter IV) represent the general exceptions which are basically exceptional circumstances where the offender can escape criminal liability.
   - Concepts that are elaborated upon in this chapter include insanity, consent and acts of children below a certain age.

Debated Provisions of the IPC

There are certain other provisions which have invited scrutiny time and again. Some of these provisions are:

Attempt to Commit Suicide—Sec. 309
- This section prescribed punishment of up to 1 year for attempting suicide.
- As per the Mental Healthcare Act, 2017, there is the presumption of severe stress on a person who attempted suicide, and such person should not be punished under Sec. 309 IPC and has been decriminalized.

Adultery*—Sec. 497
- This section, which criminalized and prescribed punishment, was criticized for treating a woman as the private property of her husband and imposing moral principles on married couples.
- Supreme Court has decriminalized adultery. However, it is a valid ground for civil offense (divorce).

Unnatural Offenses—Sec. 377
- This section provides punishment for consensual sexual acts between adults belonging to the same sex, mostly anal intercourse.
- The Supreme Court has decriminalized consensual acts of anal intercourse by adults.

The code also provides for imposing the death penalty in certain offenses like murder, rape and waging war against the government.

CRIMINAL PROCEDURE CODE

- The Criminal Procedure Code (CrPC) is a comprehensive document designed to provide due process to the accused by laying down a procedure for cognizance, arrest, bail, collection of evidence, trial and determination of innocence or guilt.
- The procedure ensures that the rights of individuals are protected against the strong State machinery.

History
- The administration of India was taken over after the rebellion of 1857 by the British crown and subsequently, the Criminal Procedure Code was enacted in the year 1861.
- The enactment of 1861 made the European natives immune from the jurisdiction of the criminal courts except for the High Court.
- The legacy of British India continued until the present code came into effect in the year 1973.

What is Investigation?
- According to Sec. 2(h) of the code, an investigation is the process of collecting evidence by either a police officer or any other person that is authorized by a Magistrate to do so.
- For the purposes of investigation, cases under CrPC have been divided into cognizable and noncognizable cases.
   i. **Cognizable offense:** It is an offense in which a police officer can arrest a person without warrant from the Magistrate, e.g., rape, murder, dowry death or attempt to murder [Sec. 2(c) CrPC].

---

*Consensual sexual intercourse between a married person and a person of the opposite sex, not being the spouse, during the continuation of marriage.

ii. **Noncognizable offense** is an offense in which the police officer cannot arrest without a warrant from the Magistrate, e.g., causing miscarriage or voluntarily causing hurt [Sec. 2(l) CrPC].
- The process of investigation starts by taking cognizance of a case and is completed when the police report is submitted.
- The process of investigation is thorough and full of intricate procedures—any irregularities in the procedure may result in the acquittal of the accused.

Arrest in CrPC and Rights of an Arrested Person

- Arrest means the apprehension of a person by the authorities, thus depriving him of his liberty.
- In criminal law, it is an essential aspect so that the accused is made to face the process of law and prevents him from absconding.

Some important rights that a person who is being arrested has are:
1. There can be no legal arrest if there is no information or reasonable suspicion that the person has been involved in a cognizable offense or commits offense(s).
2. Sec. 46 CrPC envisages modes of arrest i.e., submission to custody, touching the body physically or confining the body. In case force is required to make an arrest, it should not be any more than is actually required.
3. The arrested person must be informed of the grounds of arrest as soon as he is arrested. The arresting officer is to inform a friend, relative or nominated person of the arrestee.
4. In the case of women, the body of the person is not to be touched, unless the arresting person is also a female. A female cannot be arrested after sunset and before sunrise, except in exceptional circumstances with the prior permission of a Magistrate.
5. Sec. 54 CrPC provides for a medical examination of the accused by a medical practitioner. In case of females, the examiner has to be female too.
6. The arrestee is also entitled to be counselled and defended by a lawyer of his choice, in addition to being entitled to free legal aid.

What is Bail?

- Bail means the temporary release of an accused; it is not only the essence of criminal procedure but also a safeguard of individual liberty.
- Under CrPC, the offenses can be:
  i. **Bailable offenses** are those in which bail can be granted by the law. The court cannot refuse bail, and the police have no right to keep the person in custody. For example, causing death by rash or negligent act (Sec. 304-A IPC), causing miscarriage (Sec. 312 IPC), or voluntarily causing hurt (Sec. 323 IPC) and grievous hurt (Sec. 325 IPC).
  ii. **Nonbailable offenses** are those in which bail cannot be granted. These are serious offenses and the decision for bail is taken by a Judicial Magistrate only. For example, cases of murder (Sec. 302 IPC), attempt to murder (Sec. 307 IPC), dowry death (Sec. 304-B IPC), causing miscarriage without woman's consent (Sec. 313 IPC) or voluntarily causing grievous hurt by dangerous weapons (Sec. 326 IPC).
- The code also provides for anticipatory bail in case any person is apprehending arrest, i.e., bail even before the person is arrested.

Trial under CrPC

For the purposes of trials, the cases under CrPC can be classified in into four categories:
1. **Sessions case:** These are cases where the punishment for the offenses involved is death, life imprisonment or imprisonment for a period of ≥ 7 years. In such cases, the trial is to be handled by a Sessions Court.
2. **Summons case:** Case relating to an offense punishable with imprisonment for a term <2 years, e.g., voluntarily causing hurt, and is tried by a Magistrate. These are relatively less serious offenses and the procedure involved is also simpler.

3. **Warrant case:** Case related to an offense punishable with death, life imprisonment or imprisonment for ≥2 years, e.g., murder, dowry deaths, attempt to murder cases, etc.
4. **Summary case:** Summary trials are those kinds of trials where speedy justice has to be given, which means those cases which are to be disposed of speedily and the process of these cases is quite simplified.

Trial Procedure

- The procedure for trials is interwoven with detailed procedures; they are in place so that the guilty may be punished but also the innocent persons get every possible opportunity to prove their innocence.
- Once the innocence or guilt of an accused is determined, the aggrieved party has the option to go in appeal and challenge the decision within the stipulated statutory time.
- The appeals generally lie from a Magistrates Court to the Sessions Court, from the Sessions Court to the High Court and from the High Court to the Supreme Court.

INDIAN EVIDENCE ACT

Introduction

- Indian Evidence Act (IEA) is an Act in the Indian Constitution introduced by the Imperial Legislative Council in 1872, during British Rule in India.
- IEA defines evidence in court and states its admissibility.
- **Objectives:** Aid the courts in ascertaining the truth, to prevent inquiries from becoming prolonged and delay the judicial process, and to ensure that judges do not grow confused or muddled due to irrelevant or inconsequential evidence.
- **Purpose:** Define the sources of evidence for Indian courts.
- Evidence which does not fall under the IEA is not admissible in court, even if it is the key to determining the truth of the matter.
- Evidence law is supported by three main pillars:

1. Evidence should only consist of matters in issue
2. Hearsay evidence does not have evidentiary value
3. There should be an effort to provide the best evidence in all cases.

Salient Features

The main features of the IEA include:
a. Defining evidence
b. Provisions regarding the relevancy of evidence
c. Provisions regarding examination of evidence

Sec. 3 of IEA is an important clause that provides the definition of important terms that appear throughout the Act. It defines:
- What constitutes a court, i.e., who is authorized by this Act to collect evidence and reach a decision
- Different types of evidence, documents
- What is a fact
- What is relevant
- How a fact is proved, disproved and not proved.
- How it sets up the reading of the rest of the Act, and the interpretation of evidence law according to it?

Court: 'Court' consists of all Judges and Magistrates, and any person who is legally authorized to take evidence, with the exception of arbitrators and tribunals.

Fact: 'Fact' may be defined as "anything, state of things, relation of things that can be sensed (external fact)".

Facts in issue: Facts in issue are those facts that are sought to be proved and are also called "principal facts" or *factum probandum*. When the rights and liabilities of the parties are dependent on a fact that is in dispute or controversy, that fact is in issue.

Relevant facts: Relevant facts are those which are needed to prove or disprove a fact in issue. Relevant facts are also called evidentiary facts (*factum probans*).

Document: A document within the meaning of this Act is any writing, marks, figures inscribed on a surface for the purpose of recording a matter.

Evidence means to discover, determine or arrive at the truth.
i. **Oral evidence:** The statements made by witnesses which are allowed or needed by the court. Oral evidence must be direct i.e., the witness making the statement must have seen or heard or experienced the event first-hand.
ii. **Hearsay evidence:** Whenever information passes through indirect channels, such as rumors or gossip, it can be termed as "hearsay".
iii. **Documentary evidence:** All documents submitted to the court for scrutiny fall under the umbrella of documentary evidence. Documentary evidence holds precedence as compared to oral evidence, in terms of both credibility and permanence.

THE PROTECTION OF CHILDREN FROM SEXUAL OFFENSES (POCSO) ACT, 2012

Introduction

The POCSO Act, 2012 is an important step towards creating a safer environment for the children of our country. This Act was amended in 2019 to make better provisions that will help to provide swift justice in the form of enhanced punishments for several offenses.

Importance of POCSO Act

- This Act has been drafted to strengthen the legal provisions for the protection of children from offenses, such as sexual assault, sexual harassment and child pornography.
- Sexual offenses are currently covered under various sections of IPC (Secs. 376, 377 and 354 IPC). The IPC does not provide for all types of sexual offenses against children and, more importantly, does not distinguish between adult and child victims nor does it protect male victims from sexual offenses involving penetration.
- The POCSO Act defines a child as any person below the age of 18 years and provides protection to all children (both males and females—*the Act is gender neutral,* unlike the IPCs) under the age of 18 years from sexual abuse.
- There are multiple forms and acts of sexual abuse defined under this Act that is not just limited to pornography, harassment, or penetrative/nonpenetrative offenses.
- The Act's enactment has increased the scale of reporting sexual crimes against children.
- The crimes and cases under this Act are nonbailable in nature.

Offenses and Punishments (Flowchart 8.2)

I. **Penetrative sexual assault:** A person is said to commit 'penetrative sexual assault' if he:
   a. Penetrates his penis to any extent, into the vagina, mouth, urethra or anus of a child or makes the child to do so with him or any other person; or
   b. Inserts any object or a part of the body (not being his penis) to any extent, into the vagina, urethra or anus of a child or makes the child to do so with him or any other person; or

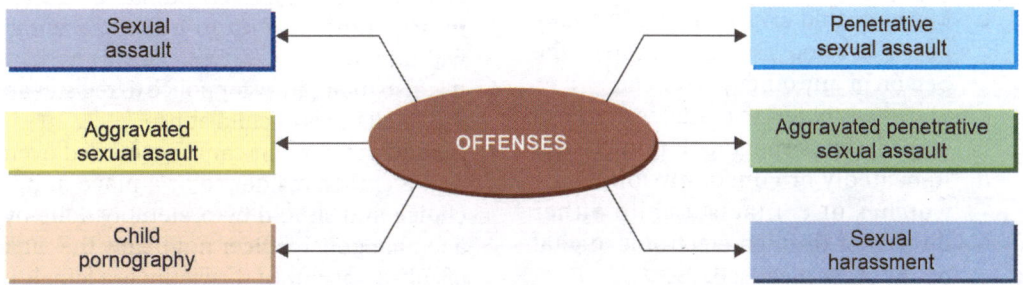

Flowchart 8.2: Offenses under POCSO Act.

c. Manipulates any part of the body of the child so as to cause penetration into the vagina, urethra, anus or any part of body of the child or makes the child to do so with him or any other person; or
d. Applies his mouth to the penis, vagina, anus, urethra of the child or makes the child to do so to him or any other person.

Offense	Punishment
For penetrative sexual assault on a child <16 years of age	Imprisonment for 20 years which may extend for the remainder of natural life + fine
For penetrative sexual assault on a child between 16 and 18 years of age	Imprisonment for 10 years which may extend for the remainder of natural life + fine
For aggravated penetrative sexual assault	Rigorous imprisonment for 20 years which may extend to a life sentence + fine or death sentence

II. **Sexual assault:** Any physical contact with sexual intent but without penetration like touching the vagina, penis, anus or breast of the child or making the child touch the vagina, penis, anus or breast of such person or any other person.
   - *Punishment:* Imprisonment for ≥3–5 years and fine.
   - *For aggravated sexual assault:* Imprisonment for ≥5–7 years and fine.

III. **Sexual harassment of the child:** It is considered sexual harassment when a person with sexual intent:
   a. Utters any word/sound, or makes any gesture or exhibits any object or part of body with the intention to be heard or seen by the child; or
   b. Makes a child exhibit her body or any part of her body, so as it is seen by the person or any other person; or
   c. Shows any object to a child in any form or media for pornographic purposes; or
   d. Repeatedly or constantly follows or watches or contacts a child either directly or through electronic, digital or any other means; or
   e. Threatens to use, in any form of media, a real or fabricated depiction through electronic, film or digital or any other mode, of involvement of the child in a sexual act; or
   f. Entices a child for pornographic purposes.
      - *Punishment:* Imprisonment for up to 3 years and fine.

IV. **Use of child for pornographic purposes:** A person is guilty of the offense if he uses a child in any form of media, for the purposes of sexual gratification, which includes:
   a. Representation of the sexual organs of a child; or
   b. Usage of a child engaged in real or simulated sexual acts (with or without penetration); or
   c. Indecent or obscene representation of a child.
      - *Punishment:* Imprisonment for 5 years and fine, and in subsequent conviction: 7 years and fine.

Salient Features (Flowchart 8.3)

- An offense is treated as "aggravated" when the abused child is mentally ill, below 12 years, or committed by a person in a position of trust or authority of child, such as a family member, member of security forces, police officer, public servant, etc.
- There is provision for punishment even in abetment or an attempt to commit the offenses defined in the Act. The punishment for the attempt to commit is up to half the punishment prescribed for the commission of the offense.
- It is mandatory for healthcare providers to report to the police about the offense. Failure to report attracts punishment with imprisonment of up to 6 months with/without fine.
- It is also mandatory for police to register an FIR in all cases of child abuse.
- A child's statement can be recorded even at the child's residence or a place of her choice and should be preferably done by a female police officer not below the rank of sub-inspector (if the victim is a female).

CHAPTER 8: Indian Judicial System and Laws

Flowchart 8.3: Salient features of the Act.

Features of POCSO Act:
- Gender-neutral act
- It is an offense not to report an abuse
- No time limit for reporting abuse
- Right to compensation for victim
- Confidentiality of victim's identity
- Periodic police verification and background check of every employee who might interact with a child
- Right to life and survival of a child

Recording a child's statement

- Statement should be recorded preferably by a woman police officer, not in uniform
- Statement should be recorded in presence of trusted adult and/or an expert, interpreter, translator or social worker
- Audio or video recording devices should be used, if available
- It should be recorded at the child's home, or any place he/she finds comfortable
- Medical examination within 24 hours in the presence of parent or trusted adult
- Police officer should read out loud the recorded statement to the child
- It should be recorded in the language of the child, as spoken by the child
- Take frequent breaks while the child narrates the incident. Don't rush the child while recording the statement
- Child/Parent must get a copy of the statement

- The child's medical examination can be conducted even prior to registration of an FIR. This discretion is left up to the Investigation Officer (IO). The IO has to get the child medically examined in a government or local hospital within 24 hours of receiving information about the offense. This is done with the consent of the child or parent or a competent person whom the child trusts and in their presence.
- The police are also required to bring the matter to the attention of the Child Welfare Committee (CWC) within 24 hours of receiving the report and should also indicate if the child is in need of care and protection; and steps taken by them in this regard.
- For speedy trial, the evidence of the child has to be recorded within a period of 30 days. The Special Court has to complete the trial within 1 year.
- There is provision for relief and rehabilitation of a child. The child must be compensated for physical and psychological trauma, and financial loss.
- The burden of proof is shifted on the accused, keeping in view the vulnerability and innocence of children, and following the principle of "guilty until proven innocent".
- To prevent misuse of the law, punishment is given for false complaints or false information with malicious intent.
- The media is barred from disclosing the identity of the child without the permission of the Special Court. The punishment for breaching this provision is imprisonment from 6 months to 1 year.

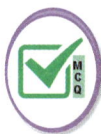

MULTIPLE CHOICE QUESTIONS

1. **The main sources of law in India are:**
   1. The Constitution
   2. Statutes
   3. Customary law
   4. Judicial decisions of superior courts
   A. 1 and 2
   B. 1, 2 and 4
   C. 1, 2 and 3
   D. 1, 2, 3 and 4

   Explanation: The sources of laws in India are—the Constitution, statutes, customary law and judicial decisions of superior courts.

2. **For the accused to be found guilty in criminal case, the prosecution must prove:**
   A. Guilt beyond all doubts
   B. Guilt beyond a reasonable doubt
   C. Guilt based on preponderance of evidence
   D. Clear and convincing guilt

   Explanation: In a criminal case, the prosecution bears the burden of proving that the defendant is guilty beyond all reasonable doubt. This means that the prosecution must convince the judge that there is no other reasonable explanation that can come from the evidence presented at trial.

3. **Example of Court of Appeal:**
   A. Sessions's court
   B. Magistrate's court
   C. SDM court
   D. High Court

   Explanation: The High Court is considered as the primary court of appeal because it is empowered to hear appeals against the judgement given by the subordinate courts within its territorial jurisdiction.

4. **Chief Judicial Magistrate can sentence a guilty for imprisonment up to:**
   A. 3 years
   B. 5 years
   C. 7 years
   D. Life imprisonment

   Explanation: The Chief Judicial Magistrate Court has the power to award imprisonment up to 7 years.

5. **A tenant who is being forced to move out of his residence files a case in court against the landlord. This is a:**
   A. Civil case
   B. Criminal case
   C. Social case
   D. Financial case

   Explanation: Civil cases involve disputes between persons or organizations in their individual capacity. Therefore, eviction of tenant is a civil case.

6. **A person breaks someone's mandible in an alleged fight. Police can:**
   A. Arrest with warrant
   B. Arrest without warrant
   C. Declare him hostile
   D. Put him in mental asylum

   Explanation: Police officer can arrest any person in cognizable offenses and does not require a warrant from Magistrate. The majority of crimes that are considered to be "cognizable" are severe in nature, such as murder, rape, kidnapping, theft, dowry deaths, etc.

7. **"Facts" under the Indian Evidence Act means:**
   A. Anything capable of being perceived by the senses only
   B. Anything not being capable of being perceived by the senses only
   C. Only any mental condition of which any person is conscious
   D. Anything capable of being perceived by the senses and any mental condition of which any person is conscious

   Explanation: "Fact" means and includes—(1) anything, state of things, or relation of things, capable of being perceived by the senses; (2) any mental condition of which any person is conscious.

8. **Warrant case means:**
   A. An offense punishable with imprisonment for life
   B. An offense punishable with death
   C. An offense for which imprisonment for ≥2 years
   D. All of these

   Explanation: Any case relating to an offense punishable with death, imprisonment for life or imprisonment for a term exceeding 2 years is a warrant case.

9. **Who is a child as per POCSO Act?**
   A. Anyone below 18 years of age
   B. Anyone below 16 years of age
   C. Anyone below 14 years of age
   D. Anyone below 12 years of age

Explanation: The POCSO Act defines a child as any person below 18 years of age. Any person, irrespective of gender, is covered under the remedies provided under this Act.

10. Which statement stands valid in regard to the POCSO Act?
    1. Every crime against children must be reported as per POCSO Act
    2. Those who do not report sexual offenses against children may be punished as per the Act

    A. Only 1
    B. Only 2
    C. Both 1 and 2
    D. None of the above

    Explanation: Every person who suspects or has knowledge of a sexual offense being committed against a child to report it to the local police. It includes offenses like sexual assault, sexual harassment and pornography, not all crime against the children.

ANSWER KEY

| 1. D | 2. B | 3. D | 4. C | 5. A | 6. B | 7. D | 8. D | 9. A | 10. B |

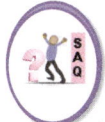

SHORT ANSWER QUESTIONS

1. Describe in brief the sources of Indian laws.
2. What are the powers of Judges and Magistrates?
3. Discuss the brief the disputed provisions of Indian Penal Code.
4. What are the differences between Civil and Criminal Cases?
5. What are cognizable and noncognizable offenses?
6. Discuss in brief the rights of arrested person as provided under Criminal Procedure Code.
7. Define bail. What is meant by bailable and nonbailable offenses?
8. What is meant by Summon case and Warrant case?
9. What is the importance of the POCSO Act? Mention the salient features of the POCSO Act.

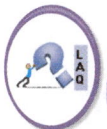

LONG ANSWER QUESTIONS

1. Give an overview of Indian Judicial System.
2. Describe in brief the Indian Penal Code.
3. Describe in brief the Criminal Procedure Code.
4. Describe in brief Indian Evidence Act.
5. What are the offenses and punishment under the POCSO Act?
6. Describe in brief POCSO Act, 2012.

SECTION II

Basic Forensic Medicine

SECTION OUTLINE

9. Legal Procedures and Nursing Jurisprudence — 117
10. Injuries — 125
11. Medico-Legal Autopsy — 136
12. Thanatology — 139
13. Identification — 151
14. Forced Anal Intercourse — 161
15. Forensic Psychiatry — 162
16. Asphyxial Conditions — 167
17. Forensic Toxicology — 172

CHAPTER 9

Legal Procedures and Nursing Jurisprudence

This section deals with basic nursing jurisprudence and forensic medicine which a forensic nurse should understand (basic know-how) so as to practice and deal efficiently with the medico-legal cases that she/he will be handling subsequently.

INQUEST

Definition: It is an inquiry or investigation by legal authorities into the cause of death where death is due to unnatural means.

Types of inquest	Conducted by
Police inquest	Police
Magistrate inquest	Magistrate
Coroner's inquest	Coroner
Medical examiner system	Medical examiner

Police Inquest—*Under Sec. 174 CrPC*

- **Definition:** The investigation or inquiry by the police into the cause of death is called police inquest.
- *Most common type of inquest in India* which is held routinely.
- Investigation is done by the police officer/investigation officer not below the rank of *senior head constable*.

Purpose of Police Inquest

To find out the:
 i. Identity of the deceased
 ii. Place of death
 iii. Time of death
 iv. Cause of death

Procedure

- Information of death is given to the police.
- Police officer informs the nearest Executive Magistrate in order to proceed with the inquest.
- Preparation of *Panchnama*
  - Investigating officer (IO) holds an inquiry into the matter, in the presence of two or more witnesses (they are called *panchas*—neighbors of that locality).
  - Then statements are recorded from the family members.
  - Finally, inquest report which is prepared is called as *panchnama*.
  - It is then signed by the investigating officer himself and by the *panchas*.
- In case of foul play/when unnatural death is suspected—investigating officer forwards the body for postmortem examination with the copy of inquest papers.
- The report is finally forwarded to the Magistrate.

Magistrate Inquest—*Under Sec. 176 CrPC*

Definition: The inquiry into the case of death conducted by magistrate is called as Magistrate inquest.

It may be conduct by Executive Magistrate or Judicial Magistrate.

Magistrate inquest is conducted in:

- Death of person in prison
- Death in custody (psychiatric hospital/mental hospital)
- Death of person due to police firing
- Rape in police custody
- Dowry death
- Exhumation (digging out of buried body)

In India, only Police and Magistrate inquest is allowed.

Coroner's Inquest

Definition: It is the inquiry into the cause of death conducted by coroner.

- Coroner is a person with medical and legal knowledge of the rank of First-Class Judicial Magistrate, appointed by State Government.
- At present, it is followed in countries such as UK, US, Canada and Australia. It no longer exists in India.
- It is similar to magistrate inquest in quality.
- Coroner is authorized only to conduct inquest; he is not authorized to conduct trial.

Medical Examiner System

- This type of inquest is conducted in the US.
- It has a board certified forensic pathologist who visits the crime scene, gather evidence and interviews the people to gather information and even conducts autopsy.
- Best system of inquest.

DYING DECLARATION

- Ideally, the Magistrate should be informed to record the dying declaration in presence of witness. But in case the person is about to die, then the statement may be recorded by a healthcare provider/forensic nurse in presence of two or more witnesses.
- The preliminary particular of the patient is noted—name, age, sex, address, Reg. No., MLC No., police station, date and time of admission, location of patient (ward, hospital), ID marks etc.
- The healthcare provider should certify that the patient is conscious and fit for giving statement (i.e. *compos mentis*)—orientation to time, place and person, GCS, BP, pulse, respiratory rate, temperature, ability to speak.
- Oath is not required (as it is believed that dying person speaks the truth).
- Statement should be recorded in simple narrative without any alterations, in patient's own words. Date and time of commencement of recording and completion of statement, mode of statement (writing/speech/gesture).
- If possible, the written statement should be read over to the patient so that it can be rechecked.
- After taking the dying declaration, it should be signed by the healthcare provider and witnesses.
- Declaration is sealed and handed over to concerned police officer along with the receipt.

Medico-legal importance: If the declarant survives, the declaration is not admitted, but has corroborative value.

SUMMONS

Definition: It is a written document issued by the court, which compels the attendance of the witness in the court of law, at a particular date and time, and place, under penalty.

- It is also known as 'subpoena' and Secs. **61-69 CrPC** deals with summons.
- It is issued by the court in writing, in duplicate signed by the Magistrate and bears the seal of the court.
- It is delivered to the witness through a police officer or an officer from the court or by any other person specifically authorized for the purpose.
- On getting the summons, the witness keeps a copy and signs on the back of the other copy of summons.
- The witness must appear before the court on the specified date and time with proper records.

- A witness must attend the court unless there are valid and urgent reasons for not attending.
A. *If a healthcare provider gets more than one summons on the same date:*
   Two different courts: He should attend the:
   1. Criminal court (given priority over civil court)
   2. Higher court

   Same type of court: Should attend the court from which he received the summons first and should inform the other court.

B. *In case witness fails to attend the court:*

With valid reason (like illness): Then message must be conveyed to the court, so that a new date of hearing will be issued to him	Without any valid reason
	• Civil cases—liable to pay damages.
	• Criminal court—court may issue notice and asks the reason tor nonattendance. In case of no justification, he may be imposed **a fine or/and imprisonment and warrant** may be issued against him.

Conduct Money

Definition: It is the fee offered or paid to a witness in civil cases at the time of serving the summons to meet the expenses towards attending the court.
- If the fee is not paid or the amount is less, the healthcare provider can bring this to the notice of the Judge. The Judge will decide the amount to be paid.
- *In criminal cases, no fee is paid to the witness at the time of serving the summons.* He must attend the court because of the interest of securing justice; otherwise charged with contempt of court. However, conveyance charges and daily allowance are paid according to the government rules.

MEDICAL EVIDENCE

Definition: It is defined as legal means to prove or disprove any medico-legal fact under inquiry.

Types
i. Oral evidence
ii. Documentary evidence

Oral Evidence

It means all statements (oral or verbal) which the court permits or requires to be made before it by witnesses, in relation to matters of fact under inquiry.

Types of Oral Evidence
i. Direct evidence
ii. Hearsay evidence/indirect evidence

Medico-legal importance: Oral evidence is more important than documentary evidence, as it permits cross-examination.

Documentary evidence is accepted by the court only after oral testimony by the person concerned.

Exceptions to oral evidence are:
i. Dying declaration
ii. Matter written in the books
iii. Evidence given by witness in lower court
iv. Reports of certain scientific experts. (ballistic expert, fingerprint expert, DNA fingerprint expert etc.)
v. Public records
vi. Hospital records, etc.

Documentary Evidence

All the documents (written or printed) that are produced for inspection of the court.

Types of documentary evidence

Medical certificates	These are issued by registered medical officer, e.g.: 1. Fitness certificate 2. Illness certificate 3. Birth certificate 4. Death certificate 5. Disability certificate 6. Mental illness certificate Doctors must retain one copy of these certificates

Contd....

Contd....

Medico-legal certificates	Reports prepared by a doctor at the request of the investigating officer/victim, usually in criminal cases, e.g.: 1. Injury report 2. Wound certificate 3. Postmortem report 4. Report after examination of victim of sexual assault These reports do not serve as evidence, until the doctor attends the court and testifies to the facts under oath
Dying declaration	**Definition:** It is written or oral statement of a person who is dying as a result of unlawful act, relating to the material facts of the cause of death or circumstances leading to his or her death. Sec. **32 IEA** deals with dying declaration.
Dying deposition	• It can only be recorded by the magistrate • In the presence of accused party/lawyer • Oath is taken • Cross examination is permitted **Medico-legal importance** • Has more legal value as acts as bed-side court • Not followed in India

PROCEDURE OF RECORDING OF EVIDENCE

Oath	• The witness has to take oath that whatever he will say, he will speak the truth, whole truth and nothing but the truth • **Medico-legal importance— Perjury:** When person gives false evidence under oath
Examination- in-chief	• **Definition:** It is the examination of witness by the party who calls him or by the prosecution lawyer (in case of criminal cases) • **Main purpose:** To place all the facts known by the witness in front of court • *Leading questions** are not asked in examination-in- chief, except when witness is declared hostile by the court

Contd....

Contd....

Cross- examination	• **Definition:** It is the examination of the witness by the opposite party or the lawyer of the accused party
	• **Main purposes**
	  1. To elicit facts favorable to the case
	  2. To test the accuracy of the statements of the witness
	  3. To modify victim's statements
	  4. To give a new look to the case
	• Leading questions are **allowed** in cross examination
	• Witnesses must be very careful while answering the questions in cross examination as defense lawyer will try to weaken the evidence of witness
	• There is **no time limit** for cross examination

Re-examination	• **Definition:** It is the examination of a witness subsequent to the cross-examination by the party who called him/ prosecutor lawyer
	• **Main purposes**
	  – To clarify the doubts that has been raised during cross-examination
	  – To explain some facts more deeply, to avoid misinterpretations
	• New points are not discussed

Court questions	Judge can ask any question at any stage of examination

*Any question suggesting the answer, which the person putting it wishes or expects to receive. For e.g. "Was kerosene used to set her on fire?"

Perjury

Definition	As per Sec. **191 IPC**, it is defined as willfully giving false evidence under oath
Punishment for perjury	As per Sec. **193 IPC**, imprisonment up to 7 years and fine
Reasons behind perjury	a. Witness may have taken bribe b. He may be under threat c. He may have personal bias towards one party

PROFESSIONAL NEGLIGENCE

Definition: It is defined as lack of reasonable care and skills on part of a healthcare provider that resulted in injury/death of the patient.

Essential elements of negligence include (4 Ds):
1. *Duty of care towards patient*
2. *Dereliction/breach in duty of care*
3. *Damage (physical, mental or financial) to the patient*
4. *Direct causation (direct relation between breach and damage)*

For a case of negligence to be established, all four conditions must be present.

Types of Negligence

1. Civil negligence
2. Criminal negligence

Civil negligence	Criminal negligence
Injury or damage is mild	More serious than civil negligence as injury is very serious
The patient goes to civil court or consumer court to ask for the compensation as the injury or damage suffered by him can be compensated by money	The patient/family reports the matter to the police Gross negligence on part of healthcare provider leads to serious injury/death of the patient
Punishment—in form of fine, no imprisonment for healthcare provider	Sec. 304 A IPC deals with criminal negligence- punishment up to 2 years of imprisonment and fine

Examples
i. Documentation errors or omissions
ii. Errors in patient's medication
iii. Neglecting to monitor patients or follow orders that have been given
iv. Giving injection intravenously when indication was intramuscular.
v. Mismanagement of delivery under the influence of alcohol/drugs.

Civil and Criminal Negligence

When a patient goes to the civil court or consumer court and reports the matter to police. In this case, negligence can be fought in both civil and criminal courts simultaneously.

Defences against Negligence

1. **No duty owed to patient:** The nurse did not treat the patient, so no duty exists.
2. **Res judicata:** The things have already been decided by the court, it cannot be tried again by the same court.
3. **Contributory negligence:** Not only healthcare provider, even patient is also found to be negligent. So, provider can take this as a defense.
4. **Therapeutic misadventure**
   – Occurrence of damage or mishap with the patient was due to some drug or procedure.
   – For example, hypersensitivity to penicillin, fatal complications with blood transfusion.
5. **Limitation period:** The case against the healthcare provider should be filed within 2 years from the date of alleged negligence.
6. **Error of judgement:** It has been recognized by the courts and law. Human fallibility is accepted in all spheres of life. Since a healthcare provider's decision turned out to be wrong, she/he cannot be liable for professional negligence.
7. **Products liability:** When a manufacturer supplies defective drug/instrument and the patient sustained injury because of that, the manufacturer is held responsible for the injury.
8. **Informed consent for the act:** The patient was duly informed of the consequences.

Punishment for Professional Negligence

i. Fine
ii. Imprisonment
iii. Warning
iv. Penal erasure

Sec. 304-A IPC deals with criminal negligence where the nurse may be punished with imprisonment for up to 2 years and fine.

Penal erasure: It is the removal of the name of a nurse from the State Nursing Register as a penalty which can be temporary or permanent.

- In a lawsuit for malpractice/negligence (civil), 'patient' is known as *plaintiff* and 'nurse' becomes *defendant*.
- To successfully sue a nurse for malpractice, the plaintiff must prove damage has been caused by the nurse's conduct.

Professional Negligence and Professional Misconduct

Features	Professional negligence	Professional misconduct
Definition	Lack of reasonable care and skills that resulted in damage/death of the patient	Conduct which is considered disgraceful and dishonorable by professional colleagues of good repute
Offense	Absence of care and skill	Violation of code of ethics
Duty of care	Should be present	Need not be present
Damage to person	Should be present	Need not be present
Trial by	Courts—civil/criminal	Nursing council
Punishment	Fine, imprisonment or both	Warning or erasure of name

Doctrine of Res Ipsa Loquitur

- Doctrine of Res ipsa loquitur means "thing/facts speaks for itself".
- Normally, in case of professional negligence, burden of proof lies with the patient, i.e., the patient has to prove the nurse's negligence
- But in some cases where rule of "Res ipsa loquitur" applies, the negligence is so gross and obvious that patient does not need to prove any negligence.
- For application of this rule three conditions must be fulfilled:
  – In the absence of negligence, the injury would not have occurred.
  – The nurse had a full control over the treatment/instrument resulting in injury the patient.
  – Patient is not guilty of contributory negligence.

Examples
i. Leaving surgical instruments or swabs in abdomen after surgery.
ii. Blood transfusions mismatch hazard.
iii. Injecting wrong drug or wrong dose.
iv. Leaving hot water bottle carelessly causing burns in elderly or child.

Vicarious Liability

- **Definition:** Employer is responsible not only for his own negligent act, but also for the negligent act of his employees by the principle of '*respondeat superior*'.
- Also called the *Master-Servant Rule* or *Captain of the Ship Doctrine*

Three conditions need to be satisfied:
1. Employer-employee relationship
2. Employee's conduct must occur within the scope of his employment.
3. Incident must occur while on the job

- In medical practice, the principal doctor becomes responsible for any negligence of his assistants. Both may be sued by the patient, even though the principal has no part in the negligent act.
- Surgeon is not liable for negligence of anesthetist, and anesthetist is not liable for negligence of operating surgeon.
- **'Borrowed servant doctrine':** Employee may serve more than one employer, e.g., the nurse employed by a hospital will be 'borrowed servant' of surgeon during operation, and servant of the hospital for all other purposes.
- Physicians and surgeons are not responsible for negligent acts of competent nurse or other hospital personnel, unless such acts are carried out under their direct supervision and control.

CONSENT

Definition: It means voluntary agreement, compliance or permission for some act.

Types of Consent

1. **Implied consent** implicitly granted by a person's actions, and the facts and

circumstances of a particular situation (or in some cases, by a person's silence or inaction).
- When a patient comes to the clinic for his medical examination and treatment, or extending the arm to receive an injection.
- It neither expressed in words nor in written form.
- Medical treatment given to an unconscious patient is implied, despite the unconscious person being unable to expressly grant consent for that treatment.

2. **Expressed consent:** It is the consent which is specifically expressed by the patient.

Oral consent	Written consent
Obtained for minor procedures	Obtained for: 1. All major diagnostic/therapeutic procedures 2. General anaesthesia

Consenting Ages

Purpose	Age
Medical examination and treatment	≥12 years
Invasive/diagnostic procedures, general anesthesia and surgical operations	≥18 years
Child <12 years of age, or unsound mind	Parent/guardian
Medico-legal examination	≥12 years (parent/guardian if <12 years)

As per the Indian Contract Act, a person is competent to contract if: (i) attained majority (≥18 years), (ii) sound mind, (iii) not disqualified by any law.

Reasons for Consent
To examine, treat or operate a patient without consent is considered: - Assault in law - Healthcare provider may be charged for negligence - Deficiency in medical services [Sec. 2(1) CPA].

Informed consent: Also called as *Doctrine of Informed Consent*

The doctor/nurse should explain:
a. The condition or nature of illness
b. The need for diagnostic tests to be done
c. All the treatment options
d. The alternative procedures
e. Risk benefit ratio of the procedures
f. Associated complications or consequences
g. Prognosis of the treatment
h. Duration and treatment cost

It should be discussed in simple patient's language so that the patient can decide if he/she wants to undergo the treatment or not.

Exceptions to informed consent (when consent is not required):

1. In case of **Emergency:** As per Section **92 IPC**, if a patient is unconscious and no guardian is available to give consent, then healthcare provider can perform emergency procedure/surgery without the consent, if it is essential to save the life of the patient
2. **Prisoners:** Convicted person has no right as any other citizen
3. Medical examination requested by the police officer of an arrested accused—under Sec. **53 (1) CrPC**
4. Treatment of notifiable diseases for community interest
5. Medico-legal postmortem—as per section **174 CrPC**

Rules for Consent

- Should be free, voluntary, clear, informed and there should not be any undue influence, fraud, misinterpretation of facts.
- All the procedures beyond routine physical examination require expressed consent.
- When written consent is obtained, it should also be signed by some other witness.
- In the case of children less than 12 years of age and in case of insane person, the consent comes from the parent or guardian.
- As per Section **90 IPC**—consent given by an insane or intoxicated person, is not valid.
- Any person of more than 18 years of age can give valid consent.
- Consent given for a diagnostic procedure cannot be considered as consent for therapeutic treatment or for some other procedure.

- No consent is required in case of medico-legal autopsies.
- Consent of both partners (husband and wife) is required for contraceptive sterilization and artificial insemination.
- Pregnant female (≥18 years) alone can give consent for termination of pregnancy.
- Husband or wife has no right to deny the treatment for his or her spouse.
- For examination of victim of a criminal case (e.g., rape), consent is mandatory.

ACTS RELATED TO NURSING PRACTICE

The Consumer Protection Act, 2019

- The Consumer Protection Act (CPA) was brought into existence for the protection of interests of the consumer and for settlement of consumer disputes within a limited time frame and with fewer expenses. This enables a patient to make a complaint to a redressal forum in respect of a defective (negligent) service, if the service has been paid for.
- The Consumer Protection Act, 2019 has replaced the previous Consumer Protection Act, 1986.
- In the Act of 1986, medical service was not included within the ambit of services. However, in 1995, healthcare was included as 'service' in Sec. 2(1) (o) of CPA by the Supreme Court (IMA vs. VP Shanta & Ors). In the new Act too, 'healthcare' has not been included in the list of services enlisted under its definition [Sec. 2(42) of the 2019 Act].
- The legislators have taken 'healthcare' out of inclusion list, but has not included in the exclusion list. The CPA 2019 defines services as '*but not limited to*' before listing the categories of services, which means that healthcare can be included under this definition.
- **E-filing of complaints:** The consumer can file complaints with the jurisdictional consumer forum located at the place of residence/work of the consumer. It also enables the consumer to file complaints electronically and for hearing and/or examining parties through video-conferencing.
- **Mediation:** There is a provision for settlement of disputes by way of mediation at the stage of complaint or at any later stage, if acceptable to both parties. In the event of failure to settle the dispute, the respective commissions shall continue to adjudicate the dispute.

Redressal Agencies

It is established at three different levels:

Redressal agencies	Headed by	Jurisdiction
1. District Commission (in each district)	District Judge	≤ ₹ 50 lakhs
2. State Commission (capital of each state)	High Court Judge	> ₹ 50 lakhs to ≤ 2 crore
3. National Commission (New Delhi)	SC Judge	> ₹ 2 crore

Limitation period: A patient can file complaint within 2 years from date which cause of action has arisen (deficiency of service has arisen/detected).

Penalties

- **Penalty for noncompliance of direction of Central Authority:** Punished with imprisonment up to 6 months with/without fine up to ₹ 20 lakh.
- **Punishment for false or misleading advertisement:** Punished with imprisonment up to 2 years with fine up to ₹ 10 lakh; and for every subsequent offense, punishment is up to 5 years with fine up to ₹ 50 lakh.

> **CPA and healthcare services**
> In the landmark decision of SC (IMA vs VP Santha, 13.11.1995), medical services were included in the Sec. 2(1) (o) of CPA.
> - Services rendered free of cost/charge for all patients are not covered under CPA.
> - Medical services delivered on payment basis fall within 'service'.
> - Hospital/nursing homes, which provide free service to some patients who cannot pay, and charges are paid by persons who are in a position to pay, are covered under this Act.
> - In case of insurance policy of patient, the service rendered by a doctor would not be free of charge.

The Medical Termination of Pregnancy Act, 1971

Indications for termination of pregnancy
1. **Therapeutic:** Risk of injury to physical or mental health of mother.
2. **Eugenic:** Risk of child being born with physical or mental abnormalities.
3. **Humanitarian:** Nonconsensual/forced sexual intercourse resulting in pregnancy (e.g., rape).
4. **Socioeconomic:** Failure of contraceptive technique.

MTP Act Rules

Emergency cases: Pregnancy can be terminated by any registered medical practitioner (RMP), even without required experience at any place, irrespective of duration of pregnancy, if it is necessary to save the life of pregnant woman.

Length of pregnancy: Under MTP Act, pregnancy cannot be terminated after 20 weeks of pregnancy. However, there are some exceptions [as per the recent MTP (Amendment) Act 2021] **(Table 9.1)**.

- The upper gestation limit of termination is up to 24 weeks for special categories of women. These include vulnerable women, such as survivors of rape, victims of incest and other vulnerable women (like differently-abled women, minors) etc.

Table 9.1: Gestation limit and doctors requirement for termination of pregnancy

Time since conception	MTP (amendment) 2021
Up to 20 weeks	One doctor¥
20–24 weeks	Two doctors for special categories of pregnant women
More than 24 weeks	Medical board, in case of substantial fetal abnormality
Any time during the pregnancy	One doctor, if necessary to save the pregnant woman's life

¥ Doctor refers to RMP with experience/training in Obs and Gyne.

- Termination can be done beyond 24 weeks in cases of substantial fetal abnormalities diagnosed by a Medical Board*.
- Opinion of only one doctor will be required up to 20 weeks of gestation and two doctors for termination of pregnancy of 20–24 weeks.
- **Consent:** Consent of woman is mandatory, except when she is minor (<18 years) or mentally ill, where consent of the guardian is obtained. Consent of husband is not necessary.
- **Maintenance of register** for 5 years and professional secrecy is maintained.
- MTPs can only be conducted at any hospital established or maintained by government, or approved by the government.

Qualification and Experience of RMP Using Medical and Surgical Methods

For RMP Conducting MTP up to 12 Weeks

The doctor should have the experience of assisting an RMP in conducting 25 cases of MTP, out of which at least five cases should have been performed independently, in an approved hospital by the Government.

For RMP Conducting MTP beyond 12 Weeks Period

The doctor should have either:
- Post-graduate degree/diploma in Obs and Gynae
- Six months of house surgery in Obs and Gynae, or
- One year or more in the practice of Obs and Gynae at any hospital.

Offenses and Penalties

- **MTP done other than RMP/or in any unauthorized place:** Rigorous imprisonment for 2–7 years. Cognizable offense.
- **Contravening of rules by government servant:** Disciplinary action including dismissal from service.

---

* Medical board will comprise of (i) A gynecologist (ii) A pediatrician (iii) A radiologist (iv) Other members as may be specified by the State Government.

- **Person willfully contravenes any regulation:** Fine of ₹ 1,000.
- **Confidentiality:** The doctor may only reveal the details of a woman whose pregnancy has been terminated to a person authorized by the law. Violation is punishable with imprisonment up to 1 year with/without fine.

The Preconception and Prenatal Diagnostic Techniques (PCPNDT) Act, 1994

- PCPNDT Act was enacted in order to check **female feticide**.
- There is **prohibition of sex selection**, before or after conception.
- '*Prenatal diagnostic techniques*' includes all prenatal diagnostic procedures and prenatal diagnostic tests (ultrasonography, fetoscopy or analysis of amniotic fluid, chorionic villi, blood).
- A recent amendment allows medical practitioners (MBBS doctors) to conduct ultrasonography on pregnant women, provided they undergo 6 months training.

Regulation of prenatal diagnostic techniques
Prenatal diagnostic techniques should be used for the detection the following abnormalities:
1. Chromosomal abnormalities
2. Genetic metabolic diseases
3. Hemoglobinopathies
4. Sex linked genetic diseases
5. Congenital anomalies.

Contd....

Contd....

Prenatal diagnostic techniques should be used in pregnant women, if any of the following conditions are satisfied:
a. Age ≥35 years.
b. Undergone ≥2 spontaneous abortions or fetal loss.
c. Has been exposed to teratogenic agents (drugs/radiations/infections/chemicals).
d. Family history of mental retardation or physical deformities (spasticity or any other genetic disease).

- *Written informed consent* of pregnant woman is taken. A copy of consent is given to her.
- Healthcare provider **should not communicate** the sex of fetus.
- Records are preserved for a period of 2 years.
- Any person or genetic counseling center/laboratory/clinic should not issue any advertisement in any manner regarding facilities of prenatal determination of sex.

Penalties
- **Doctor contravening the provisions of Act:** Imprisonment up to 3 years and fine up to ₹ 10,000,
    - Subsequent conviction: Imprisonment up to 5 years and fine up to ₹ 50,000.
    - Penal erasure for 5 years for first offense and permanently for subsequent offense.
- **Any person who contravenes provisions of Act:** Imprisonment up to 3 years and fine up to ₹ 50,000, and on subsequent conviction with imprisonment up to 5 years and fine up to ₹ 1 lakh.
- Every offense is cognizable, nonbailable and noncompoundable.

CHAPTER 10

Injuries

Definition of Injury

As per section **44 IPC**, injury is defined as any harm, whatever illegally, caused to any person in **M**ind, **R**eputation, **B**ody or **P**roperty.

Classification of Injury

Medical (Based on Causative Factors)

1. **Mechanical injuries**

Caused by blunt force	Caused by sharp force
a. Abrasion	a. Incised wound
b. Bruise	b. Chop wound
c. Laceration	c. Stab wound
d. Fracture/dislocation	

2. **Thermal injuries**

Caused by heat	Caused by cold
a. Burns	a. Frostbite
b. Scalds	b. Trench foot
c. Heat cramps and heat stroke (systemic effects)	c. Hypothermia (systemic effect)

3. **Other injuries**
   a. Electric injuries
   b. Blast injuries
   c. Radiation injuries

Legal (Based on Nature of Injuries)
a. Simple
b. Grievous

Medico-legal (Based on Manner of Injuries)
a. Suicidal
b. Homicidal
c. Accidental
d. Fabricated injuries

> *Blunt force trauma* causes abrasion, contusion, laceration and fracture/dislocation of bone of tooth. *Sharp force trauma* causes incised, chop and stab wounds.

ABRASION

Definition: Abrasion is caused by the removal of superficial epithelial layer of the skin, usually the epidermis by friction against a rough surface.

Types of Abrasions

1. **Scratch/linear abrasion**
   - Caused by a pointed object passing across the skin, such as fingernails, thorn or pin **(Fig. 10.1A)**
   - Fingernail abrasions are seen in throttling
2. **Graze abrasion**
   - Caused by horizontal or tangential friction between the skin and the hard rough surface
   - Seen in road traffic accidents **(Fig. 10.1B)**
3. **Pressure abrasion**
   - Caused by linear pressure of a rough object over the skin
   - Ligature mark in hanging and strangulation
4. **Imprint abrasion**
   - Caused by force applied perpendicular to the skin and bears the imprint of the object causing it
   - Tire-tread mark, imprint of bicycle chain

Most common type of abrasions is graze abrasions.

Healing of Abrasion

Produces minimum bleeding, heals rapidly (takes 1 week), with *no permanent scarring on healing*.

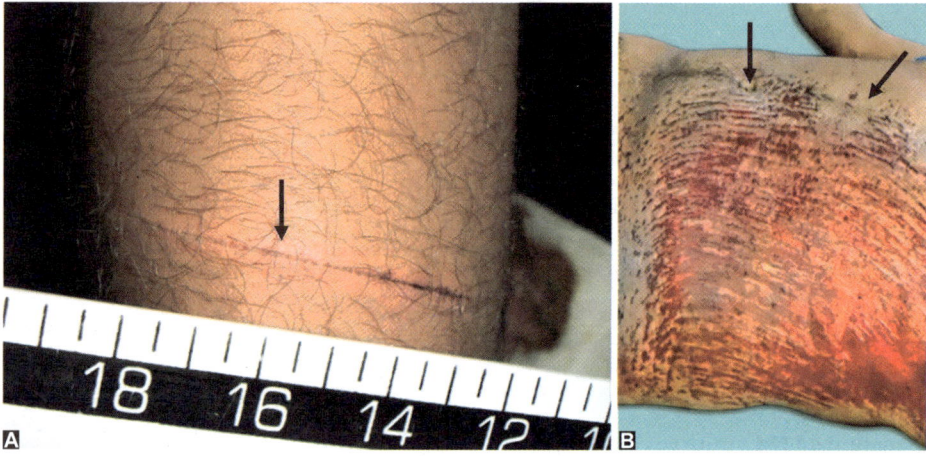

Figs. 10.1A and B: Abrasions: (A) Scratch (arrow); (B) Graze (arrows).

Duration	Healing changes
Fresh	Bright red, oozing of serum and blood
2–24 hours	Exudation dries to form a reddish scab
2–3 days	Reddish-brown scab
4–5 days	Dark brown scab
5–7 days	Brownish black scab, starts falling off, epithelium grows and covers defect

Medico-legal Importance

- Usually, abrasions are seen in accidents and assaults.
- Abrasions on the face or body of the victim/assailant indicates struggle.
- Abrasions give an idea about the site of impact and direction of force.
- **Nature of injury:** Abrasions are superficial injuries and simple in nature. Abrasions over the cornea may cause corneal opacity, which may cause grievous hurt **(Sec. 320 IPC)**.
- Patterned abrasions are helpful in connecting the wound with the causative weapon.
- Age of injury can be determined from healing changes.
- Character and manner of injury may be known from its distribution. For example, in throttling, crescentic abrasions made by fingernails are found on the neck.

BRUISE/CONTUSION

Definition: Extravasation of blood in the subcutaneous/subepithelial tissues due to rupture of blood vessels as a result of blunt force.

Ectopic Bruise/Migratory Bruises

When extravasated blood at point of impact by a blunt weapon tracks down due to gravity along the fascial planes and may appear where the tissue layers become superficial.

Examples

Anterior cranial fossa fracture	Black eye/ Raccoon eye **(Fig. 10.2A)**	Collection of blood in periorbital region
Middle cranial fossa fracture	Battle sign	Collection of blood in mastoid region

Patterned Bruise

The bruise which reflects the pattern of the object causing it.

Examples

i. Railway track bruise—caused by stick **(Fig. 10.2B)**
ii. Six penny bruise—seen in throttling
iii. Steering wheel impact injury in car accidents

Delayed Bruise

- **Definition:** Bruise which takes some time to appear at the point of impact; also called as **deep bruise**.
- In this, bleeding occurs deeper to subcutaneous tissues. Since it is deeper, it

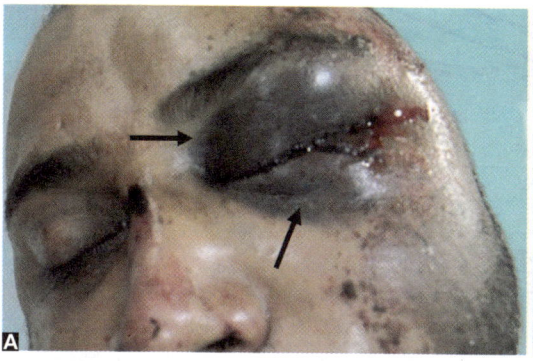
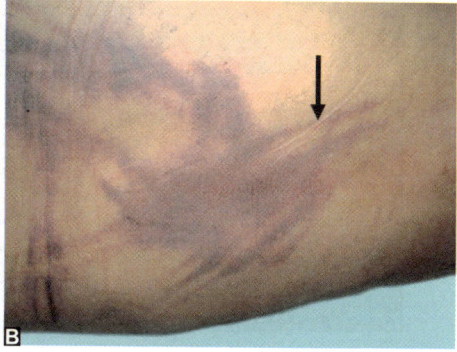

Figs. 10.2A and B: Bruise: (A) Black eye (arrows); (B) Patterned bruise (railway line/tram-line type) on the back caused by blows with a rod/stick (arrow).

may take hours to 2 days to appear at the surface.
- Therefore, it is very important to reexamine the person 1–2 days after first examination.

Estimation of Age of Contusion (Bruise)

On the basis of color changes (mnemonic- **VIBGYOR**)

Duration	Color	Reason (Due to)
Fresh	Red	Oxyhemoglobin
Few hours to 3 days	Violet/Blue	Deoxyhemoglobin
4–5 days	Brown	Hemosiderin
5–6 days	Green	Biliverdin
7–12 days	Yellow	Bilirubin
≥2 weeks	Original/Normal	Normal

Medico-legal Importance

- Age of bruise helps in determining time of infliction of injury.
- Artificial bruise can be produced by applying juices of marking nut or calotropis on the skin in order to charge somebody of assault.
- Contusions/bruises near genital areas may be due to sexual assault.
- Multiple bruises in various stages of healing in case of child suggest child abuse/battered baby syndrome.
- Character and manner of injury may be known from its distribution. For example, six-penny bruises on the neck are produced by forcible pressure of fingertips as in case of throttling.

LACERATED WOUND/LACERATION

Definition: Tearing of skin, mucous membrane, muscle or internal organs caused by blunt force impact producing shearing or crushing force.

Weapons used: Blunt weapons (cricket bat, hammer, iron rod, hockey stick, etc.)

Characteristics (Fig. 10.3)

1. **Margins**—irregular
2. **Bruise and abrasion**—present around the margin
3. **Hair bulbs**—crushed
4. **Blood vessels**—crushed
5. **Hemorrhage**—less (due to crushing of blood vessels)
6. **Tissue bridges**—present, and is the hallmark of lacerated injury

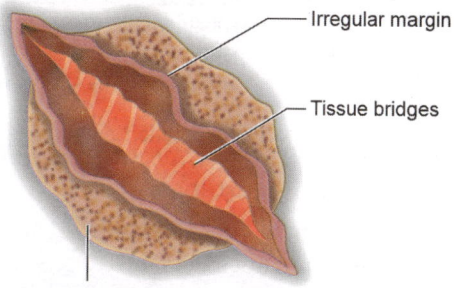

Fig. 10.3: Characteristics of laceration.

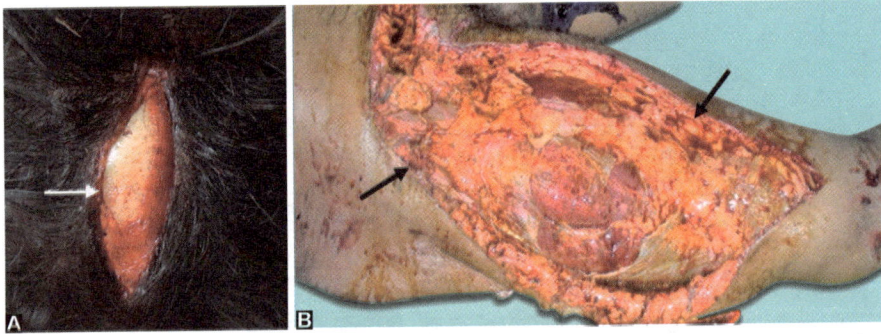

Figs. 10.4A and B: Laceration: (A) Spilt laceration on scalp (arrow); (B) Avulsion of skin, subcutaneous tissues and fascia of thigh in road traffic accident (arrows).

Types of Lacerated Wounds

1. **S**plit laceration (Fig. 10.4A)	• When blunt force is applied at the **bony prominence**, skin gets sandwiched between bone and object causing split laceration • Usually seen at—scalp, forehead, zygomatic process, shin • As margins look regular, these lacerated wounds are called as **incised looking lacerated wounds** (looks like incised wounds)
2. **S**tretch laceration	• Occurs due to overstretching of skin and subcutaneous tissue • Caused by heavy forceful impact • Seen in—run over injuries, compound fractures

3. **A**vulsion laceration (Fig. 10.4B)	• Produced by a tangential force/shearing force
	• Seen in case of run over by vehicles
	• **Leads to**
	  – *Flaying:* Due to rotational force of wheel leading to detachment of skin and subcutaneous tissue over a large area
	  – *Degloving injury:* Entire skin comes out
	  – Amputation injury

Medico-legal Importance

- Laceration is usually homicidal or accidental but not suicidal.
- Laceration over face can result in extensive scar formation on healing resulting in disfiguration of face—grievous injury
- Avulsion laceration/flaying helps in determining the direction of force.

INCISED WOUND

Definition: Clean cut wound through the tissue which *longer than its depth*.

Weapons used: Knife, box cutter, glass, razor or scalpel.

Characteristics (Fig. 10.5A)

1. **Margins:** Edges are clean cut, well-defined, free from contusions and abrasions, and usually everted.
2. **Length:** Greater than its width and depth.
3. **Width/breadth:** Greater than edge of weapon.
4. **Shape:** Spindle-shaped.
5. **Depth and direction:** Usually deeper at commencement *(head end), except in suicidal cut throat*. Towards termination, cut becomes shallow *(tailing)*. Depth and tailing will suggest the direction of force.
6. **Hemorrhage:** More since vessels are cut clean.
7. **Beveled cuts** are seen if the blade of the weapon enters obliquely.

Medico-legal Importance

- Helps in determining the **type of weapon.**
- **Nature of injury** can be determined—as incised wounds usually are not fatal as they do not penetrate deep enough to damage large blood vessels. However, they are highly fatal if present over the neck as veins of neck are present superficially.

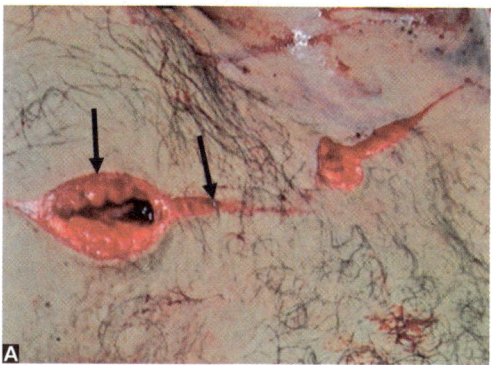 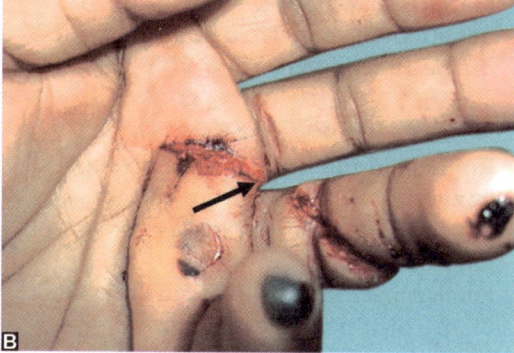

Figs. 10.5A and B: (A) Incised wound over chest (arrows); (B) Defense wounds on palm (arrow).

- Helps in determining **direction of force** (tailing present at end of incised wound).
- Helps in determining **age of injury** from healing changes.
- Relative position of assailant and victim can be determined.
- **Manner of injury** can be determined:
  - *Suicide:* Fatal wounds are present over accessible areas, such as front of neck, groin, chest, back of legs. Multiple incised wounds of varying depths and usually do not injure the face. *Hesitation cuts are seen.*
  - *Homicidal wounds:* Deep and deliberate and are seen on head, front of neck and trunk. *Incised wounds on nose, ears and genitals are usually homicidal,* and may result from sexual jealousy.
  - *Accidental wounds:* Commonly seen around hands.
  - *Defense wounds:* Injuries are seen on the forearm and palm, when the victim may try to ward off an attack by raising hands and arms in defense or by grabbing the weapon **(Fig. 10.5B).**

STAB WOUND

Definition: Clean cut wound through the tissue which is *deeper than its length and width.*

Weapons used
- **Sharp:** Knife, dagger, scissors, pens, needle
- **Blunt:** Screw driver, iron rod, cricket stump

Types of stab wound: Two types—penetrating (only entry wound is present) and perforating (both entry and exit wounds are present).

Various shapes of stab wounds

Weapon	Shape	
Single edged	Wedge/triangular	▷
Double edged	Spindle shaped	⬳
Arrow	Circular	○
Fork	Circular wounds (3–4 in no.)	●●●
Square pointed	Cruciate	✦

Characteristics (Fig. 10.6)

1. **Depth**—is the greatest dimension.
2. **Breadth**—is more than the thickness of blade due to gaping.
3. **Length**—is usually less than the width of stab wound because of stretching of skin.

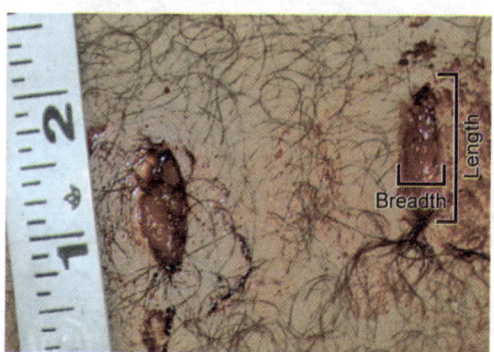

Fig. 10.6: Stab wound.

4. **Margins**—are clean cut. But in case of full penetration—patterned abrasion/bruise can be seen (hilt mark).

Medico-legal Importance
- Concealed punctured wounds suggest homicide.
- Depth of the wound suggests amount of force used.
- Foreign material can be seen in the wound.
- Shape of the weapon suggests type of weapon.
- Manner of production can be determined.

CHOP WOUND

Definition: Deep gaping wound caused by *moderately sharp cutting edge of a heavy weapon*, applied with significant degree of force.

Weapon used: Axe, chopper, hatchet, butcher's knife

Characteristics (Fig. 10.7)
1. A chop wound is a combination of blunt and sharp force injury.
2. **Margins:** Sharp and may show abrasion, bruise or laceration with severe injury to underlying tissues.
3. Presence of incised wound with underlying bone fracture.

Medico-legal Importance
- Mostly homicidal in nature.
- Sometimes, accidental or suicidal.

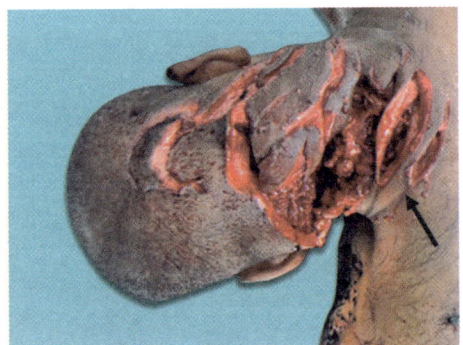

Fig. 10.7: Chop wounds (arrow).
(*Courtesy*: Dr Murugesa Bharathi, IGMC, Puducherry)

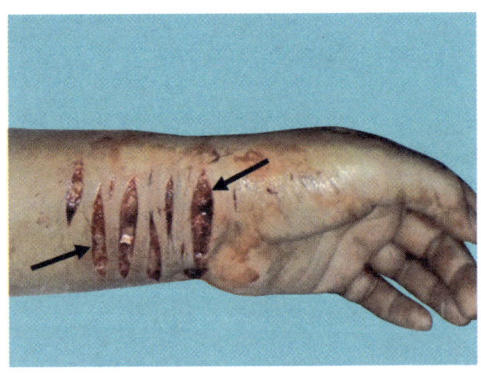

Fig. 10.8: Hesitation cuts over wrists (arrows).

- Proper wound examination can give clue about the causative weapon.

HESITATION CUTS

Definition: Multiple, small, superficial incised wounds; seen in *suicidal wounds* **(Fig. 10.8)**.
- These are seen at the beginning of the incised wound.
- They are also called as tentative cuts, trial marks.
- It shows hesitation while gaining courage to make a final decisive cut.
- Seen on accessible parts of body.

Usual Sites of Hesitation Cuts
• Front of wrist
• Front of elbow
• Front and sides of neck
• Back of legs

Medico-legal Importance
- It suggests suicidal attempt/tendency.
- These are caused by light sharp edged weapons (knife/razor).
- It indicates direction of cut (deeper at the beginning and superficial at end).

PATTERNED INJURIES

Definition: Patterned injuries are one which has a distinct pattern that may reproduce the characteristics of the object causing the injury.
- Most common are patterned abrasion and patterned bruise.

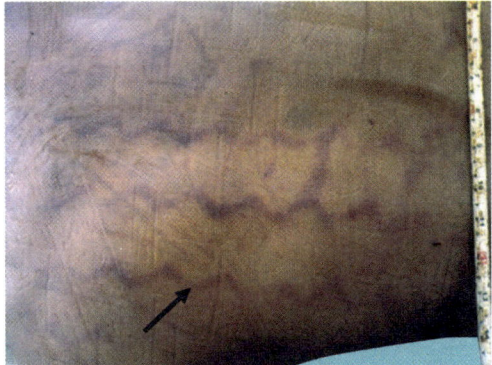

Fig. 10.9: Patterned injury (Tire tread bruise) (arrow).

- For example, "Railway track bruise"—by stick, "six penny bruise"—in throttling, tire mark pattern in RTAs **(Fig. 10.9)**, etc.

Medico-legal Importance

Connect a particular weapon or object to an injury, which may connect an assailant with the crime.

SELF-INFLICTED INJURY/FABRICATED INJURIES

Definition: These are defined as the wounds produced by a person deliberately on his own body or by another person with his/her consent.

Types

i. Self-inflicted injuries	Produced by person on his body
ii. Self-suffered injuries	Produced by another person with his/her consent

Diagnosis

Based on the:
i. Clinical history
ii. Features

History

- History of assault incompatible with injuries.
- No defence injury despite history of assault.

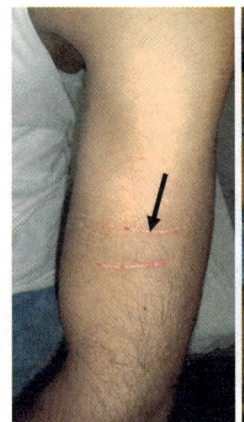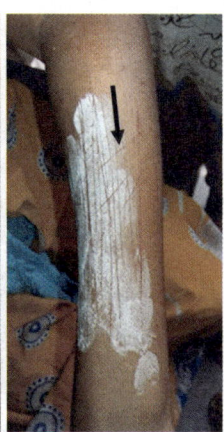

Fig. 10.10: Self-inflicted injuries (superficial incised wounds on left arm and forearm) (arrows).
(*Courtesy:* Dr Parmod Goyal, AIMSR, Bathinda)

Features (Fig. 10.10)

Type of injury	• Incised wounds (mostly)—multiple, superficial, parallel • Abrasions • Burns
Sites	• Front of forearm • Outer side of upper arm • Front of chest and abdomen • Outer sides of thigh
Clothes	• Are not cut (usually) • If cut—not compatible with nature of injuries
Injuries produced by	Knife, razor, glass piece, scissors, ice pick

Medico-legal Importance

These are produced with an intention:
- To make false charge against another person with assault or attempt of murder
- To make simple injuries grievous
- By women, to bring a charge of rape
- By prisoners, to bring charge of beating by officers
- To avoid hard duties by employees
- By an assailant to pretend self defense.

FIREARMS INJURY

Entry Wound in Firearm Injury

Entry wound is one that results when a projectile enters a body.

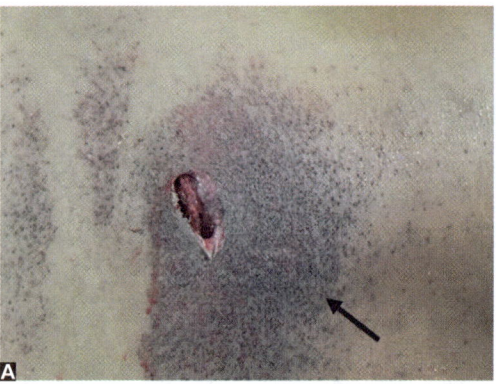 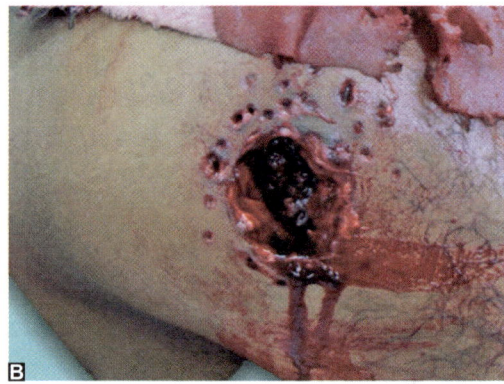

Figs. 10.11A and B: Entry wound: (A) Bullet (tattooing can be seen around the entry —close range) (arrow); (B) Shot gun (satellite pellet wounds can be seen around the main entry wound—"rat hole appearance" —mid range).

Characteristic features (Figs. 10.11A and B)

1. In skull, entry wound is clean cut on outer table and beveled in the inner table.
2. Smaller than the diameter of the bullet (except contact shot).
3. Edges are inverted.
4. Bruising, abrasion and grease collar, burning, blackening, tattooing can be seen **(Fig. 10.12)**.
5. Bleeding is less as compared to exit wounds.
6. Singeing of hair will be there (close range)
7. Wound track is cherry-red due to COHb and/or carboxymyoglobin.
8. Fibers of clothes are turned in.

Entry wound and exit wound in firearm injuries (Figs. 10.13A and B)

Features	Entry wound	Exit wound
1. Size	Smaller	Larger
2. Margins	Inverted	Everted
3. Clothes/fibers	--do--	--do--
4. Abrasion and grease collar[¥]	Present	Absent
5. Singeing, blackening and tattooing*	--do--	--do--
6. Bleeding	Less	More
7. Fat protrusion	Absent	Present
8. Wound track	Cherry red color (due to COHb)	No color change

[¥]**Abrasion collar:** Narrow rim of abrasion surrounding the bullet entry wound caused by friction and indentation.
[¥]**Grease collar:** Black colored ring lining the entry wound caused from removal of substances from bullet as it passes through skin.
***Tattooing:** Consists of unburnt gun powder particles that are embedded in skin.
***Blackening:** Deposition of powder soot produced by combustion of gunpowder.

- The characteristics of firearm injuries can be varied and dependent upon several factors, such as distance, clothing, etc.
- Forensic nurse may limit their interpretation of such injuries to include only what they observe. For example use of terms such as entry and exit wound can be easily misinterpreted and challenged.

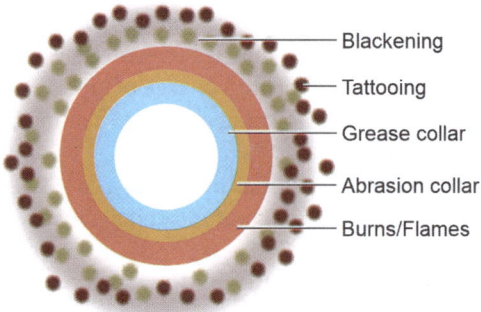

Fig. 10.12: Characteristics of close shot firearm entry wound.

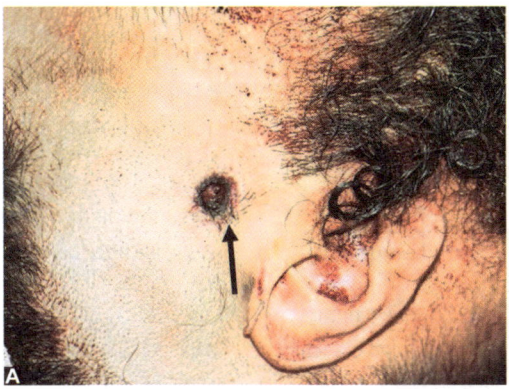 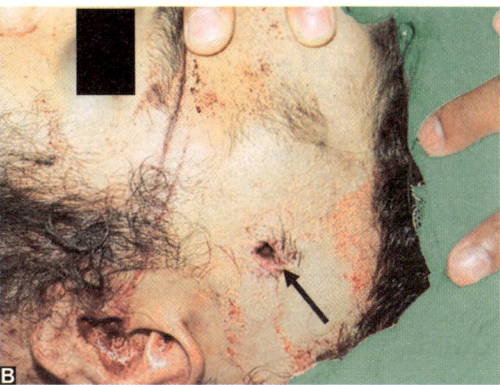

Figs. 10.13A and B: Suicidal firearm wounds (bullet): (A) Entry wound (arrow); (B) Exit wound (arrow).

- It is better to describe it as "lacerated wound" and then mention its size, shape, number, location, abrasion around it, soot soiling and tattooing which can be interpreted later by trained experts.

Features of Suicide by Firearm

- Common in males with history of previous psychiatric illness, financial loss.
- Most of the suicidal firearms have shot distance as contact or very close range shot wound with sites of entry as:
  - Temple—the most common site
  - Center of forehead
  - Mouth
  - Midline behind the chin
- The person uses his dominant hand to press the trigger, steadying the muzzle against the head with the non-dominant hand.
- Presence of powder soot may be seen on the non-dominant hand.
- Only one wound is present.
- Presence of powder residue on hand pressing trigger.
- Cadaveric spasm may be seen with the weapon firmly grasped in the hands.
- Presence of weapon at crime scene (mostly house).
- Presence of suicide note at crime scene.

THERMAL BURNS

Definition of burns: Burn is an injury caused by heat, or by a chemical or physical agent having an effect similar to heat.

Classification of Burns (Figs. 10.14A and B)

Table 10.1 depicts the classification of burns.

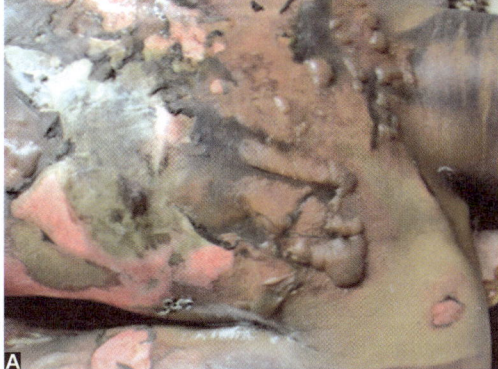
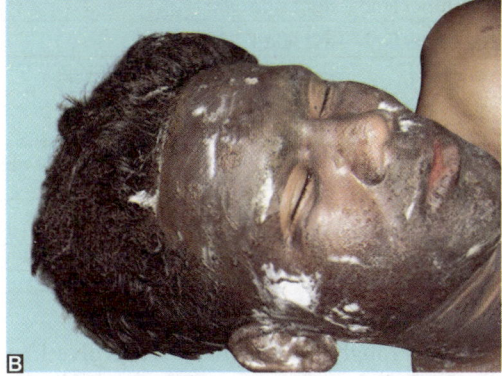

Figs. 10.14A and B: Burn injury: (A) 2nd degree burn, blisters can be seen; (B) Blackening and singeing of hair.

Table 10.1: Classification of burns.

	1st degree	2nd degree superficial	2nd degree deep	3rd and 4th degree
Depth	Involves only epidermis	Involves epidermis and papillary dermis	Involves epidermis and whole of dermis	Till subcutaneous layer (3rd degree) even muscles (4th degree)
Color	Red	Red	Red	Black and charred
Pain to stimuli	Tender	Tender	Less painful	Painless (since nerves are destroyed)
Blisters	Present (+/–)	Present	Less in number	Absent
Blanching	Present	Present	Varied blanching	Absent
Healing	Heals spontaneously in 3–5 days	Heals within 2 weeks	Heals within 3 weeks	Difficult to heal, contracture seen
Scar	Absent	Absent	Hypertrophic scar and keloid formation	Hypertrophic scar and keloid formation
Seen in	Sunburns	Scalds, flash burns	Scalds, flash burns	Prolonged contact with flame, hot surface, hot liquids

Rule of 9

It is a method used to estimate percentage of **total body surface area (TBSA)** that has burnt.
- It is also called **Wallace Rule of 9**.
- As per the rule, body is divided into 11 anatomical regions and each represents 9% of TBSA. Remaining 1% area is for perineum **(Table 10.2 and Fig. 10.15)**.

Table 10.2: Rule of 9.

Region	% TBSA
1. Head and neck	9
2. Upper limb—right side	9
3. Upper limb—left side	9
4. Chest	9 (Front) + 9 (Back)
5. Abdomen	9 (Front) + 9 (Back)
6. Lower limb—right side	9 (Front) + 9 (Back)
7. Lower limb—left side	9 (Front) + 9 (Back)
8. Perineum	1
Total	(9 × 11) = 99 + 1 = 100

Medico-legal Importance

1. Gives rough estimate of TBSA involved.
2. Helps to know prognosis in case of burns (as >33% TBSA burns has poor prognosis)

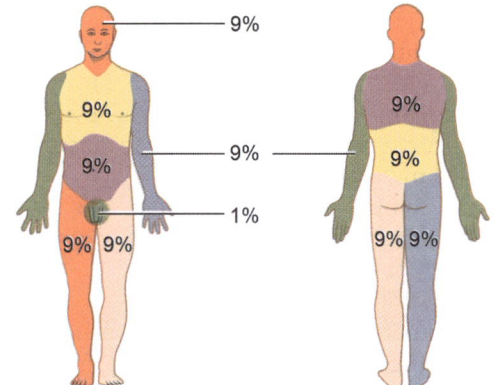

Fig. 10.15: Rule of 9.

3. Helps in calculating amount of fluid required for resuscitation by Parkland formula.

ELECTRICAL INJURY

Joule Burns

Definition: The point where electric current enters the body is usually characterized by presence of electric mark. This electric mark (entry point) is called as Joule burn.

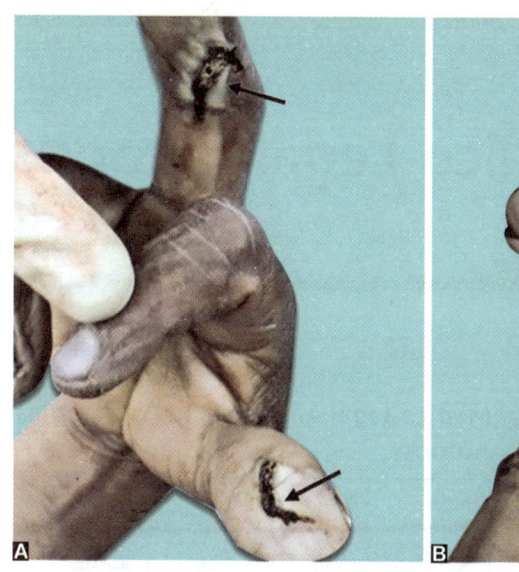 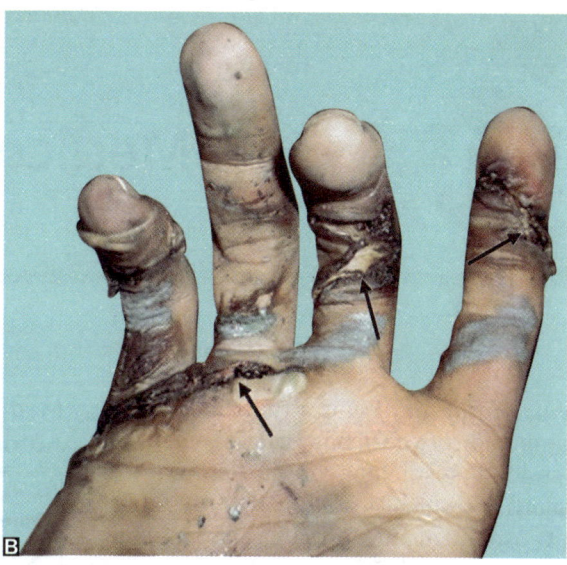

Figs. 10.16A and B: Joule burn (arrows).

Characteristics of Joule Burns (Figs. 10.16A and B)

- Chalky white in color, shallow, centrally collapsed blister, from few millimeters to 1–1.5 cm in diameter and have a raised border
- If contact is prolonged, skin mark become brown or charred.

Sites

Seen on exposed parts of body, especially on palmer aspect of hand.

Medico-legal Importance

The presence of Joule burns is not itself a proof of electrocution as similar marks can be produced even after death except for the zone of hyperemia.

CHAPTER 11

Medico-Legal Autopsy

Medico-legal autopsy is a type of scientific examination of a dead body carried out in case of sudden, suspicious, obscure, unnatural, litigious or criminal deaths in order to establish the cause and manner of death, and time since death.

A complete autopsy should be done (all the body cavities should be opened and every organ must be examined).

Objectives of Medico-legal Autopsy

1. To find out the cause of death (natural or unnatural).
2. To find out time since death, mode of death and place of death.
3. To find out manner of death (accidental, suicidal or homicidal).
4. To establish identity of deceased when not known/not identifiable.
5. To identify if the injuries are antemortem or postmortem in nature.
6. In case of newborns, to determine the question of live birth and viability of the baby.
7. To find out if any treatment was given to deceased before death.
8. To investigate into the case so that, it can help in identifying the criminal (e.g., foreign materials, fingerprints).

Medico-legal Autopsy and Pathological Autopsy

Features	Medico-legal autopsy	Pathological/ clinical autopsy
Done in	Unnatural deaths	Natural deaths
Purpose	Determine cause of death and time since death	To know pathophysiology of disease causing death
Done by	Forensic medicine experts	Pathologists
Consent	From State	From relatives
Body handed over to	Investigating officer	Relatives

Types of Skin Incisions (Figs. 11.1A to C)

Skin incisions are of following types:

1. **I-shaped incision:** *Most common method*. It extends from the chin down to the symphysis pubis and avoiding the umbilicus.
2. **Y-shaped incision:** The straight line of Y corresponding to the xiphisternum to pubis incision of I-shaped incision. The forks of Y run down medially to the chest and extending from the acromion process.
3. **Modified Y-shaped incision:** It is used to study the neck, such as in hanging or strangulation. An incision is made

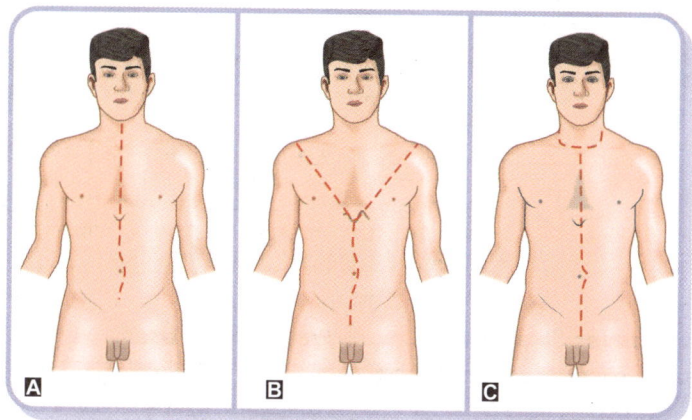

Figs. 11.1A to C: Types of skin incisions: (A) I-shaped; (B) Y-shaped; (C) Modified Y-shaped.

in midline from suprasternal notch to symphysis pubis. The incision extends from suprasternal notch over the clavicle to its center on both sides and then passes upwards over the neck behind the ears.

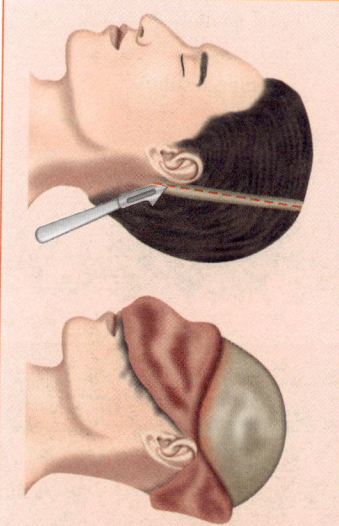

Scalp and Skull
- An ear-to-ear bone deep incision is made along the vertex of the scalp.
- The scalp is reflected forwards to the superciliary ridges, and backwards to a point just below the occipital protuberance.
- Look for hematoma, edema or any fracture.
- Saw skull by making a saw-line in slightly V-shaped direction (angle of 120°).
- Skull cap is removed and dura is exposed which is examined from outside for epidural hemorrhage, then dura is cut from periphery followed by falx cerebri, and examined for subdural and subarachnoid hemorrhages, and other pathology.

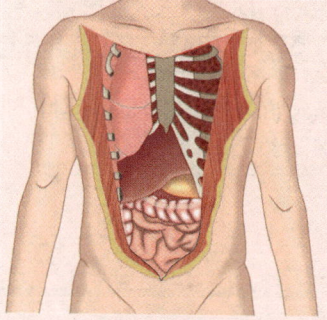

Chest
- The skin and muscles of the chest are dissected sidewise and carried back to the midaxillary line, down to the costal margin and up over the clavicles.
- Examine the ribs and sternum for fractures.
- Open the chest by cutting the costal cartilages from second rib onwards close to the costochondral junctions with help of cartilage knife.
- Sternoclavicular joints are finally disarticulated on both sides.
- Sternum is removed.
- Pleural cavity is examined for presence of any blood, pus, adhesions.

Contd....

Contd....

	Abdomen • An incision to rectus abdominis is made till 5 cm above pubis symphysis. • A small nick is made in the fascia to admit the left index and middle fingers with palmar surfaces up. • Peritoneum is cut up to the xiphoid and abdominal cavity is looked for presence of any blood, pus, fluid or perforation. • Finally, evisceration of the organs is done.

Viscera Preservation for Chemical Analysis in Case of Suspected Poisoning after PM Examination

Viscera Preservation (in Routine) (Figs. 11.2A to C)

Bottle 1	Stomach along its contents and upper part of small intestine (30 cm) along with its contents
Bottle 2	**Liver:** 300 g along with gallbladder **Kidneys:** Half of each kidney
Bottle 3 (vial)	**Blood:** 10 mL
Bottle 4	**Urine:** 100 mL
Bottle 5	Sample of the preservative

Preservatives Used

Saturated solution of NaCl	Most commonly used *Contraindicated* in corrosive poisoning (except carbolic acid)
Rectified spirit	Best preservative Used in corrosive poisoning *Contraindicated* in carbolic acid poisoning
Formalin	For histopathological examination
Sodium fluoride (NaF)	For detecting cocaine, CO, cyanide, alcohol

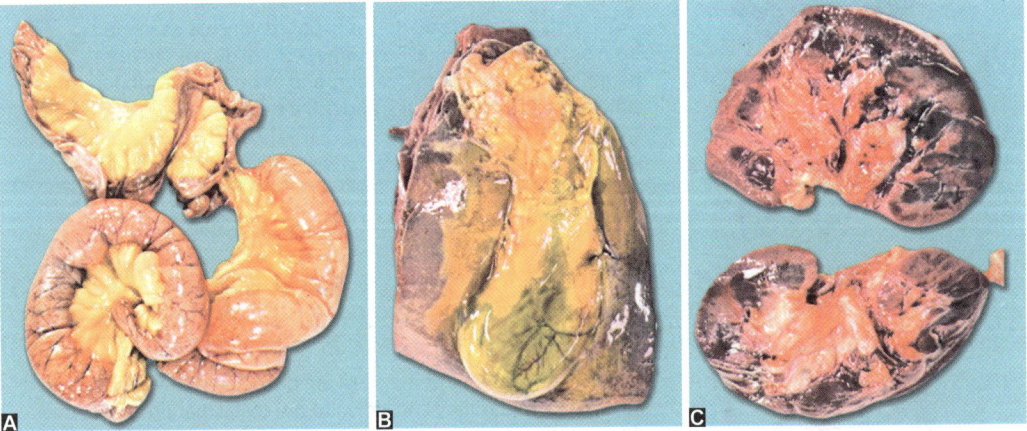

Figs. 11.2A to C: Viscera preservation: (A) Upper part of small intestines; (B) Part of liver along with gallbladder; and (C) Half of each kidney.

CHAPTER 12

Thanatology

Thanatology is the scientific study of death in all its aspects including its cause and phenomena.

Definition of Death
Permanent and irreversible cessation of functions of brainstem.

Types of Death (Diff. 12.1)
1. **Somatic death:** It is defined as complete and irreversible cessation of brainstem functions.
2. **Molecular death:** It is defined as progressive disintegration of body cells and tissues which occurs after somatic death.

Diff. 12.1: Somatic death and molecular death.

Features	Somatic death	Molecular death
Definition	Complete and irreversible cessation of brainstem functions	Progressive disintegration of body cells
Occurs	Before molecular death	After somatic death
Cells	Alive	Dead
Response to external stimulus	Present	Absent
Conditions simulating	Suspended animation	No condition resembles it
Confirmed by	Flat ECG and EEG, absent pulse and absent breath sounds	Rigor mortis, algor mortis, PM staining

Suspended Animation/Apparent Death
Definition
Condition in which vital signs of life (such as heart beat and respiration) cannot be detected by routine clinical methods, as the functions are reduced to a minimum.

Mechanism
BMR is greatly reduced so that the requirement of the oxygen decreases but dissolved oxygen in body fluids is enough to satisfy the demands of the body.

Types

1. Voluntary	Seen in yoga practitioners
2. Involuntary	**D**rowning, **E**lectrocution, **N**ewborn, **T**yphoid, **I**nsanity, **S**unstroke

Medico-legal Importance
- The patient can be resuscitated by cardiac massage and artificial respiration.
- Before certifying death, ECG or EEG should be done to rule out suspended animation.

Modern Concept of Moment of Death
- The **moment of death** is the exact time when the person dies. The concept of the moment of death has changed through the years. The traditional cardiopulmonary standard (cessation of heartbeat and breathing) was the measure used during most of the 20th century to determine the presence of life.
- As ventilator technology advanced, circulation and respiration could be maintained

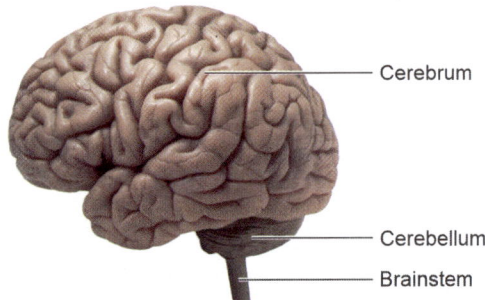

Fig. 12.1: Parts of brain.

by means of a mechanical respirator, despite loss of all brain functions, and thus have brought the concept of **brain death**, i.e., irreversible loss of cerebral functioning.

- **Harvard criteria of brain death:** Laid stress on determining the activity of only brain to determine death (**Fig. 12.1**).
- **Minnesota criteria of brainstem death:** Mohandas and Chou suggested that the most important part is brainstem and one must consider only brainstem death (**Fig. 12.1**).

Legal Concept of Death and Diagnosis of Brainstem Death

The legal concept of death is "Brainstem death".

- The traditional cardiopulmonary standard (cessation of heartbeat and breathing) is not considered currently, since circulation and respiration could be maintained by means of a mechanical respirator, despite loss of all brain functions.
- *Brain death* is the complete and irreversible cessation of functioning of the brain. Brain includes all the central nervous system (CNS) structures, except the spinal cord (**Fig. 12.1**).
- Brain death is now accepted as brainstem death. The respiratory center which controls respiration lies within the brainstem. If this area is dead, the person is unable to breathe spontaneously or regain consciousness.
- Since a normal functioning reticular formation within the brainstem is essential for the proper functioning of the cortex, brainstem death is considered to be sufficient for brain death.

The two essential requirements for the diagnosis of brain death are:
- **Establishment of cessation of all brain functions**, i.e., cerebral and mainly brainstem functions, determined clinically and confirmed by laboratory tests which include EEG (flat isoelectric EEG).
- **Demonstration that cessation of these functions is irreversible:**
  Irreversibility is established by:
  - Determination of the cause of loss of brain function.
  - Exclusion of reversible conditions, such as hypothermia, electrolyte imbalance, drug intoxication, shock, hypotension, etc.

Brainstem Death Certification

1. Two medical practitioners of which one should be neurologist or neurosurgeon must perform the brainstem death tests.
2. Patient's attending physician should participate in determination of death.
3. Such tests *should not be performed* by transplant surgeons or any doctor in the transplant team.

The three important findings seen in brain death are coma, absence of brainstem reflexes and apnea:

1. **Coma or unresponsiveness:** No cerebral motor response to pain in all extremities.
2. **Absence of brainstem reflexes:**
   - Absent pupillary response to bright light.
   - No oculocephalic reflex or absent oculovestibular reflex.
   - No corneal reflex to touch with a cotton swab or no grimacing to deep pressure on nail bed, supraorbital ridge.
   - No gag reflex or cough response to bronchial suction.
3. **Apnea test:** It is based on the fact that loss of brainstem function definitively results in loss of centrally controlled breathing, with resultant apnea.
   - It involves disconnection of ventilator from the patient and documenting absence of respiratory efforts.

CAUSE OF DEATH, MECHANISM OF DEATH, AND MANNER OF DEATH

1. **Cause of death** is any injury or disease producing physiological derangement, briefly or over a prolonged period, which results in the death of the individual, e.g., a gunshot wound to the abdomen, adenocarcinoma of the lung or coronary atherosclerosis.
2. **Mechanism of death** is the physiological derangement produced by the cause of death that results in death, e.g., hemorrhage, septicemia, metabolic acidosis, or respiratory paralysis. A particular mechanism of death can be produced by multiple causes of death and vice versa. Thus, if an individual dies of hemorrhage, it can be produced by a gunshot wound or a stab wound or a malignant tumor of the lung eroding into a blood vessel. A cause of death, e.g., a gunshot wound of the abdomen can result in many possible mechanisms of death, such as hemorrhage or peritonitis.
3. **Manner of death** explains how the cause of death came about. Manner of death can generally be categorized as natural (death due to disease), homicide, suicide, accident or undetermined **(Flowchart 12.1 and Table 12.1)**.

A cause of death may have multiple manners of death. An individual can die of massive hemorrhage (mechanism of death) due to stab wound of heart (cause of death), with the manner being homicide (someone stabbed him), suicide (stabbed himself), accident (fell over the weapon) or undetermined (not sure what happened).

Flowchart 4.1: Manner of death.

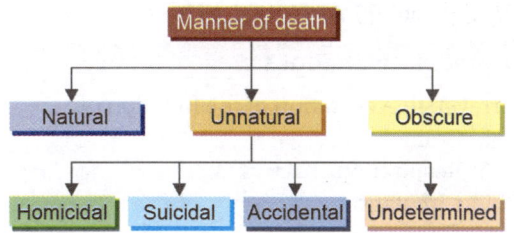

Table 12.1: Description of manners of death.

Manner	Definition
Natural	Death resulting from disease
Homicide	Death resulting from the deliberate action of another
Suicide	Death intentionally self-inflicted
Accident	Death as a result of an environmental influence

- For some deaths, the manner may be "undetermined" because the circumstances are unclear, e.g., whether drowning was accidental or suicidal.
- Deaths from alcohol and drug abuse are difficult to classify and are sometimes described as 'unclassified'.

Natural deaths: Death is due to aging process, disease or illness not directly influenced by external forces.
- If the doctor is unsure of cause and manner of death, he will not certify the death and will inform the police.
- The police can then ask for postmortem examination which can help in determining the cause of death.
- If it reveals that the death is from natural causes, then no further inquiry is needed.

Unnatural deaths: All deaths that cannot be described as death by natural causes are categorized as unnatural deaths.
- This includes road traffic accidents, falls, drowning, poisoning, hanging, gunshot injuries, stabbing, etc.
- The police will ask for a postmortem examination and depending on the circumstances of the death, further investigation will take place.

DEATH CERTIFICATE

International format of certifying the cause of death is defined by the WHO. The system divides the cause of death into two parts:
1. **Part I** describes the condition(s) that led directly to death (immediate cause). It is divided further into subsections—(a), (b), (c) and (d).
2. **Part II** is for other conditions, not related to those listed in Part I, that have also contributed to death (contributory cause).

SECTION II: Basic Forensic Medicine

■ MODE OF DEATH

Definition: Abnormal physiological state existing at the time of death, e.g., coma, congestive cardiac failure, cardiorespiratory failure, cardiac arrest or pulmonary edema.

There are three modes of death depending upon the system most obviously affected are:

1. Coma

Definition: State of deep unconsciousness from which a person cannot be roused, with minimal or no detectable responsiveness to stimuli.

Seen in cases of:
i. Disease of the brain
ii. Systemic disorders—diabetic ketoacidosis, uremia, eclampsia
iii. Intoxication—alcohol, opium

2. Syncope

Definition: Death from failure of the function of the heart resulting in hypoxia and hypoperfusion of the brain.

Seen in cases of:
i. Heart disease
ii. Hemorrhage
iii. Vagal inhibition
iv. Poisoning, such as digitalis, aconite, etc.

3. Asphyxia

Definition: Death due to failure of functioning of lungs.

Seen in cases of:
i. Hanging
ii. Strangulation
iii. Drowning, etc.

■ SUDDEN DEATH

Definition: Death occurring instantaneously or within 1 hour of the onset of morbid symptoms (as per WHO, if death occurs within 24 hours).

It is the sudden and unexpected death of a person, who prior to death was not suffering from any dangerous disease, poisoning or injury.

1. **Cardiovascular diseases** (*most common cause*)
   - Myocardial infarction
   - Coronary artery disease
   - Congenital heart disease
   - Valvular heart disease
   - Cardiomyopathies
   - Aortic aneurysm
2. **Respiratory system**
   - Pneumothorax
   - Acute epiglottitis
   - Air embolism
   - Pulmonary embolism
   - Obstruction of respiratory passage by foreign body
3. **Gastrointestinal system**
   - Appendicitis
   - Pancreatitis
   - Strangulated hernia
   - Peritonitis
   - Massive GIT hemorrhage
4. **Central nervous system**
   - Subarachnoid hemorrhage
   - Intracerebral hemorrhage
   - Stroke (CVA)
   - Brain tumor
   - Meningitis
5. **Genitourinary and reproductive system**
   - Ruptured ectopic pregnancy
   - Uterine hemorrhage
   - Tumors of bladder and kidney
   - Chronic nephritis
6. **Endocrine causes**
   - Diabetic coma
   - Pheochromocytoma
   - Adrenal insufficiency
7. **Miscellaneous**
   - Anaphylaxis
   - Drug abuse
   - Mismatched blood transfusion

■ CHANGES AFTER DEATH

Immediate Changes

Irreversible cessation of the function of:
i. Brain
ii. Respiration
iii. Circulation

Early Changes

i. Facial pallor
ii. Primary flaccidity of muscles
iii. Loss of elasticity of skin
iv. Changes in the eye
v. Algor mortis
vi. Livor mortis (PM staining)
vii. Rigor mortis

Late Changes

i. **D**ecomposition/Putrefaction
ii. **A**dipocere
iii. **M**ummification

Immediate Signs of Death

1. **Irreversible cessation of the function of brain:** Tests to confirm cessation of brain and brainstem functions:
   – Loss of reflexes
   – Dilated pupils
   – Loss of muscle tone
   – Flat EEG
2. **Irreversible cessation of respiration:** Tests to confirm cessation of respiration:
   – *Inspection:* Chest movements not visible.
   – *Palpation:* Chest movement cannot be felt.
   – *Auscultation:* Breath sounds not heard.
3. **Irreversible cessation of circulation:** Tests to confirm cessation of circulation:
   – Pulsations—absence of radial, femoral and carotid pulses
   – Absence of the heart beat on auscultation
   – Flat ECG for 5 min

Early Changes

Changes in the eyes after death (Figs. 12.2A and B):

1.	Loss of corneal reflex	Not a reliable sign
2.	Cornea	Become hazy and opaque in 6–8 hours after death
3.	Pupils	Become dilated and fixed
4.	Eyeball	Becomes flaccid due to fall in IOP (from 10 mm Hg to 0 mm Hg) within 4–6 hours after death
5.	Sclera	**Tache noire** • Deposition of dust particles over sclera giving dark brown-black color. • Occurs within 3–6 hours after death
6.	Retina	**Kevorkian sign/Trucking of blood vessels** • Segmentation of retinal blood vessels • Occurs immediately after death • Seen with ophthalmoscope
7.	Vitreous humor	Increase in—K^+, hypoxanthine Decrease in—Na^+, Cl^-, glucose

ALGOR MORTIS

Definition: Cooling of body after death.
- *Algor mortis is the first sign of death;* then followed by rigor mortis.

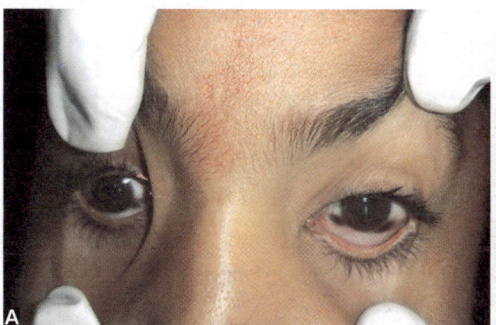 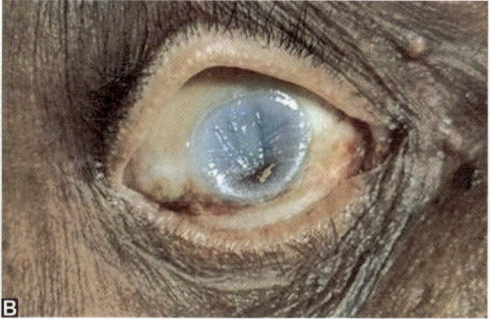

Figs. 12.2A and B: Changes in eyes after death: (A) Tache noire; (B) Opaque and sunken sclera.
(*Courtesy:* Dr Lishu Chaure, BRLSABVM Medical College, Chhattisgarh)

- Body temperature of cadaver starts falling. After some hours, it equals the temperature of environment due to cessation of energy production and inactivity of heat regulating center.
- Surface temperature falls more rapidly than inner core temperature.
- For estimation of time since death (TSD), the measurement of inner core temperature is taken.
- Method is useful in temperate climates, because in tropical countries (such as India) there is minimal fall in body temperature, and in deserts the temperature may even rise after death.
- Curve of cooling pattern is **sigmoid or inverted 'S' shaped** and 3 phases are seen (Fig. 12.3).
- Average rate of fall of body temperature is 0.4–0.7°C/hour and attains environmental temperature in 15–18 hours after death.
- **Rule of thumb:** Temperature falls at about 1.5°F/hour.

Recording of Temperature after Death

Site	Method
• Rectum • Subhepatic space • External auditory canal	Thermocouple Thanatometer—25 cm long thermometer

- **High rectal temperature:** Seen in struggle or exercise prior to death.
- **Low rectal temperature:** Seen in congestive cardiac failure, hemorrhage, collapse and secondary shock.

Medico-legal Importance

- Helps in estimation of TSD.
- It is a sign of death.
- Rapid cooling of a dead body delays the processes of rigor mortis and decomposition.

Postmortem Caloricity

Definition: Initial rise of body temperature for first two hours after death.

Causes of PM caloricity	Mechanism
1. Infectious diseases/septicemia	Due to increased bacterial activity
2. Hot temperature (Tropical countries)	As dead body absorb heat from the environmental temperature
3. Convulsions (tetanus, strychnine poisoning)	Due to increased muscular contractions
4. Pontine hemorrhage	Due to loss of heat regulation center

Medico-legal importance: PM caloricity leads to wrong estimation of TSD.

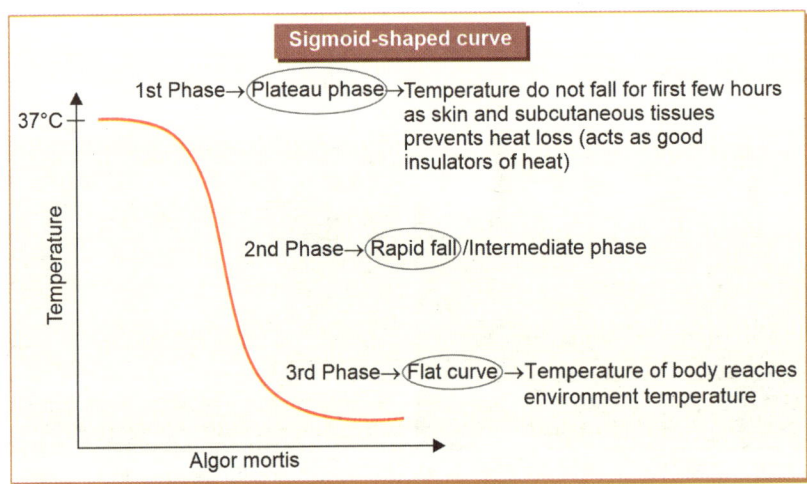

Fig. 12.3: Rate of fall of temperature after death.

RIGOR MORTIS

Definition: Stiffening of muscles of body after death (**Fig. 12.4**).
- It involves both voluntary and involuntary muscles.
- Seen after primary flaccidity of muscles.
- It is due to the formation actin-myosin complex and loss of ATP generation.

Rule of 12 (Fig. 12.5)

1st phase	Appearance of rigor mortis	Take 12 hours but involves only proximal parts
2nd phase	Persistence of rigor mortis	Take next 12 hours (12–24 hours), rigor mortis present at distal parts
3rd phase	Passing off rigor mortis	Takes another 12 hours (24–36 hours)

Order of Appearance
- First appears in heart muscle (involuntary) within 1 hour after death.
- Among *voluntary muscles*, rigor mortis develops sequentially and follows a descending/proximo-distal progression (**Nysten's/Shapiro's rule**): *First appears in muscles of eyelids and last in fingers and toes.*

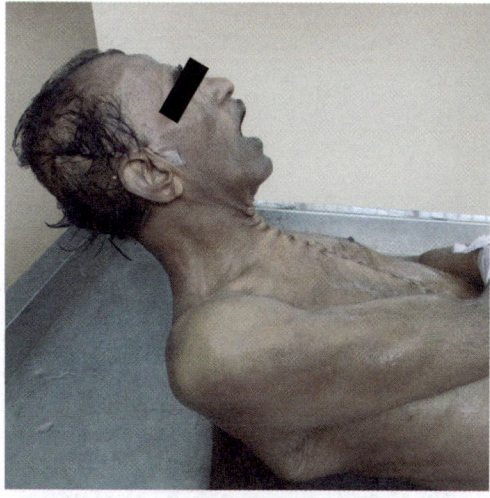

Fig. 12.4: Rigor mortis.

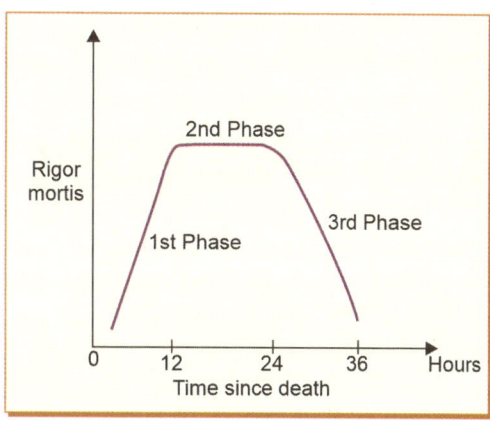

Fig. 12.5: Rule of 12.

Testing and Breaking Rigor Mortis
Tested by lifting the eyelids, depressing the jaw, and gently bending the neck and joints of all four limbs.

Medico-legal Importance
- Sign of death and indicates molecular death.
- **TSD:** During summer, if rigor mortis has not set in, death might have occurred within 2 hours. If rigor mortis has involved the whole body then death might have occurred between 12–24 hours. In winter season, the above timings are roughly doubled.
- Position of body at the time of death, e.g., if body is lying on its back with its lower limbs raised in air, it indicates that it reached full rigidity elsewhere.

CONDITIONS SIMULATING RIGOR MORTIS

1. Heat stiffening
2. Cold stiffening
3. Cadaveric spasm
4. Gas stiffening

Cadaveric Spasm
Definition: Condition in which the muscles of the body that were in state of contraction at the time of death continue to be in contracted state even after death without passing through the stage of primary relaxation.

The other muscles of the body are in stage of primary relaxation.

Involvement of Muscles

Spasm of voluntary group of muscles	Involvement of whole body (rare)
• Presence of grass and weeds in hands—in case of drowning • Weapon clenched in hands—in case of suicides	E.g., soldiers shot in battle

Cadaveric spasm continues till rigor mortis appears, then vanishes off with rigor mortis.

Medico-legal Importance

- Indicates **sudden death** with great emotional stress (excitement, exhaustion, fear, fatigue).
- It suggests **manner of death**
  - *Suicidal death:* Weapon/pistol held clenched tightly in hand.
  - *Homicidal death:* Clothing, hair or buttons of assailant may be held firmly in hand.

PM STAINING

Definition: Bluish-red or purplish-red discoloration of the skin over the dependant body parts after death **(Fig. 12.6)**. It is also known as livor mortis, hypostasis, or PM lividity.
- **Mechanism:** After death, blood stops flowing and due to force of gravitation gets collected in vessels and capillaries of dependant body parts resulting in PM staining.
- **Development of PM staining**

Onset	30 min
Well developed	4 hours
Completely develops	6 hours

- **Fixation of PM staining:** Time taken for fixation—8 hours.
  If position of body is changed before fixation—position of lividity also changes.
- **Testing for fixation**
  - Firmly press the area with thumb for 30–45 seconds.

- *If PM staining disappear:* PM staining not fixed.
- *If PM staining remains:* PM staining fixed.

Staining fixed	TSD >8 hours
Staining not fixed	TSD <6 hours

Areas of Contact Pallor

PM staining is not seen in areas which are in direct contact with the ground, i.e., staining is not seen over pressure areas. For example, in case of supine position—pressure points are at back of head, shoulder blade, gluteal region, back of foot **(Fig. 12.6)**.

Distribution and Extent of PM Staining

Supine position	Back of head, and neck, back of trunk except areas of contact pallor
Prone position	On front of face, chest and abdomen
Hanging	Lower parts of forearm and legs (glove and stocking distribution)
Drowning	• In stagnant water—found on face, upper part of chest, hands and legs • In moving water, PM staining not seen as body moves continuously

Color of PM Staining

Color of PM staining	Cause of death
Bluish-purple	Normal
Cherry red	Carbon monoxide
Bluish-green	Hydrogen sulfide
Black	Opiates
Brick red	Cyanide poisoning

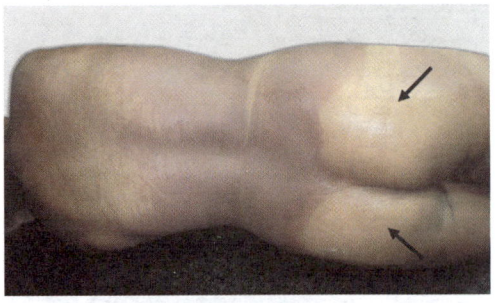

Fig. 12.6: PM staining at back with contact flattening (arrows).

Medico-legal Importance
- It is a sign of death.
- It helps in estimation of TSD.
- Helps in determining position of body after death.
- Helps in determination of cause of death.
- Sometimes, PM staining is mistaken for bruise.

DECOMPOSITION/PUTREFACTION

Definition: Process by which complex organic body tissue breaks down into simpler inorganic compounds or elements *due to the action of saprophytic microorganisms or due to autolysis* (Figs. 12.7A to D).

Putrefaction usually follows the disappearance of rigor mortis. During hot season, it may commence before rigor mortis has completely disappeared from lower extremities.

Autolysis
- Immediately after death, cell membranes become permeable and breakdown, with release of cytoplasm containing enzymes.
- Proteolytic, glycolytic and lipolytic action causes autodigestion and disintegration of organs, and occurs without bacterial influence.
- Earliest autolytic changes occur in parenchymatous and glandular tissues, and in the brain.
- In dead born infants, *maceration*—an aseptic autolysis is seen.

Bacterial Action
- **Microorganisms involved:** *Clostridium perfringens* (most common) which produces enzyme 'lecithinase', *Staphylococcus*, non-hemolytic *Streptococcus*, *diphtheroids*, and *Proteus*.

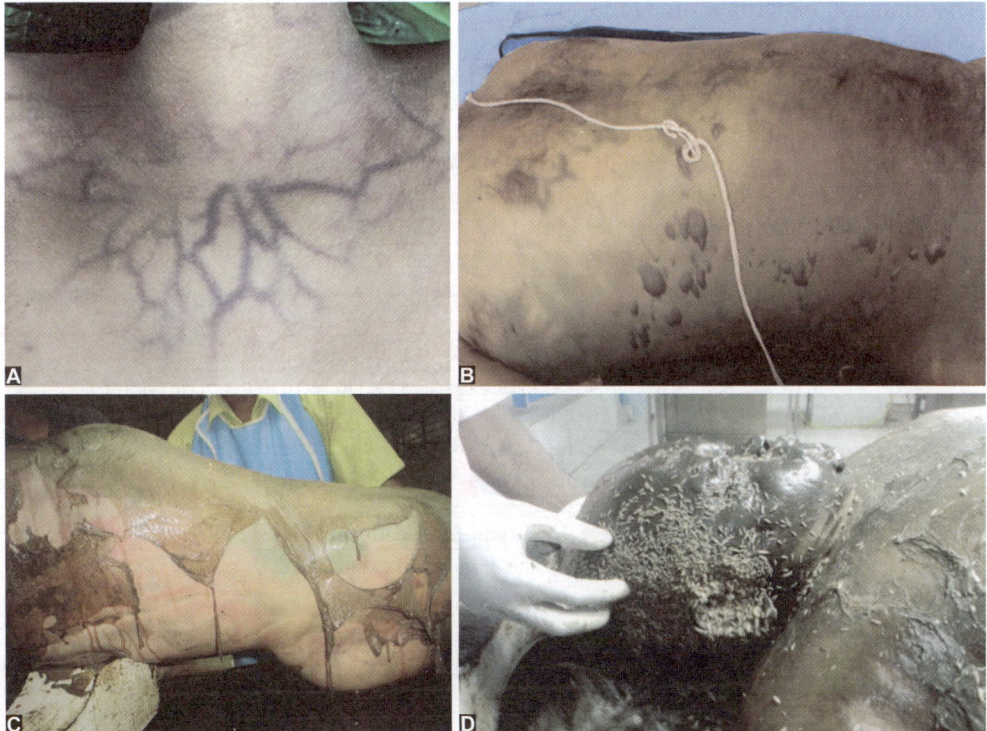

Figs. 12.7A to D: Putrefactive changes after death: (A) Marbling of veins; (B) Discoloration and blisters formation; (C) Peeling off of skin; (D) Puffiness of body and maggots.

(*Courtesy:* Dr Viswakanth B, KIMS, Mangaluru)

- **Gases produced:** H$_2$S *(major gas)*, phosphorylated hydrogen, ammonia, CO$_2$, CO, mercaptans and methane.

External Signs

Decomposition changes ('4 Ds'): Discoloration (greenish), distension, degradation *(skin slippage and degloving)* and dissolution.

- **First external sign of decomposition:** *Greenish discoloration over the right iliac fossa.* Contents of cecum are full of bacteria which lies underneath this area. *C. perfringens* are most abundant at the ileocecal zone.
  - *Onset:* 12 hours after death in summer, and 36–48 hours in winter. Discoloration gradually spreads all over the abdomen, external genitalia, face, neck and thorax, and lastly on the limbs.
  - In temperate conditions, discoloration is seen in 24–48 hours after death.
- **First internal sign of decomposition:** Discoloration of aortic intima followed by undersurface of liver (as it is in contact with transverse colon).
- **Marbling of skin:** Blood vessels are visible as greenish-black patterns and results in skin discoloration ranging from green to black.
  - *Areas involved:* Shoulder, roots of limbs, thighs, sides of abdomen, neck and chest **(Fig. 12.7A)**.
  - *Onset:* 36–48 hours.

Internal Changes due to Putrefaction

Organs with muscular and fibrous tissue resist putrefaction than the parenchymatous organs, with the *exception of the stomach and intestine*, which decompose rapidly because of their contents.

- **Liver** softens and becomes flabby in 12–24 hours, and blisters appear on its surface in 24–36 hours.
- **Brain** becomes soft, discolored pinkish-gray within 72 hours, and liquefies in 5–10 days.
- **Heart** is moderately resistant.
- **Prostate and uterus:** *Last organs to decompose*—help to identify sex of dead bodies in advanced state of decomposition.

Medico-legal Importance

- Helps in estimation of TSD.
- Identification of deceased is impossible in advanced decomposition.
- No opinion can be given as to cause of death, except in case of poisoning, fractures and firearm injuries in advanced putrefaction.

DETERMINATION OF TIME SINCE DEATH

Refer to **Tables 12.2** and **12.3,** and **Fig. 12.8**.

Table 12.2: Estimation of TSD.

1. **Changes in eye**	1. Eyeball	Becomes flaccid due to fall in IOP (from 10 to 0 mm Hg) within 4–6 hours after death	
	2. Sclera	**Tache noire:** Occurs within 3–6 hours after death	
	3. Cornea	Hazy and opaque in 6–8 hours after death	
2. **PM staining**	Mottled patches	30 min–1 hour after death	
	Coalesce	4–6 hours after death	
	PM fixation	8–12 hours after death	
3. **Algor mortis**	Not a reliable method; the body attains environmental temperature in about 16–20 hours after death in temperate climates.		
4. **Rigor mortis**	Starts	Within 1–2 hours after death	
	Appearance of rigor mortis	Takes 12 hours to develop	
	Persistence of rigor mortis	Persists for next 12 hours	
	Vanishes off	In next 12 hours	

Contd....

Contd....

5. **Putrefaction**	Greenish discoloration of right iliac fossa	12–24 hours after death
	Marbling	36–48 hours after death
	Skin slippage	36–48 hours after death
	Peeling of skin	48–72 hours after death
	Loosening of hair	>72 hours after death

Table 12.3: Time scale of postmortem changes (in tropical countries).

Time scale	Significant changes
Around 15 min	Trucking of blood within retinal blood vessels (Kevorkian sign)
30 mins–1 hour	Retina pale, dull patches of PM staining develop, no fall in rectal temperature
2 hours	Opacity of cornea and rigor mortis start developing, postmortem caloricity may be seen.
3–4 hours	Tache noire develop in eyes, confluence of PM staining. Body cold to touch (algor mortis)
4 hours	Well developed PM staining
4–8 hours	Intraocular tension falls to zero
5–6 hours	Complete PM staining, optic disk outline is hazy
7–10 hours	Blurred optic disk outline, flies lay eggs
8–12 hours	Fixed PM staining, cornea permanently hazy, rigor mortis fully developed, architecture of kidney maintained
16–20 hours	Body temperature attains environmental temperature (temperate counties)
12–24 hours	Cornea white and flattened, rigor mortis present in the body, greenish discoloration is seen in right iliac fossa (in summers), liver soft and flabby, distension of abdomen, postmortem purge, larvae or maggots of flies appear in body, disturbed architecture of kidneys
24–36 hours	Rigor mortis passes off, blisters appear on surface of liver, marbling of veins seen, marked changes in kidneys
36–48 hours	Tongue protrude out, prominent marbling of veins and distention of abdomen, blisters on lower surface of trunk and thighs, putrefactive odor is noticeable. Body completely flaccid and rise in body temperature (warm to touch)
48–72 hours	PM staining gets displaced, eyes protrude, fish-mouth like appearance of face, hair and nails become loose, brain is soft, pinkish-gray, autolytic changes in kidneys, steady increase in vitreous potassium (till 100 hours)
3–5 days	Teeth become loose, skin of hands and feet come off, innumerous maggots, pupa seen, body lice die
5–10 days	Abdomen bursts open, puffiness of body passes off, brain and other tissues liquefy, complete life cycle of fly
7–15 days	Adipocere (hydrolysis and hydrogenation of body fats, and preserves the features of the body)
3–12 months	Mummification (drying and dehydration of tissues of the body)
12 months	Skeletonization (In soil buried bodies)

Other changes which are used in determining TSD:

- **Insect activity (Forensic entomology):** By about 18-36 hours, flies lay their eggs. The eggs hatch into maggots or larvae in about 12-24 hours. In 4-5 days, maggots develop into pupae, and by 8-12 days pupae into adult flies. Lice usually die within 3-6 days after the death of the individual.
- **Stomach contents:** From the state of digestion of food and quantity of food in the stomach, TSD can be estimated.

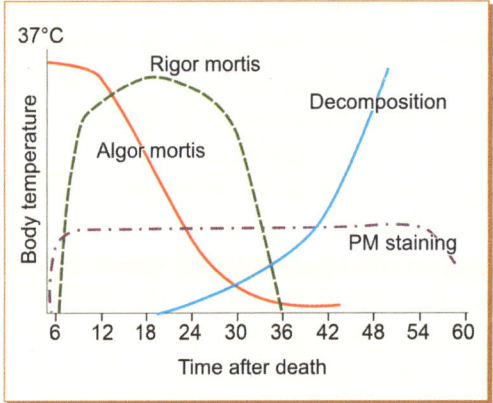

Fig. 12.8: Time since death.

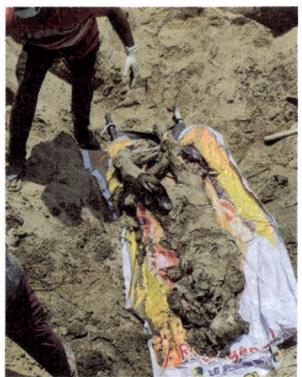

Fig. 12.9: Exhumation.
(*Courtesy:* Dr Murugesa Bharathi, IGMC, Puducherry)

If the quality, quantity and the time of the last meal taken can be known, the TSD can be estimated. If the stomach is full and contains undigested food, then death occurred within 2–4 hours of eating of the last meal.

- **Intestinal contents**: From the content of the pelvic colon and the rectum, it can be said if the person attended the nature's call within last few hours or not. If it contains feces, death may have occurred in the night and if empty, sometime after evacuation in the morning (depending upon the person's habit).
- **Contents of urinary bladder:** The amount of urine in the bladder may give some idea of TSD. If a body is found in the morning with the bladder full, then he might have died before the usual time of leaving his bed.
- **Vitreous humor:** Potassium, magnesium, urea, creatinine, uric acid and lactic acid increase after death.
- **Facial hair growth:** If the time of his last shave is known, then survival time can be calculated, and the TSD can be estimated indirectly.
- **Circumstantial evidences:** Pocket articles mobile, diary, cinema tickets, etc., may indicate the date and time up to which the person survived.

Exhumation

Definition: It is the lawful digging out of an already buried body from the grave for postmortem examination **(Fig. 12.9)**.

- It is not frequent in India because mostly the bodies are cremated. But there is no time limit for exhumation.
- **Authorization:** Exhumation orders are only given by the Magistrate.

Purpose for Exhumation

1. For identification of the diseased
2. To determine the cause of death, time since death and manner of death
3. For doing autopsy for the second time when the first autopsy was not done properly
4. To retrieve some vital objects (bullets) from the body
5. When the body has been disposed off without conducting any autopsy and later on foul play is suspected

CHAPTER 13

Identification

Identification is the determination of the individuality of a person by recognizing certain characteristics that are unique to that person.

Types

1. **Complete/Absolute identification:** Ascertaining identity with full certainty can be done by dactylography or DNA
2. **Incomplete/Partial Identification:** Race, age, sex, height etc., provides limited information about the person

Data of Identification

General	Miscellaneous	Forensic study
Age	Anthropometry	Dactylography
Sex	Superimposition	DNA fingerprinting
Race	Tattoo marks	Hair
Religion	Scars	
Stature		
Bones		
Teeth		

The surest method of identification is dactylography and the best method is DNA fingerprinting.

EXAMINATION OF SKELETAL REMAINS

1. **To determine whether it is a bone or not?** Forensic expert with his anatomical background can differentiate a bone from any object that may look like bone, e.g., wood, plastic.
2. **If it is a bone, does it belong to human or animal?**

Fragmented bones	
1. Old/burnt/cremated bones	• Gross anatomical characteristics • Microscopic characteristics (Haversian system) • Chemical analysis of bone ash may be done
2. Fresh ones which still has some blood constituents	Serological test (Precipitin test) can be done

But it is very easy to identify the species, if whole skeleton is available.

3. **Whether the bones belong to one individual or not?**

Bones available are placed in anatomical position of articulation:
- If all the available and separate parts fit to each other, and
- If age, sex and race of all the bones is same

} It belongs to the single individual

4. **Determining the stature of individual**
   Hepburn's osteometric board is used to measure length of the long bones.
   Best bone to determine stature—femur
   Methods:
   – Regression formula
   – Percentile formula
   Karl Pearson's formula is used for Americans.
5. **Determining the race of the individual**
   Race can be determined from the **cephalic index (C.I.)**.

$$C.I. = \frac{\text{Maximum transverse breadth of skull}}{\text{Maximum anterio-posterior length of skull}} \times 100$$

The Indian skull is Caucasian with few Negroid characters, and the value is 75–79.9.

6. **Determining the age of the individual**
   a. Eruption of teeth helps in estimation of age **(Table 13.1)**
   b. Ossification centers of bones (studied by means of X-rays) **(Table 13.2)**.

Table 13.1: Age estimation from dentition.

Tooth	Deciduous teeth (in months)	Permanent teeth (in years)
Central incisor	6–8 (lower, 1st to erupt) 7–9 (upper)	6–8
Lateral incisor	7–9 (upper) 10–12 (lower)	7–9
First premolar	—	9–11
Second premolar	—	10–12
First molar	12–14	6–7 (1st to erupt)
Canine	17–18	11–12
Second molar	20–30 (2–2½ years)	12–14
Third molar	—	17–25

Table 13.2: Ossification centers of bones (studied by means of X-rays).

Bone	Centers of ossification	Age of appearance	Age of union
Clavicle	Medial end	15–17 years	20–22 years
Humerus	Head Greater tubercle Lesser tubercle Capitulum Trochlea Lateral epicondyle Medial epicondyle	1 year 3 years 5 years 1 year 9–10 years 10–11 years 5–6 years	At 5–6 years, the three fuses together (*conjoint epiphysis*) and at 17–18 years, fuses with the shaft At 14–15 years, all three fuses with the shaft 16 years
Radius	Upper end Lower end	5–6 years 1–2 years	15–17 years 17–19 years
Ulna	Upper end Lower end	8–9 years 5–6 years	15–17 years 17–19 years
Carpals	Pisiform	9–12 years	—
Hip bone	Ischiopubic rami Triradiate cartilage Iliac crest Ischial tuberosity	— — 15–16 years 16–17 years	7 years 12–14 years 19–21 years 20–22 years
Femur	Head Greater trochanter Lesser trochanter Lower end	1 year 4 years 14 years 9 months IUL	17–18 years 14–15 years 15–17 years 17–18 years
Tibia	Upper end Lower end	At birth 1 year	17–18 years 16–17 years
Fibula	Upper end Lower end	4 years 2 years	17–18 years 16–17 years

c. Closure of cranial sutures (studied by means of X-rays) **(Table 13.3)**.
d. Symphyseal surfaces of pubic bone.

Age estimation	Age (years)	
Site for X-ray required	Female	Male
Elbow	13–14	15–16
Wrist	16–17	18–19
Shoulder	17–18	18–19
Iliac crest	18–19	19–21
Ischial tuberosity and inner end of clavicle	21–22	21–23

Table 13.3: Closure of cranial sutures.

Suture closure	Age
Posterior fontanelle (occipital)	At birth to 6 months
Anterior fontanelle (bregma)	1½–2 years
Two halves of mandible	1–2 years
Metopic suture	1 year (3–9 months), may remain unfused
Basiocciput with basisphenoid	18–20 years (females) 20–22 (males)
Lambdoid suture	45–50 years
Parietotemporal	60–70 years

Age Estimation from Mandible

Features	Infancy	Adult	Old age
Body	Shallow	Thick and long	Shallow
Ramus	Obtuse angle with body	Almost right angle	Obtuse angle (about 140°)
Mental foramen	Near the lower margin	Opens midway	Near the alveolar margin
Condyloid process	Lower level than coronoid process	Above coronoid process	Neck is bent backwards

Medico-legal Importance of Age

- **Criminal responsibility:** Child <7 years is not held criminally responsible.
- **Employment:** Child <14 years cannot be employed for any type of work (factory/mine, etc.).
- **Consent:** Can give valid consent for general physical and medico-legal examination (≥12 years); any major diagnostic or operative procedure, donating organs and consent for sexual intercourse (≥18 years).
- **Attainment of majority:** Person attains majority at 18 years (21 years if under guardianship of Court of Wards).
- **Kidnapping:** Taking away a person (boy <16 years, girl <18 years) by illegal means is considered as kidnapping.
- **Statutory rape:** Sexual intercourse with any girl <18 years with her consent is rape **(Sec. 375 IPC)**.
- **Judicial punishment:** No juvenile (<18 years) will be sentenced to death or life imprisonment.
- **Marriage:** Female <18 years and male <21 years cannot marry.
- **Casting of vote** (18 years).
- **Testamentary capacity:** Mentally sound person can make a valid will (18 years).
- **Evidence:** Child of any age can give evidence, if the court is satisfied that the child is truthful **Sec. 118 IEA**.

7. **Determining sex of the individual:** Sex is determined from skeleton based on sexual characteristic of skull, pelvis, mandible, sacrum and long bones (seen after puberty). Krogman's degree of accuracy in sex determination from bones:

Whole skeleton	100%
Pelvis + skull	98%
Pelvis	95%
Skull	92%
Long bones	80%

Male and Female Skull (Figs. 13.1A and B)

Features	Male skull	Female skull
Forehead	Sloping/receding	Vertical
Glabella and supraorbital margins	More prominent	Less prominent
Orbits	Square shaped and small	Round shaped and large
Mastoid process	Large, round and blunt	Small and pointed
Frontonasal junction	Presence of angulation	Smoothly curved
Zygomatic arch	More prominent	Less prominent
Nuchal crest	Well-defined ledge or hook	Absent or slight expression
Partial eminence	Less prominent	More prominent
Frontal eminence	Less prominent	More prominent
Palate	U-shaped	Parabola-shaped
Suprameatal crest	Present	Absent

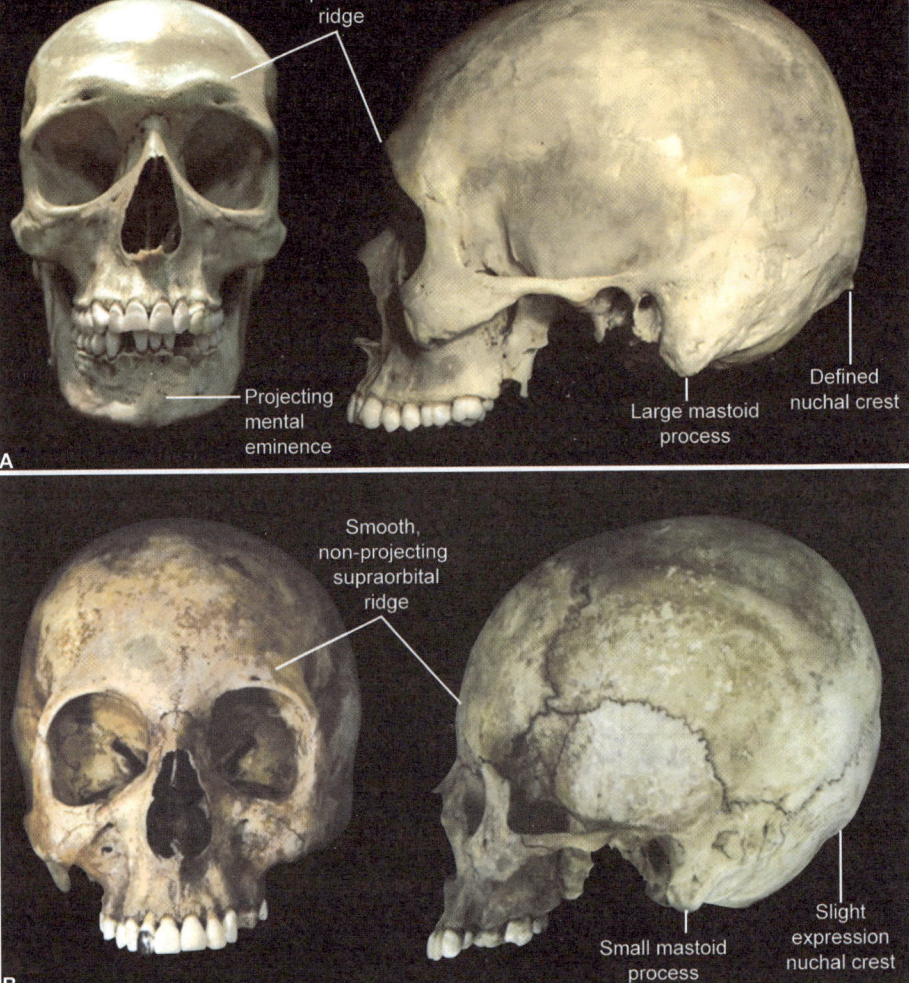

Figs. 13.1A and B: Skull: (A) Male; (B) Female.
(*Courtesy:* Dr Carolyn Isaac, Western Michigan University Homer Stryker MD School of Medicine, Michigan)

Male and Female Mandible

Features	Male mandible	Female mandible
Chin	Square	Rounded
Ascending ramus	Greater breadth	Smaller breadth
Angle of mandible	Everted	Inverted
Angle of body with ramus	Less obtuse	More obtuse
Condyles	Large	Small
Ramus flexure	Rearward angulation of posterior border	Straight ramus
Muscular markings	Prominent	Not prominent

Male and Female Pelvis (Figs. 13.2A and B)

Features	Male pelvis	Female pelvis
Preauricular sulcus	Narrow, shallow	Broad, deep
Subpubic angle	V-shaped (70–75°)	U-shaped (90–100°)
Sciatic notch	Small, narrow, deep	Large, wide, shallow
Pubis body	Narrow and triangular	Broad and square
Ischial spines	More prominent	Less prominent
Ischial tuberosity	Inverted	Everted
Obturator foramen	Oval	Triangular, apex forwards
Pelvic inlet	Heart shaped	Circular/elliptical
Pelvic cavity	Funnel shaped	Broad
Pelvic outlet	Smaller	Larger
Sacroiliac joint surface	Large, less angulated	Small and L-shaped

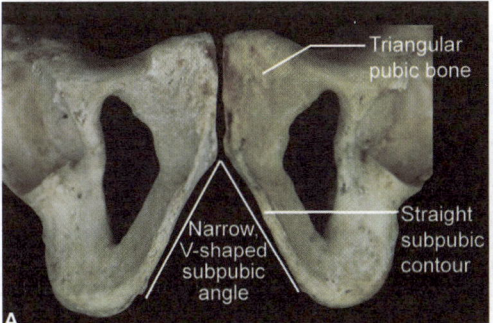 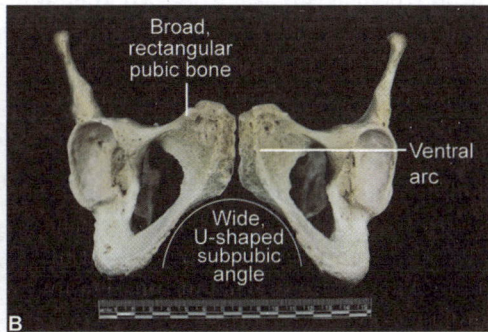

Figs. 13.2A and B: Pelvis: (A) Male; (B) Female.
(Courtesy: Dr Carolyn Isaac, Western Michigan University Homer Stryker MD School of Medicine, Michigan)

8. **Identification of the individual**
   It can be determined from—
   - DNA analysis.
   - *Teeth:* Extractions, artificial dentures.
   - Superimposition.
   - Neutron activation analysis.
   - Radiological investigations.
9. **Determining cause of death**
   - Fractures of bones.
   - Foreign body (bullet).

- Chemical analysis for detection of metallic poison.
10. **Determining time of death:** It may be determined from the condition of parts and decomposition changes.
11. **Determining type of weapon:** From antemortem injuries, it may be possible to determine whether a hard blunt weapon, a light or heavy sharp cutting weapon, a pointed weapon or a firearm was used.

Bite Marks

- Bite mark is semicircular or crescentic pattern caused by the front teeth (incisors and canines) with a gap on either side due to separation of upper and lower jaw.
- These may be abrasions, bruises and lacerations or a combination of all these.

Medico-legal Importance

Bites marks are commonly seen in cases of:
- **Sexual assault:** Marks are usually seen on breasts, neck, shoulders, thighs, abdomen, pubis or vulva.
- **Child abuse:** Marks are seen anywhere on the body, such as arms, hands, shoulders, cheeks, buttocks and trunk.
- Bite marks on foodstuffs (apples, cheese or chocolate), leather (key rings or belts) and wood (pencils) in cases where a perpetrator might have taken a bite out of something in the victim's home and left it behind.
- Police officers may be bitten by the resisting offenders.
- In assaults, bite marks may be found anywhere on the body.
- **Self-inflicted bite marks** are present on accessible parts of the body, e.g., shoulders or arms; seen in psychiatric patients or teenage girls.
- **In sexual assault**, sucking action during bites produces multiple petechial hemorrhages due to rupture of small capillaries and venules.
- **Accidental marks** resulting from falls on to the face and during fits, biting of tongue and lips may also be there.

Human Hair and Animal Hair (Figs. 13.3A and B)

Features	Human hair	Animal hair
Texture	Thin and fine	Thick and coarse
Root	Bulb shaped	Brush like
Cortex	Broader	Narrow
Medulla	Narrow/non-continuous/fragmented/may be absent	Broad/continuous
Medullary index	<1/3	>1/3
Tip	Cut/frayed	Tapered
Pigment granules	Uniformly distributed	Mostly present around the medulla

SCARS

- Scar is formed, if injury is at the level of dermis and below.
- Most superficial wounds which involve the epidermis (superficial burns/abrasions) will heal by epithelialization without scar formation.

Age of Scars

- **Firm union, reddish:** 5–6 days.
- **Pale, soft, tender:** 2 weeks–2 months.
- **Brownish, glistening, little tender:** 2–6 months.

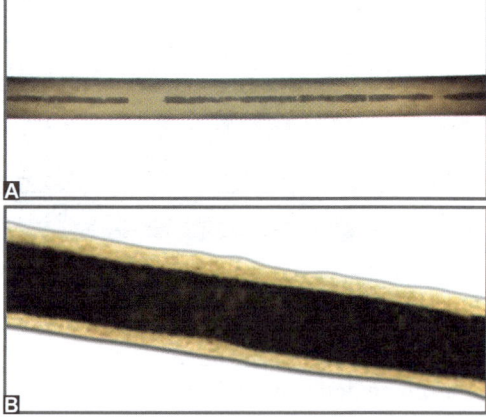

Figs. 13.3A and B: Hair: (A) Human; (B) Animal.

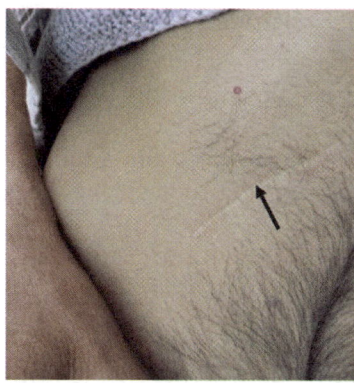

Fig. 13.4: Scar on the abdomen (arrow).

- **White, glistening, corrugated, non-tender:** >6 months.

Erasure: Can be erased by excision and skin grafting.

Medico-legal Importance

- Helps in identification of a person.
- Shape may indicate the type of weapon or agent that caused injury **(Fig. 13.4)**.
- Age of scar indicates time of infliction of injury.
- Disfiguration by scar constitutes grievous hurt **(Sec. 320 IPC)**.
- Striae gravidarum and linea albicantes indicate previous pregnancy.
- May be used to charge an enemy with assault (scar may originally be due to disease).
- Linear scars on wrist or throat (hesitation cuts) indicate previous attempts at suicide.
- Linear needle scars indicate an IV drug abuser, and depressed scars a skin popper.

TATTOO MARKS

- Designs made in the skin by multiple small puncture wounds with needles dipped in coloring matter which is attached to an oscillating unit.
- **Dyes used:** Indigo, cobalt, carbon, vermilion, cadmium, selenium, Prussian blue and India ink.
- **Permanent tattoos are obtained:**
  - Using black, blue and red dyes.
  - When the dye penetrates dermis.
  - Tattooed area is protected by clothing.
- **Visibility of latent tattoo:** Rub the area and examine with magnifying lens.
- **Identification of faded tattoos**
  - Infra-red photography.
  - UV lamp.
  - High contrast photography.
  - Computer image enhancement.
- Can be recognized in decomposed/drowned bodies when the epidermis is removed.
- Tattoos can be identified by *pigmentations of regional lymph nodes*, since some pigment migrates from the site to lymph nodes.

Complications: Sepsis, abscess, gangrene, syphilis, hepatitis B, AIDS, leprosy and tuberculosis.

Erasure of tattoo: Surgical methods using Q-switched Nd:YAG laser, complete excision and skin grafting, or scarification; electrolysis; or using caustic or corrosive substances.

Medico-legal Importance

- Helps in identification of a person.
- **Religion and nationality:** Designs of flags, Cross, Lord Hanuman or Krishna provides clue to a person's religion or nationality **(Fig. 13.5)**.

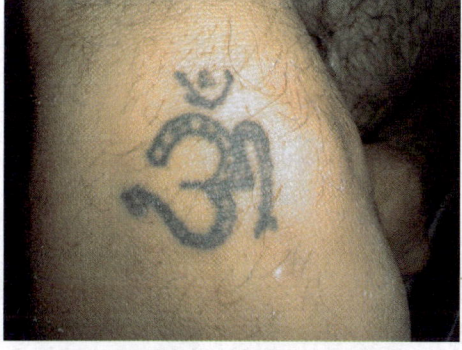

Fig. 13.5: Tattoo on upper arm.

- Political affiliations of a person can be known, e.g., hammer and sickle, lotus or right hand.
- **Race:** Tattooing on chest and limbs, common amongst Japanese.
- **Profession/occupation:** Gangs or coal miners have specific tattoo marks.
- **Behavioral characteristics:** Some tattoos may indicate high-risk behaviors including alcohol and drug use, violence, carrying weapons, sexual activity, eating disorders and suicide.
- Social status.

DACTYLOGRAPHY

Definition: It is the study of fingerprints as method of identification.
- It is the surest data of identification/most reliable method of identification as:
  - Patterns are not inherited
  - Different even in identical twins
- **Fingerprints** are impression of ridge patterns on fingers due to secretion of oils from the glands in the skin.

History

- First person to use fingerprinting—William Hershel.
- Systematized by—Sir Francis Galton.
- Improved by—Sir Henry, hence called as **Henry and Galton System.**

Classification of Fingerprints (Figs. 13.6A to D)

Loop (most common)	70%
Whorls	25%
Arches	5%
Composite (least common)	1%

Types of Fingerprints

1. Visible print—seen with naked eye. For example, fingerprints made from grease, blood.
2. Latent print—not visible to naked eye, therefore needs to developed to make it visible.
3. Plastic print—impressions over soft materials, such as soap, cheese.

Latent Finger Prints

- Latent fingerprints are friction skin impression made of moisture, eccrine gland secretions and sebaceous oils.
- They are generally not visible to the unaided eye.
- Latent prints are the most prominent example of Locard's principle of exchange.
- Most crime scene fingerprint impressions are commonly latent prints.
- Latent print requires additional processing to be rendered visible and suitable for comparison. Processing of latent prints to render them visible and suitable for comparison is called *development, enhancement* or *visualization*.
- Most methods for the development of latent prints were developed on the basis of knowledge about the latent print residue composition.

Recording of Fingerprints

Before recording the fingerprints, hands are washed, cleaned and dried and then fingerprint is taken using Printer's ink on an unglazed paper.

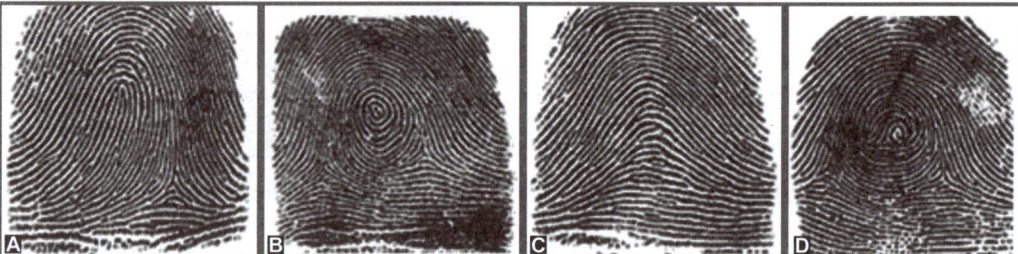

Figs. 13.6A to D: Fingerprints: (A) Loop; (B) Whorl; (C) Arch; (D) Composite (or mixed).

It is done by two methods:
1. Plain impression—by gently pressing the inked fingertips on paper.
2. Rolled impression—by rolling thumb/finger from side to side.
   It is customary/conventional to take left thumb impression in males and right thumb impression in females.

Removal of Fingerprints

- Fingerprints can be erased permanently and deliberately by criminals to reduce their chance of conviction.
- Alteration of fingerprints are seen in—eczema, celiac disease.
- Permanent impairment of fingerprints are seen in—leprosy, electric injury, radiation.

Medico-legal Importance

- Identification of a person.
- Identification in case of accidental exchange of newborn infants.
- Identification of victims of mass disaster.
- Properties and legal documents.
- Identification in mummified bodies.
- Identification of licensing procedure.
- **Sex determination:** The amino acid content in fingerprints can be used to determine sex.
- **Drug abuse:** The secretions in fingerprint contain residues of various chemicals and their metabolites, which can be detected.

DNA FINGERPRINTING

- DNA fingerprint was first developed in England in 1985 by *Alec Jeffreys*.
- Primary method for identifying and distinguishing individual human beings based on their unique DNA pattern.
- Two methods of DNA analysis are:
  1. Restriction fragment length polymorphism (RFLP): Most common method of DNA typing is RFLP analysis of VNTR loci.
  2. Polymerase chain reaction (PCR)
- Method of detecting DNA fragments—separating them by gel electrophoresis and then transferring them to a nitrocellulose/nylon membrane—is called **Southern blot,** named after its inventor, *Dr Edward Southern*. Similar blotting techniques are used to study RNA *(Northern blot),* and proteins or polypeptides *(Western blot).*
- Due to large number of distinguishable alleles in most populations, it is possible to establish a *'DNA signature'* for almost any individual and establish as link between a suspect and biological evidence in a criminal investigation.
- PCR was discovered by *Kary B Mullis* (got Nobel Prize in chemistry).

Requirements for PCR

i. Heat resistant DNA polymerase *(Taq polymerase).*
ii. Primers.
iii. Deoxynucleoside triphosphates.
iv. DNA-fragments.

Specimen Selection and Preservation

Living Subjects

i. **Blood** (*most common sample*). 5 mL of venous blood is collected in EDTA tube. Heparin is not used as an anticoagulant since it interferes with PCR. Sample can be preserved at 2–8°C (not frozen).
ii. **Buccal swabs** are considered a convenient alternative for collecting genetic material.
iii. **Hair follicles with roots** (plucked hair), about 10–20 from head. Root of hair contains nuclear DNA *(keratinocytes)*, and shaft contains mitochondrial DNA.

Dead Bodies

- **Best sample in fresh bodies:** Unclotted 10 mL of blood (EDTA anticoagulated in a sterile tube). Due to settling out of WBCs, clotted blood is not a good source of DNA.
- **In advanced decomposition:** Hard tissue (bone and vascular pulp of teeth)
  - Best material is muscle or spleen if decomposition is establishing; bone marrow (from femur) and teeth (usually molars) in advanced decomposition.

Uses of DNA Fingerprinting

1. Identification of a person.
2. Diagnosis and developing cures of inherited disorders, such as cystic fibrosis, hemophilia, Huntington's disease, familial Alzheimer's, sickle cell anemia and thalassemia.
3. Establish paternity in custody and child support litigation.
4. Identifying remains of soldiers.
5. Biologists routinely use it, particularly to protect endangered species.
6. Accidents/mass disaster investigations and postmortem identification of skeletal remains/mutilated bodies.

CHAPTER 14

Forced Anal Intercourse

Sodomy is the anal intercourse between two males (homosexual sodomy) or between a male and a female (heterosexual sodomy).

Findings seen in victim of anal intercourse are:

Non-habitual passive victim	Habitual passive victim
Examination is done in left lateral decubitus position	Examination done in knee chest position
1. Pain and tenderness during digital rectal examination (DRE) 2. Substances found in/around anus—fecal matter, lubricants, semen, loose foreign hair 3. Inflammation around anus 4. Bleeding due to laceration 5. Loss of normal anal tone 6. **Injuries** – Perianal abrasions—due to frictional shearing force by penetrating penis – Bruises—may be mistaken for hemorrhoids – Laceration – Anal fissures—wedge shaped, present in posterior quadrant and radially towards the anal canal Swabs taken from inside and outside anus for FSL examination	1. No pain and tenderness during DRE 2. No inflammation around anus 3. Shaving of anal hair may be present 4. Lateral traction test—external anal sphincter relaxes reflexly during bimanual traction of buttocks 5. Loose foreign hair and lubricants 6. Perianal skin—thickened, keratinized due to constant regular friction 7. Anal sphincter—lax and patulous and dilated anal canal with old, healed fissures 8. Anal opening—deeply situated giving funnel-shaped depression of buttocks 9. Evidence of venereal disease — Veneral disease — Large fissure — Lax sphincter — Small fissures

■ OPINION

1. Findings of examination are consistent/not inconsistent with the history of alleged sexual assault.
2. There is evidence/no evidence of recent/anal penetration.
3. The injuries on the body could be/could not be suggestive of resistance from the victim.
4. There is evidence/no evidence of recent anal coitus. (Based on laboratory results).

CHAPTER 15

Forensic Psychiatry

Insanity and Mental Illness

Insanity
It is the disease of the mind, which affects the personality, mental status, critical faculties, emotional processes and interaction with the social environment.

Mentally-ill Person
Any person who is in need of treatment by reason of any mental disorder other than mental retardation.

Psychosis
Gross impairment in reality-testing (withdrawal from reality), as if living in a world of fantasy.

Neurosis
Patient suffers from emotional or intellectual disorders which causes subjective distress, but does not lose touch with reality.

Psychosis and Neurosis

Features	Psychosis	Neurosis
Insight*	Absent	Present
Empathy¥	-do-	-do-
Delusions/hallucinations	Present	Absent
Dealing with reality	Impaired	Preserved
Behavior	Not within socially acceptable norms	Within acceptable norms

Contd....

Features	Psychosis	Neurosis
Examples	Schizophrenia	Anxiety, phobia

*Patient's awareness and understanding of his illness and need for treatment.
¥Showing the capacity to feel and understand the psychological and emotional state of another.

Delusion

- Delusion is false but firm belief in something which is not a fact despite proof to the contrary.
- It is a disorder of content of thought.

Types

Hypochondriacal delusion	Patient believes of having some serious disease (such as cancer) based on his own interpretations of physical signs and symptoms.
Delusion of infidelity (Othello syndrome)	• Patient believes that his partner is unfaithful to him or her. • Seen in patients with alcohol dependence.
Delusion of reference	Person believes that everyone is looking at him or talking about him. For example, if patient sees anyone smiling then he believes that they are laughing at him.
Nihilistic delusion	• Patient denies the existence of their body, their mind or even world in general. • Seen in patients of depression.

Contd....

Contd....

Delusion of influence	Patient complains that his thoughts, feelings and actions are being influenced and controlled by some outside agency, e.g., radio/mobile/internet.
Delusion of love/Erotomania	• Patient believes that a person of higher socioeconomic status is in love with her/him. • Usually common in females.
Delusion of persecution	• Most common delusion. • The person thinks that people around him are trying to kill him/harm him/making conspiracy against him. • Commonly seen in schizophrenia
Delusion of grandiosity	• Person imagines himself to be very rich/powerful although in reality he may be poor. • Seen in patients with mania and schizophrenia

Medico-legal Importance

The doctrine of diminished responsibility is applicable to an insane person who does an unlawful act due to delusion, which reduces his power of reasoning and understanding capacity, e.g., if he commits some act which is not directly related with the effect of the delusion, but has an indirect bearing, such person cannot be regarded as fully responsible for his illegal acts.

Hallucination

- Hallucination is false perception by senses without any external object or stimulus.
- Seen in insanity, high fever, drug intoxication and during withdrawal from drug addiction.

Types

Auditory hallucination	• False perception of sound (noises, music) without any source, e.g., hearing sound when there is none. • Seen in schizophrenia • Most common hallucinations

Contd....

Contd....

Visual hallucination	• Patient observes something without anything being present. • Seen in delirium tremens.
Olfactory hallucination	• False sense of smell (pleasant/unpleasant) without any source. • Seen in medical disorders (temporal lobe), schizophrenia.
Gustatory hallucination	• Patient experiences different tastes (sweet/bitter/sour) without any food or drink. • Seen in temporal lobe epilepsy.
Tactile hallucination (touch)	• Patient experiences crawling of insects/rats over his body. • Seen in cocainism, schizophrenia.

Medico-legal Importance

Hallucinations are not under voluntary control and a person will not be responsible if he is incited to commit homicide.

Illusion

Illusion is a false interpretation by the senses of an external object or stimulus which has a real existence.

Types

Universal illusions	Found in all individuals and same for all individuals, e.g., the rail tracks appear to be converging to all of us.
Personal illusions	Differ from individual to individual, e.g., a person sees a dog and mistakes it for lion, or imagines a string hanging in his room to be snake.

A sane person may experience illusion, but can correct the false impressions. An insane person continues to believe in the illusions, even though the real facts are clearly pointed out.

Impulse

Impulse is an uncontrolled, sudden and irresistible urge which compels the person to conscious performance of an act. A sane person is capable of controlling an impulse, but an insane person cannot.

Diagnosis of Impulsive Control Disorder

- Failure to resist the impulse, which is harmful to self or others.
- Before the act—feeling of increased tension.
- After performing it—person has sense of relief, and finally feels guilty.

Types

Kleptomania	An irresistible desire to steal articles of low value
Pyromania	Impulse to set the things on fire
Oniomania	Impulse of shopping
Dipsomania	An excessive desire to drink alcohol
Mutilomania	A desire to maim animals

Obsession-Compulsion

- **Obsession:** Persistent and recurrent idea, image, thought, or emotion that cannot be eliminated from consciousness by logic or reasoning.
- **Compulsion:** Repetitive behavior or mental acts that the person feels driven to perform in response to an obsession.
- It is a disorder of content of thought and is regarded as senseless by the patient (*insight is present*).

Phobia

Phobia is morbid and irrational fear in the presence of stimulus, and the person tries to avoid the situation.

Types

Agoraphobia	Social phobia	Specific (simple) phobia
Morbid fear of places from which escape is difficult	Fear of socially demanding situations and fear of embarrassment	Strong, persistent and irrational fear of an object or situation (most common type of phobia)
E.g., crowd, market, stores	E.g., stage fear, public speaking	E.g., claustrophobia, hydrophobia, zoophobia

Lucid Interval

Lucid interval is a period in insanity during which all the signs and symptoms of insanity disappear, i.e., it is a period of sanity in between two periods of insanity.

- Common in mania and melancholia.
- Can make his will (testamentary capacity) during this period.
- Responsible for all his acts performed during the period of lucid interval.
- If he commits a crime, then he may take the plea of previous insanity.

CIVIL RESPONSIBILITY OF INSANE

Management of self and property	The court may appoint a guardian to take care of the mentally ill, and may appoint a manager to manage the property.
Contracts	A contract made by mentally-ill person, who does not understand the nature and quality of the contract will be considered invalid. However, he is liable for contracts if made during lucid interval.
Marriage and divorce	Marriage is invalid, if one of the parties, at the time of ceremony, was suffering from mental illness.
Adoption	Taking/giving adoption of a child is not allowed, if either of the parents is mentally-ill.
Witness	A mentally-ill person cannot be considered as competent to give evidence in the court of law. He can be regarded as competent during lucid interval.
Consent	The consent given by a mentally-ill person is not valid because he is unable to understand the nature and consequence of that to which he gives the consent.
Testamentary capacity	Will made by mentally-ill person is considered invalid because mentally-ill person does not have the capacity to make a valid will.
Guardianship	A mentally-ill person is not considered as a legal guardian of a minor.

Testamentary Capacity

This means the capacity of a person to make a valid will. The law defines it as the possession of a sound disposing mind *(compos mentis)* which must be certified by a doctor.

- **Will made by mentally-ill person:** Considered invalid because mentally-ill person does not have the capacity to make a valid will.
- **Will made in lucid interval:** Considered valid because in lucid interval the person is normal (i.e., of sound mind) and is able to judge and foresee the consequences of his acts.
- **Will made by drunk person, or under insane delusions:** Invalid, as the testator is incapable of understanding the nature and consequences of his own judgements.

Salient features of a valid will:
1. Should be executed by a testator
2. Should be sound mind
3. Should be major (age ≥18 years)
4. Should be signed by testator in the presence of at least two witnesses.

CRIMINAL RESPONSIBILITY OF INSANE

McNaughton's Rule

- McNaughton's rule deals with criminal responsibility of an insane person.
- Under this, a person is not criminally responsible, if at the time of the crime, he did not know the nature of the act or that it was wrong. It has the following requirements:
  1. There should be evidence of mental disease.
  2. This mental disease or defect must exist at the time of commission of crime.
  3. It should be of such degree that the person is unable to understand that the act is wrong and/or contrary to the law.

It means, if a person accused of a crime is found to be a normal, sound person, he will be punished. But if a person is found to be mentally ill, then the person is not punished.

- This is the legal test of insanity and is also known as the **'Right or Wrong' test**.
- McNaughton rule is incorporated **under Sec. 84 of IPC in Indian law**. It states that "Nothing is an offense which is done by a person who, at the time of doing it, by reason of unsoundness of mind, is incapable of knowing the nature of the act or what he is doing is either wrong or contrary to the law."

FEIGNED INSANITY/MALINGERING

- Feigned insanity means that the person is pretending to be mentally-ill/insane in order to deceive and for gain.
- A *malingering patient* intentionally produces false or exaggerated physical or psychological symptoms to obtain incentives.

The person has some motive behind this act, e.g.,
a. To avoid inquiry
b. To avoid trial
c. To avoid conviction
d. To avoid punishment
e. To avoid going to prison

Hence, it is the duty of the psychiatrist/forensic nurse to distinguish between two.

- It is also necessary that no sane person is confined to a psychiatric hospital.
- Strongly suspect malingering when there is a medico-legal presentation. For example, a lawyer refers a patient or a patient is seeking compensation for injury.

To differentiate true insanity from feigned insanity, salient points are highlighted in **Diff. 15.1**.

Role of Forensic Psychiatric Nurse

Forensic psychiatric or mental health nurses deal with mental health issues of victims and offenders. The forensic psychiatric nurse assesses:
1. Perpetrator's ability to plan intent.
2. Risk for violence and for committing additional crimes.
3. Competency to stand in trial.

Diff. 15.1: True and feigned insanity.

Features	True insanity	False insanity
Onset of disease	Gradual/slow	Sudden
Predisposing factor	Usually present, history of insanity	Absent
Motive	Absent	Present (history of crime)
Facial expression	Peculiar vacant/agitated look	Normal/exaggerated
Fatigue on exertion	Does not get fatigued	Easily fatigued
Insomnia	Present	Absent
Dressing up	Poorly dressed/careless	Reasonably dressed up
Habits	Dirty and filthy	No ill habits
Whether examining or not	Features always present	Features exaggerate on examination
Repeated examination	Not worried	Resists

4. Writes and submits formal reports to the court.
5. Serves as expert and fact witness.
6. Consults with attorneys and law enforcement personnel.
7. Provides therapy.

Nurses in non-forensic mental health settings can use knowledge of these roles and functions in providing care to offenders.

CHAPTER 16

Asphyxial Conditions

Asphyxia is a condition when there is reduced or no supply of oxygen to body tissues.

Cardinal Signs of Asphyxia

1. Congestion of organs
2. Cyanosis of ear, lips, nail beds } **Asphyxial triad**
3. Petechial hemorrhages/Tardieu spots on face, neck, chest
4. Right ventricular enlargement
5. Increased fluidity of blood

Classification of Asphyxial Deaths

A. Mechanical Causes

1. **Hanging:** Form of violent asphyxial death produced by suspending the body with ligature tied around the neck. The constricting force is the weight of the body or part of body weight.
   a. **Based on degree of suspension**
      - *Complete:* Body is fully suspended and no part touches the ground.
      - *Partial:* Part of body is touching the ground, in sitting, kneeling or prone position.
   b. **Based on position of knot**
      - *Typical:* When knot is at nape of neck on the back.
      - *Atypical:* Knot of ligature is anywhere other than on occiput.
2. **Strangulation:** Form of violent asphyxial death caused by constriction of air passage at the neck by any means other than suspension of the body (**Diff. 16.1**).

Classification of Strangulation

1. Ligature strangulation	Ligature is used to compress the neck
2. Manual strangulation (Throttling)	Compression of neck by hands
3. Bansdola	Strangulation by bamboo or stick
4. Mugging	Strangulation by compressing neck in bend of elbow or knee
5. Garrotting	Compression of neck by a ligature which is tightened by twisting it with a lever (rod, stick)

3. **Suffocation:** Form of asphyxia caused by mechanical obstruction to the passage of air into the respiratory tract by means other than constriction of neck or drowning.
   a. **Smothering:** Form of asphyxia caused by mechanical occlusion of external air passages, i.e., the nose and mouth by hand, cloth, plastic bag or other material.
   b. **Gagging:** Form of asphyxia which results from pushing a gag (rolled up cloth or paper balls) into the mouth, sufficiently deep to block the pharynx. It combines features of smothering and choking.
   c. **Choking:** Asphyxia caused by an obstruction within the air-passages by a foreign object, like coin, fruit seed, candies or any other material.
   d. **Overlaying:** Overlaying results due to compression of the chest, nose and mouth so as to prevent breathing.

Diff. 16.1: Hanging and strangulation (Figs. 16.1A and B).

Features	Hanging	Strangulation
Signs of asphyxia	Less marked	More marked
Protrusion of tongue	Less marked	More marked
Bleeding from nose, ear	Rare	More common
Ligature mark a. Direction b. Continuity c. Level in neck d. Base e. Abrasions and bruise around ligature f. Tissues beneath ligature mark	• Oblique • Incomplete • Above the level of thyroid • Hard, dry, parchment-like • Less common • White, glistening	• Horizontal • Complete • Below the level of thyroid • Soft, reddish base • More common • Shows hemorrhage and ecchymosis
Fracture of thyroid cartilage	Less common	More common
Fracture of hyoid bone	More common	Less common
Stains of saliva	Common	Rare
Discharge of urine and feces	Less common	More common
Seminal discharge	Common	Rare
Manner of death	Suicidal > Homicidal	Homicidal (mostly)

e. **Burking:** Combination of homicidal smothering and traumatic asphyxia.
f. **Traumatic asphyxia:** Asphyxia resulting from respiratory arrest due to mechanical fixation of chest preventing normal movements of chest wall.

4. **Drowning**
   a. **Typical (wet):** Obstruction of air passages and lungs by inhalation of fluid.
   b. **Atypical:** Type of drowning in which water or fluid does not enter the lungs but death of the person occurs immediately.

B. Pathological Causes

When oxygen is not able to enter lungs due to diseases of upper respiratory tract/lungs; e.g., laryngeal edema, stridor, tumor, etc.

C. Environmental Causes

Asphyxia due to lack of oxygen. Seen in high altitude, inhalation of CO, sewer gas.

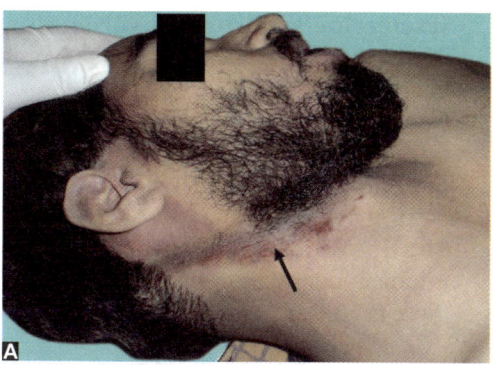
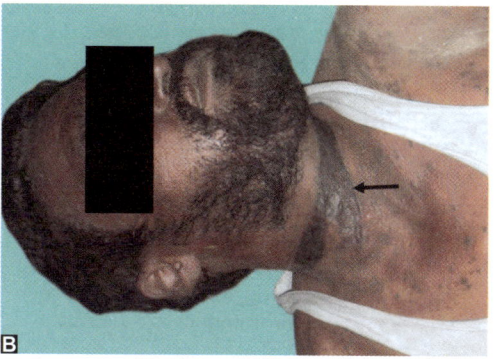

Figs. 16.1A and B: Ligature mark: (A) Hanging (arrow); (B) Strangulation (arrow).

D. Positional Asphyxia

Asphyxia due to abnormal position. Seen in Jack-knife position.

Antemortem and postmortem Hanging (hanged after death with other means to simulate suicide).		
Features	Antemortem hanging	Postmortem hanging
Ligature mark a. Direction b. Continuity c. Level in neck d. Base	• Oblique • Non-continuous • Above thyroid • Dry, hard, parchment-like	• Circular • Continuous • At/below thyroid • No changes seen
Le facie sympathique*	Present	Absent
Stain of saliva	Present	Absent
Fecal/urinary/seminal discharge	Present	Absent
Stretching of neck	Present	Absent
Signs of asphyxia	Present	May be present/absent
PM staining	Glove and stocking pattern	Absent
Suicide note	Present	Absent

* If the knot presses on cervical sympathetic, eye of same side may remain open and pupil is dilated.

Specimens to collect and preserve
i. Ligature material
ii. Clothings
iii. Viscera
iv. Fingernail scrapings
v. Blood (grouping, alcohol, drugs)
vi. Vaginal swabs (in females)
vii. Any other stains

The ligature is preserved and should be cut away from knot and reconstructed by joining cut ends with tape or another cord. This is done to verify and corroborate with the findings of autopsy subsequently.

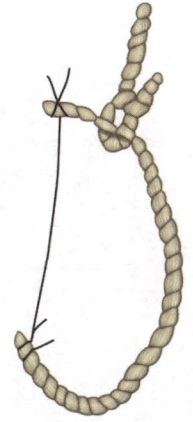

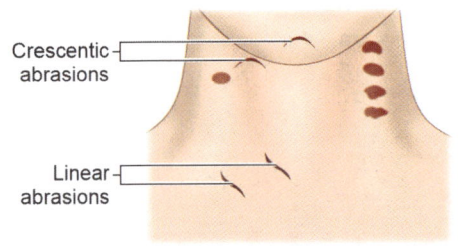

Fig. 16.2: Fingertip bruising and nail scratches seen in throttling.

Throttling
- The cause of death in throttling is asphyxia due to obstruction of respiration.
- Findings seen in case of throttling/manual strangulation are shown in **Figure 16.2**.

Drowning
Type of violent asphyxial death where entry of air into lungs is prevented due to submersion of mouth and nostrils into water or any liquid medium.

Types

Typical drowning (Wet drowning)	Atypical drowning
• Fresh water drowning • Sea water drowning	• Dry drowning • Immersion syndrome • Near drowning • Shallow water drowning

Atypical Drowning
1. **Dry drowning:** As soon as water enters the lungs, laryngeal spasm occurs leading to asphyxia.
2. **Immersion syndrome (hydrocution):** Cold water stimulates the vagus resulting in cardiac arrest.
3. **Near drowning (2° drowning):** Person does not dies of drowning, rather dies of complications, such as pneumonia, electrolyte imbalance.
4. **Shallow water drowning:** When an unconscious person drowns even when there is little amount of water.

Near Hanging/Attempted Strangulation

- Near-hanging is a situation in which patients survive a hanging injury long enough to reach the ED **(Figs. 16.3A and B)**.
- Several populations are at risk of hanging or strangulation like *toddlers* (neck may get caught and strangled in ill-constructed cribs) *adolescents* (accidental hanging, throttling or strangulation due to 'choking game' or in playground), *adults* (autoerotic accidents, sex-related assaults and suicidal depression, and in prisons) and in *elderly* (suicidal hanging due to depression).

Signs and Symptoms
The clinical presentations in near hanging can vary according to the age and sex of the victim, and the method, force and duration of asphyxiation.
a. Dysphonia or hoarseness of voice.
b. Dysphagia or difficulty in swallowing
c. Dyspnea is very common, but often a late development.

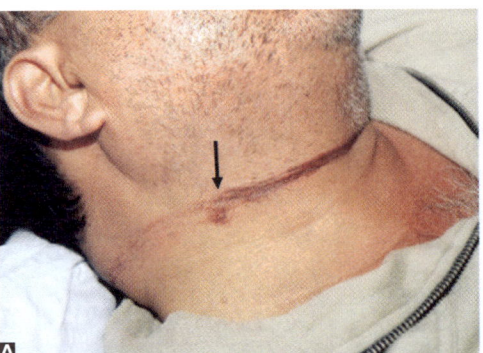
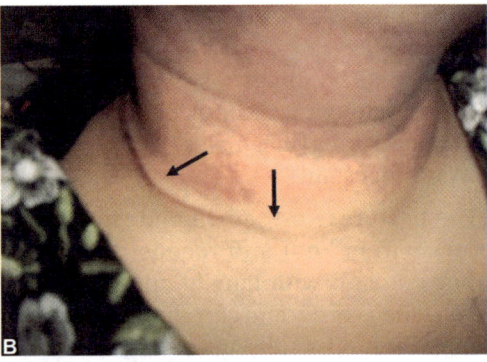

Figs. 16.3A and B: (A) Survivor of near hanging (arrow shows the point of knot); and (B) Survivor of chain-snatching (arrows show the impression mark of chain that she was wearing).

d. Pain and swelling in the throat or neck is common after attempted strangulation.
e. **Altered mental status:** Restlessness, confusion, loss of orientation or combativeness due to cerebral hypoxia.
f. **Neurologic symptoms** such as changes in vision, tinnitus, ptosis, facial droop, or unilateral weakness, paralysis or loss of sensation.
g. **Petechiae** can occur at or above the area of compression, and are most frequently seen on the face, periorbital region, eyelids, scalp and conjunctiva.
h. **Neck:** Injury to the soft tissues in the neck may manifest with abrasions (scratches), hyperemia, ecchymoses and edema.
   - *Attempted manual strangulation:* Fingertips may produce faint oval or discoid bruises 1.5–2 cm in size (may be more in case of continued bleeding or confluent bruises).
   - *Attempted ligature strangulation or hanging:* Ligature marks may be subtle or hidden within the natural skin folds of the neck.
i. **Lungs:** Aspiration pneumonitis may occur due to inhalation of vomitus. Pulmonary edema is common in comatose hanging victims.
j. Involuntary urination or defecation, expulsion of fetus (if pregnant) may occur.

Medico-legal Importance

- Healthcare practitioner who examine such cases in the emergency have to follow a protocol regarding the documentation of medico-legal formalities, besides imparting treatment in order to save the life of patient.
- Injuries due to assault are required to be informed to the police (if police is not accompanying) to ensure safe disposition of the patient. In case of suspected child abuse, child protective agency should be notified.

Autoerotic Asphyxia/Sexual Asphyxia

Definition: It is a paraphilia, when a person develops partial asphyxia in his own body by means to enhance sexual arousal.

Methods of Producing Sexual Asphyxia

- **Hanging:** Most frequent method
- Suffocation by plastic
- Manual pressure on carotid vessels
- Degree of asphyxia is produced by mechanical means is controlled (as after experiencing orgasm, constricting force around the neck is released but death may occur in some cases).
- It is seen in association with masochism.

CHAPTER 17

Forensic Toxicology

Definition of Poison

Poison is any substance in any form (solid, liquid, gas) which if introduced into the body through any route (injection, ingestion, inhalation, contact) will produce ill health or death by its local or constitutional effects or both.

Legal Aspects in Relation to Poisoning

- In law, the real difference between a medicine and a poison is the intent with which it is given. If the substance is given with the intention to save life, it is medicine, but if it is given with intention to cause bodily harm, it is a poison. The law does not make any difference between homicide by means of poisons and homicide by any other means (punishment is under **Sec. 302 IPC**).
- **Sec. 284 IPC** states that whoever causes hurt/injury with rash or negligent conduct with respect to poisonous substance shall be punished with imprisonment up to 6 months with/without fine (up to ₹ 1000).
- **Sec. 328 IPC** deals with administering of any poison, stupefying or intoxicating agent with the intent to cause hurt and facilitate the commission of an offense. Punishment is imprisonment up to 10 years and also fine.

Classification of Poisons

Poisons can be classified into six types as given below:

1. **C**orrosives	Strong acids	Mineral acids: HCl, HNO$_3$, H$_2$SO$_4$ Organic acid: Oxalic acid, carbolic acid (phenol)
	Strong alkalis	NaOH, KOH
	Metallic salts	Zinc chloride, ferric chloride
2. **I**rritants	Inorganic	Metallic: As, Pb, Hg, Cu Nonmetallic: Phosphorus
	Organic	Plants: *Abrus precatorius*, Castor, *Croton* Animals: Snakes, scorpions
	Mechanical	Powdered glass, diamond dust
3. **N**eurotics	Cerebral	Somniferous: Opium Inebriants: Alcohol Deliriants: *Datura*, cocaine, cannabis
	Spinal	Strychnine
	Peripheral	Curare

Contd....

Contd....

4. **C**ardiac	Digitalis, oleander, aconite, hydrocyanic acid			
5. **A**sphyxiants	CO, H_2S, CO_2			
6. **M**iscellaneous	a. **Agrochemicals**			
	Pesticides	Fumigants	Herbicides	Rodenticides
	OPC Carbamates	Alphos	Paraquat	Thallium sulfate Zinc phosphide
	b. **Drugs of dependence:** Antidepressants, hallucinogens c. **Petroleum products:** Kerosene, petrol d. **Food poisoning:** Bacterial, chemical			

Legal Duties of a Healthcare Provider in Case of Poisoning

- **In suspected case of poisoning:** It is the duty to inform the police in all cases (*in case of government medical officer*).
- **In case of private hospital/nursing home/clinic:** The healthcare provider should inform police/Magistrate only in case of **homicidal poisoning:** But he is not bound to inform police in case of suicidal/accidental poisoning *(but should inform all cases for his safety).*
- If the provider does not inform the police—he will be punished under **Sec. 176 IPC**.
- Note the preliminary particulars of the patient (name, identification marks, age, sex, occupation, etc.)
- **History:** He should take proper history of poisoning, if it is suicidal, homicidal or accidental or how much quantity taken.
- He should inform his senior doctor about the case.
- **Collection of evidence:** The forensic nurse should collect gastric lavage, food, vomitus, blood, urine, feces and preserve and then seal it properly, and then send it for chemical analysis in FSL. Failure to do so is punishable under **Sec. 201 IPC** (destruction of evidence).
- He should prepare MLC report with consent.
- If condition of patient is serious and about to die, he should inform the police and should make arrangements for Dying Declaration.
- In case the patient dies, he should not issue Death Certificate but instead send the body for postmortem examination.
- Any opinion regarding the nature/type of poison should be given only after getting the report from FSL.

General Principles of Treatment in Case of Poisoning

a. **Immediate resuscitation of the patient and maintain vitals**

A—Airway	Chin lift, suctioning of secretions to clear airway
B—Breathing	O_2 supply by bag and mask ventilation, ventilators, ET tube
C—Circulation	Measure BP, pulse, continuous ECG monitoring
D—Disability/CNS Depression	Corrected by drugs and IV fluids

b. **Removal of unabsorbed poison**

Injected poison	- Remove the sting in case of bee, wasp - Apply tourniquet or ice locally - Treat allergy and anaphylaxis
Contact poison	- Remove clothes - Wash the affected area with soap and water
Inhaled poison	- Remove the patient into fresh air - Start O_2 supplementation
Ingested poison	Gastric lavage with water/$KMnO_4$/activated charcoal is done to remove the unabsorbed poison from stomach with the help of Ryle's tube or orogastric tube

c. **Administration of antidotes:** Antidotes are substances that act specifically to counteract the action or poisonous effects of a toxic agent. The various types of antidotes are:

1. Physical antidotes	They neutralize the poison either by its mechanical action or by preventing its absorption. • *Activated charcoal:* It acts by adsorbing the poison on its surface; dose—50–100 g • *Demulcents:* Forms a protective layer over the gastric mucosa, thus preventing absorption of poison, e.g., aluminum hydroxide, magnesium hydroxide, milk
2. Chemical antidotes	They neutralize the poisons by reacting with it and forming a harmless compound. • $KMnO_4$ (1:5000)—oxidizes the poison and reduces itself (losing pink color). Effective against most of the alkaloids (opioids, barbiturates) • *Tannic acid*—used in lead, mercury, zinc poisoning • *Albumin*—used in mercury chloride and copper poisoning • *Tincture Iodine*—used in lead, mercury poisoning
3. Physiological antidotes	Antidotes act on the target cell and produces pharmacological effects exactly opposite to the action to those produced by poison, e.g., atropine for OPC poisoning
4. Chelating agents	They inactivate the metallic ions by forming a complex with the metallic poison which is soluble in water and excreted through urine, e.g., BAL, EDTA, desferrioxamine, penicillamine, etc.

d. **Removal of poison by excretion**

1. Forced diuresis by urine alkalinization	• Urine is made alkaline by use of sodium bicarbonate • Helps in promoting excretion of acidic drugs through urine • Done in salicylate, barbiturate poisoning
2. Forced diuresis by urine acidification	• Urine is made acidic by use of ammonium chloride • Helps in promoting excretion of alkaline drugs through urine • Done in poisoning/overdose of TCA, amphetamines, quinine
3. Whole bowel irrigation	Polyethylene glycol is given by nasogastric (NG) tube
4. Hemodialysis	Hemodialysis is done in: Lithium Alcohol Barbiturates Salicylates
5. Hemoperfusion	• Blood is circulated extracorporeally from an arterial source through a filter filled with activated charcoal and then back to patient's venous blood • Done in case of poisoning due to caffeine, barbiturates, mushroom
6. Diaphoretics	Increases excretion of drugs by increasing perspiration leading to increased excretion of toxic agents
7. Exchange transfusion	This involves slowly removing the poisoned patient's blood and replacing it with fresh donor blood or plasma, useful if antidote is not available

Gastric Lavage

- Gastric lavage is a method used for removal of unabsorbed poison from stomach (also called as *stomach wash*).
- Most effective—if used within 3 hours of ingestion of poison
- **Tubes used for gastric lavage**

Ryle's tube	Children
Ewald/Boas tube	Most commonly used in adults

- **Agents used for gastric lavage**

In case of children	Normal saline
In case of adults	• Tap water • 1: 5000 $KMnO_4$ • 4% Tannic acid

Procedure

Position of the patient	Left lateral position/Trendelenburg position (to reduce the chances of aspiration)
Insertion of tube	Till 50 cm mark (in case of adults) And 25 cm mark (in case of children)
Checking position of tube	Little air in a syringe is forced down the tube • Gurgling sounds heard through stethoscope placed over the stomach • If hissing sounds heard on other end—tube has entered trachea
Pouring of fluid	• After confirmation of tip of tube in the stomach, 250 mL of warm water is poured through the funnel • The first wash is preserved for chemical analysis

Contraindications of gastric lavage

Absolute contraindications	Relative contraindications
Corrosive poisoning—risk of perforation **(except carbolic acid poisoning)**	1. Convulsant poison (strychnine) 2. Comatose patient 3. Compromised unprotected airway 4. Kerosene/Volatile poisons 5. Esophageal varices

Whole Bowel Irrigation

- It is a method of removal of absorbed poison from GIT by excretion.
- In this method, PEG (polyethylene glycol) solution is given via NG tube (2 liters).
- While performing this, patient has to sit on the toilet seat.
- This method can flush out our entire GIT within 5 hours.
- **Criteria for its use**
  i. When activated charcoal is not able to adsorb the ingested poison
  ii. When enteric-coated drugs have been ingested
  iii. When some drug is ingested by body packers for illegal transport.

Body Packers

- **Definition:** The person who conceals and transports illicit/illegal drugs for the purpose of smuggling across countries by ingesting or inserting them into body cavities.
- For smuggling, drugs of high quality are packed commonly in condoms, foils, balloons. After reaching destination, the smuggler takes laxatives, defecates and then retrieves the packets from feces to deliver them to drug dealers.
- The body packers are usually detected and arrested at the airports and sent for the examination.

Medico-legal Importance

- Risk of toxicity in case drug packets rupture
- Acute intestinal obstruction

Drunkenness

Drunkenness is a consequence of drinking intoxicating liquors to such extent so as to reduce his capacity for rational action and conduct, and can be dangerous to himself or to others.

Preservation of Blood Sample in Case of Drunkenness

The blood alcohol concentration (BAC) is the most useful measure, as there is rapid equilibration across the blood-brain barrier; BAC reflects the concentration of alcohol currently affecting the brain.

- Soap and water (instead of spirit swab) is used to clean the site to be venepunctured.
- The blood is collected from antecubital or femoral vein using a disposable syringe.
- Blood container should be tightly stoppered to prevent loss of alcohol by evaporation, and labeled with name, date, time of taking the specimen and signature of the medical personnel.

Case Study Worksheets

Case Study 1

Mrs JS, a 29-year-old female presented to the ED two days after delivery. She complained of abdominal pain and some vaginal bleeding. The pregnancy was uncomplicated and baby was born through a normal vaginal delivery at a primary health center. On examination, the patient was pale and weak. Her vitals were: pulse 100/min feeble, BP was 80/60 mm Hg, temperature 37.1°C, RR 24/min. The attendant helped Mrs JS to the bathroom and noted the sanitary pad saturated with bright red blood. She and her husband both appeared very anxious.

Q1A. What do you think is happening to the patient?

_____
_____
_____
_____

Q1B. What should you anticipate and do in this situation? Why?

_____
_____
_____
_____

Case Study 2

Mr KM, a 65-year-old male, presented to the ED with chest pain which started about 20 mins after dinner. He described the pain as a "crushing pressure" located behind the mid of sternum and radiating down his left arm and to his back and lasted for few minutes. He rated the pain as 5/10. On examination, the patient was sweating profusely and pale, and complained of shortness of breath.

Q2A. What do you think the patient condition is due to? What intervention should you perform right away?

_____
_____
_____
_____

Q2B. Do you consider that failure to respond to the patient's complaints would amount to negligence?

_____
_____
_____
_____

Case Study 3

Mr LS, a 22-year-old male patient was brought to the ED after falling from a hostel balcony. He tried to jump from one balcony to another but fell down two stories. Upon arrival to the ED, he is awake, alert, and oriented. There are various abrasions and bruises from head to toe and a large swelling near his left temple.

Q3A. What assessments should you perform to best assist the patient and the police?

_____
_____
_____
_____

Q3B. What should the nurse be cognizant (knowledgeable) of caring for this patient?

_____
_____
_____
_____

Case Study 4

a. A 20-year-old girl was killed when she was caught in the crossfire between two rival gangs at war. The girl was crossing the road when the two groups started to fire indiscriminately. Another bystander was also injured in the shootout.

b. A 78-year-old elderly patient admitted in the psychiatric ward verbally abused a nurse, pulled her hair and scratched and bruised her, when she prevented him from leaving the hospital to go home in the middle of the night.

Q4A. How do you classify this act of violence?

a. _____

b. _____

Q4B. Briefly describe the types of violent acts.

_____
_____
_____
_____

Case Study 5

A 30-year-old female was stabbed to death in a garage. One bloodstained handkerchief was also found near the victim. Based on the bloodstain patterns and other evidence at the scene of crime, it was apparent that the killer had been injured during the incident.

Q5A. What precautions must be taken in collecting and preserving biological evidence?

_____

_____

_____

_____

Q5B. Why bloodstains need to be preserved?

_____

_____

_____

Case Study 6

Ms CK went to a fresher's party where she befriended Mr LK. She felt a little dizzy after consuming few drinks. LK offered her lift to the hostel. He had been really nice during the first few weeks of college, so CK was happy to have his help. In the car, which was parked in secluded place, LK pushed her down and proceeded to pull at her clothing. CK tried to protest but felt dizzy and could not seem to get any strength behind her protests. She remembered nothing after getting back to the hostel room. When CK's roommate came in, she narrated the incident to her who urged her to go to the hospital for an exam. She was reluctant, but eventually agreed to get an exam done. The nurse's made a complete documentation of CK's condition, and statements about the incident. She then took samples for a toxicology test in addition to other samples in the SAFE kit. The FSL report showed presence of semen and toxicology report found blood alcohol level of 80%. LK was accused of raping CK, but he claimed that she consented to, in fact initiated, sex after they left the party.

Q6A. Would you consider CK's incident as rape or sexual assault, or both? Explain.

_____

_____

Q6B. Do you consider the consent of CK as valid consent for sexual intercourse?

_____

_____

_____

_____

Case Study 7

"At about 11 pm, we went to bed and my husband who was drunk began to accuse me of cheating on him. He took a pillow and put it over my face. I could not breathe. I gasped for air. He then hit me over my face and took a rope and tried to strangle me. It hurt. He said he was going to kill me. He kept saying he was going to kill me and my family and our two daughters. I kicked him hard and ran out. He then sobered up asked for forgiveness repeatedly." The forensic nurse who took the history of this woman noted various abrasions, bruises and swelling, and included her statement in the treatment notes.

Q7A. Is this a case of interpersonal violence? If so, what type?

_____
_____

Q7B. What can be expected from the forensic nurse while appearing for the testimony?

_____
_____
_____
_____

Case Study 8

Ms AT a 16-year-old student goes to a government school in your locality. Her mother is a housekeeper and often leaves her to fend for herself in the evenings. Her father has passed away when she was very young and she has no siblings. Ms AT has been the victim of sexual abuse and assault by her mother's live-in partner. She came to visit the local clinic because she found out that she is pregnant as a result of the assaults. She did not want to address the issue of the sexual assault however, she wanted to get an abortion. Ms AT does not want to charge her mother's partner with anything and she definitely does not want the police involved. She also expressed how important it is that her mother does not find out about the incidents.

Q8A. What elements would you include in the patient's care plan? Mention in brief.

_____
_____
_____
_____

Q8B. How are the legal obligations of forensic nurse in reporting this incident?

_____
_____

Case Study 9

A 21-year-old pregnant female presented to the ED in critical condition following a car accident. She exhibited signs and symptoms of internal bleeding and was advised to have a blood transfusion and emergency surgery in an attempt to save her and the fetus. She refused to accept blood or blood products. Her refusal was based on a fear of blood transfusion due to her religious beliefs and faith.

Q9A. Do you think patient's autonomy should be respected, or ignore the patient's wishes and provide life-saving measures?

_____
_____

Q9A. What should the nurse do in such a situation?

Case Study 10
A 17-year-old girl came to the OPD and was diagnosed with a sexually transmitted infection (STI). She had relationships with few boys in the last 6 months. Although the doctor told her about her diagnosis privately, her mother who was in the waiting room and wanted to know what the doctor said. She told the doctor and nurse that she does not want anyone to know about the STI, including her mother.

Q10A. Do you think patient's confidentiality should be respected?

Q10B. Should the nurse discuss reproductive health and provide sex education to her?

Case Study 11
A 65 year old illiterate elderly lady was admitted for hysterectomy. The nurse on duty was instructed by the surgeon to have her signature in the consent form before the scheduled operation as he has already informed her of the operation. As she went to the ward with the consent form and met the patient, she noticed that the lady seemed confused about the operation and was unsure where or how to sign the paperwork. There was no near relative with the patient.

Q11A. Do you think the nurse should take her signature/thumb impression without delaying the procedure further as it is a busy day?

Q11B. What should the nurse do in such a situation?

Case Study 12

Mrs XY a 77-year-old elderly female diagnosed as stage 4 breast cancer with metastasis to the lungs was admitted in the ward with bronchopneumonia. Her condition is not very assuring. Mrs XY spoke with the nurse and conveyed her wishes for no life-saving measures including a DNR (Do Not Resuscitate). She does not have an Advance Directive in place. However, her children cannot agree on what treatment or life-saving measures are appropriate. Her family members want staff to exhaust all efforts to save her.

Q12A. What is an Advance Directive?

_____
_____
_____
_____

Q12B. What should the nurse do in such a situation?

_____
_____
_____
_____

Case Study 13

Mr MK was diagnosed with lung cancer 2 years ago. After chemotherapy, he experienced a brief remission but recently the cancer has recurred. His doctor informed his family that treatment will likely be unsuccessful and it may offer a few more months of life. His wife and their children are sceptical about telling Mr MK how bad his condition is, and the doctor has made no effort to talk to the patient about it. After his family left the hospital, he called for the nurse and asked her to tell him what the doctor said. Mr MK believes that he is not being told about his condition properly.

Q13A. Do you think the nurse should tell the patient's about his condition that could cause greater distress or use blanket answers to help decrease anxiety?

_____
_____
_____
_____

Q13B. What is "veracity" in context of ethical obligations of nurses?

_____
_____

Case Study 14

Mr KT a 20-year-old male college student came to the psychiatry OPD with complaints of sexual preoccupations. During adolescence, he developed a liking for observing others engage in sexual activity and followed couples to their homes in the hope of witnessing sexual intercourse. He masturbates on seeing that and achieves sexual gratification which he is incapable of experiencing otherwise. Mr KT informs that he has not yet been caught, but he expresses concern and embarrassment related to his actions. He came to consult as the frequency of this behavior has steadily increased.

Q14A. How do you classify this behaviour as?

Q14B. As a forensic nurse, are you going to report the patient to the police?

Case Study 15

A 79-year-old male patient was brought to the ED for evaluation after he fell down in the bathroom. He had a medical history of osteoporosis and dementia. The patient was irritated, confused, uncooperative and was able to walk independently but was unsteady. The nursing assessment was done and specific instructions to implement fall interventions, such as bed side rails up, call bell within the reach of patient and putting the patient close to nursing station were documented. The patient was sent for diagnostic CT scan head and X-rays of chest, pelvis and limbs. The results of diagnostic tests were negative. Following his return to the ED, the nurse helped the patient to the bathroom and left the room after returning the patient to his bed but forgot to put the side rails up and placing the bell within the reach of the patient. After about one hour, the housekeeping staff found the patient groaning in pain and laying on the floor next to his bed. The patient complained of pain in his left hip and left leg which was shortened, flexed and externally rotated. The patient was again sent for X-rays which confirmed fracture neck of left femur. Following his return, the patient was moved to a bed closer to the nursing station.

Q15A. What could have been done at the first place to prevent such an accident?

Q15B. Do you consider this as negligence on the part of nursing personnel?

Case Study 16

A patient who is a designer by profession was undergoing a surgical procedure under anesthesia. The patient informed that he had a carpal tunnel release operation of right hand (dominant hand) few weeks ago so he requested that the intravenous (IV) line be placed on his left hand. There were seven unsuccessful attempts made (documentation was not there) to insert the IV by two different nurses in the left hand. Ultimately, a cannula was successfully placed in volar aspects of the patient's right wrist. The patient complained of tingling pain and numbness of the wrist immediately after the insertion. The nurse did not verify or check whether the IV site was red, swollen or flushed easily. Following the procedure, the patient complained of pain and the IV cannula was removed. The following day, he noted difficulty in using his right hand and forearm, increased pain and decreased range of motion. He was diagnosed with complex regional pain syndrome. Since it was his dominant hand, he was unable to work and sued the nurse. There was lack in documentation concerning multiple attempts of cannula insertion.

Q16A. What should be done by the nurse in such a scenario?

_____
_____
_____
_____

Q16B. Do you consider this as negligence on the part of nursing personnel? Explain.

_____
_____
_____
_____

Case Study 17

Mr BK a 43-year-old alcoholic presented to the OPD with history diarrhea, abdominal cramping, and stomach pain. He is diagnosed with intestinal amebiasis. He is prescribed Tinidazole 2 g orally each day for 3 days. His previous medical notes indicated that he is allergic to metronidazole.

Q17A. What should be done by the nurse in such a scenario?

_____
_____
_____
_____

Q17B. What advise should the nurse give to the patient?

_____
_____

Case Study 18

Mr RM was coming back from his factory when his car was stopped and was attacked with rods and weapons by 2–3 persons wearing masks. They fled with his car leaving him bleeding profusely on the road. One of the passersby brought him to the hospital. He suffered the following injury on his head (**image**).

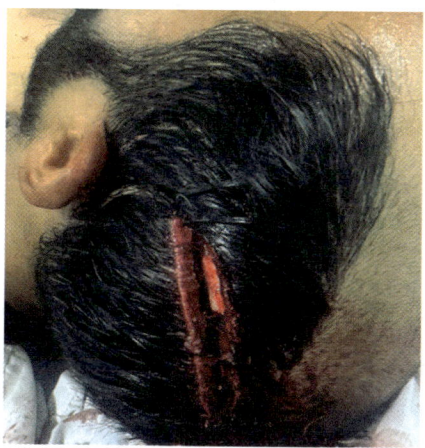

Q18A. Describe the injury seen in the image.

_____

_____

Q18B. What kind of weapon may have caused it and what is the nature of injury?

_____

_____

Case Study 19

Mr SN a 36-year-old tech personal was found unconscious in his bedroom which was bolted from inside. He recently had been laid off by his company and was having financial troubles. The following injuries were seen on his person when he was examined in the ED.

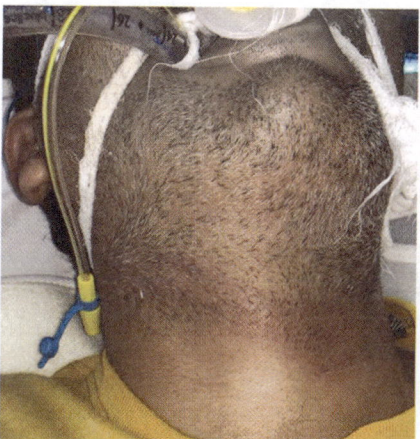
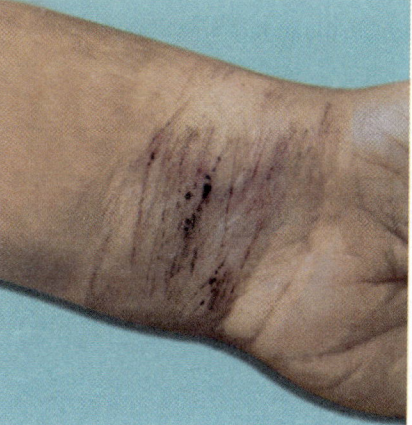

Q19A. Describe the injuries seen in the images. What do you think these injuries represent?

_____
_____
_____
_____

Q19B. Do you think the case is reportable to the police? If yes, why? If no, why not?

_____
_____

Case Study 20

Mrs RK a 31-year-old female presented to the ED after sustaining 2nd to 3rd degree burns when her clothes caught fire while working in the kitchen. She was unable to provide the history and the history was narrated by her sister-in-law. There was a strong smell of gasoline coming from her body and clothes. The diagram shows the surface area burnt.

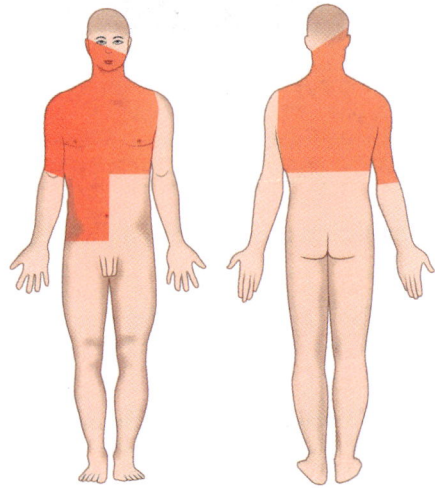

Q20A. Calculate the surface area involved using the rule of nine.

_____
_____

Q20B. What should be the legal duties of the forensic nurse?

_____
_____
_____
_____

Hint

1. The patient was bleeding per vaginum–she might have a tear or rupture in her uterus from her delivery 2 days ago. She was showing signs of shock because she is pale and weak and her pulses were feeble.

   Ms JS was decompensating due to hemorrhage. So, cross matching should be done immediately and arrangement for blood, blood products particularly packed RBCs and fluids are a must. Oxygen should be given.

2. Angina or myocardial infarction. Make him lie on bed and start oxygen—this can be done quickly and easily and can help to prevent further complications from low oxygenation. Oxygen helps to improve oxygenation as well as to decrease the myocardial oxygen demands. Often it takes a few minutes or more for medications to be available from the pharmacy, so it makes sense to take care of this intervention first.

   Yes, not responding immediately to the situation may lead to worsening of patient's condition.

3. Full head-to-toe assessment noting all injuries and documenting it properly along with photographs. Glasgow Coma Scale (GCS) and pupillary check and a focused neurological exam along with alcohol and drug screen. Also, assessment for suicidal ideation in case his fall was intentional.
   - To identify immediate neurologic emergencies (i.e., concussion and epidural hemorrhage which may have early symptoms of headache, dizziness, bloody or watery discharge from, nose or ear, lack of awareness of surroundings, and nausea and vomiting; these may immediately follow the head trauma or evolve gradually over several minutes to hours)
   - Recognition of neurologic sequelae (such as aphasia, ataxia, hemiplegia and quadriplegia)
   - Prevention of further injury and deterioration (use of cervical/neck collar)

4. a. Community violence. b. Workplace violence.
   - Who committed the violence—self-directed, interpersonal and collective
   - Nature—physical, sexual, family, domestic, workplace, etc.

5. Observe universal (standard) safety precautions and not to contaminate the samples. On clothing, wrap the item in clean paper, place the article in a brown paper bag and seal and label. Do not attempt to remove stains from the cloth. Place only one item in each bag. Do not use plastic containers. Blood in liquid pools should be picked up on a gauze pad or other clean sterile cotton cloth and allowed to air dry thoroughly, at room temperature. It should be refrigerated or frozen as soon as possible.

   Blood grouping can be done. DNA can be extracted from the stains and PCR analysis can be conducted. STR profiles generated from these samples can identify the culprit.

6. Both rape and sexual assault.

   A person cannot give consent if they are under the influence of alcohol or drugs. In such circumstances, even if the woman consents to a sexual relationship, it will not be considered valid or as an "excuse for committing rape." The court said in the case of rape, when a woman says "No" to sexual intercourse even once, it must signify she is unwilling.

7. Yes. Family violence—domestic violence—intimate partner violence.

   In addition to questions about the physical injuries, the nurse may be asked questions about the cause of the injuries and about battered woman syndrome. It will be primarily a fact-based testimony and sometimes can be confusing courtroom experience. Complete pretrial preparation with the public prosecutor would be more helpful. The victim may sometimes withdraw her statement.

8. Consider physical, mental, and emotional healthcare.

   The POCSO Act, and the Criminal Law Amendment Act, 2013 mandate healthcare providers to report sexual assault to the police and provide free treatment to the victim. Failure to do so shall evoke punishment with fine or imprisonment or both. So, the nurse needs to inform the police. Although mandatory disclosures by law are not considered to be professional misconduct, it may led to feeling of betrayal by the patients, breach of trust and rapport with the healthcare provider, deterrence from treatment, dropout from follow-up, stigmatization, and discrimination.

9. If a patient is major, alert, oriented, and understands the consequences of accepting or rejecting medical care or treatment, she/he may refuse that care.

   The nurse should document all the necessary information provided (in case of refusal of treatment) and the patient's response, including her reason for declining treatment. Proper documentation will protect the nurse from legal consequences if the patient or her family later feels treatment should have been provided.

10. It is common when nurses must determine whether it is appropriate to discuss a patient's medical information with a parent or guardian. Parents and guardians are allowed access to medical records for any patient under the age of eighteen. Currently, in many Western countries some laws allow minors to consent to care under certain conditions without parental knowledge, consent or access to their medical records. When an adolescent is old enough to give consent for healthcare, information pertaining to that care is typically considered confidential. In Indian context, information needs to be shared with mother as consent for MTP can be given by parents or guardian of patients who are below 18 years. Moreover, a registered medical practitioner (RMP) is obliged under the POCSO Act to report to the police when a minor approaches him/her for an abortion. In a recent ruling, the Supreme Court has stated that doctors are exempted from disclosing the identity of minors who have come in for an abortion to the police. The court opined that it is necessary to harmonize the provisions of the MTP and POCSO laws, thereby enabling minors to approach an RMP for abortion without the fear of exposure.

    Yes. Definitely, developmentally appropriate evidence-based sexual health education should be provided by the nurse that promotes healthy sexual development for adolescents.

11. No. All patients have the right to be fully explained and informed, and understand the treatment options and procedures before they are provided in a language he/she understands.

    Since, the patient appears to be confused and not sure, the nurse should again provide information in a way the patient understands, allowing her to ask questions and have the option to allow or refuse treatment. If the patient does not fully understand what the nurse is saying, the nurse should notify the doctor and ask him to explain the procedure, including anticipated outcomes and risks once more.

12. A legal document that states a person's wishes about receiving medical care if that person is no longer able to make medical decisions because of a serious illness or injury.

    If the patient is of sound mind and clearly understands her prognosis with and without treatment, she has the right to decide what treatment she does or does not want. The healthcare provider should encourage the patient to prepare an Advanced Directive. But the healthcare provider, patient or any relative cannot take any decision for DNR on their own. When patients have an Advanced Directive, healthcare providers know what the patient's wishes are if they become unresponsive and need interventions to sustain life. It also helps take the weight of difficult decisions from family members, which is important as loved ones may be influenced by emotions. In cases where there is no Advanced Directive in place, laws are there that allow for authority to be given to parents, guardians, a spouse, or another person who may apply for the same through the treating doctor. The nurse's primary responsibility is to her patient. Nurses must advocate for the autonomy and rights of patients. If an Advanced Directive is made, the responsibility of following her wishes is easier.

13. Treating doctors are recognized as the decision-makers for patients and determine whether to withhold information based on whether they thought the information would cause undue stress or more harm than good. However, patients have a right to know about their own diagnosis and prognosis. The doctor is responsible for notifying the patient of his diagnosis. But, nurses are more likely to encounter the patient face-to-face and are often the ones the patients look to for clarification. It is best to answer questions as carefully and caringly as possible. If the nurse is unsure of the appropriate answer, the question should be deferred to the patient's doctor.

    Veracity is the principle of telling the truth and is related to the principle of autonomy. Veracity is the basis of trust in the "nurse-patient" relationship. Veracity enables meaningful treatment goals and expectations.

14. Paraphilic disorder.

    Although he admitted to stalking and voyeurism, the healthcare provider need not inform the police as no crime has been committed and there is no section of IPC or CrPC so as to make it reportable.

15. The patient should have been shifted closer to the nursing station along with placement of side rails of bed and call bell by his side, when it was anticipated that some untoward incident may happen with elderly patients.

    Yes. The patient needed close monitoring and additional staff should be there to take care of such high risk patients. In this case, documentation showed that the patient was difficult to handle and there's was the need for additional monitoring to minimize the risk of fall and keep the patient safe.

16. Due care should have been taken as he was a high-risk patient. There was no need to use the right hand for IV cannula. The nurse should have checked to ensure proper insertion of IV cannula and addressed the patient's complaints with adequate documentation.

    Yes. The nurses were unable to locate the vein to put the cannula and multiple attempts made which was not documented. This may show as lack of competency. There was breach in nursing standard of care and deviation in patient care. There was overall lack of proper and concise documentation. But whether the complex regional pain syndrome is due this cannula needs to be justified.

17. The nurse has an ethical obligation to advocate for the patient's safety and well-being. Administering a medication that is contraindicated could cause harm to the patient. The nurse should notify the physician of the history of allergy and to suggest an alternative medication.

    The nurse should advise the patient that she is verifying the doctor's order because of his drug allergy and ask him to wait until the order is confirmed or changed.

18. Chop wound.

    Moderately heavy sharp weapon/object. Grievous in nature (fracture pieces of bone can be seen).

19. Faint ligature mark of hanging and superficial incised wound. Suicidal intent.

    In case of Government Medical Officer: It is the duty of the doctor to inform the police in all cases, whether suicidal, accidental or homicidal. In case of private medical practitioner, he should inform Police/Magistrate only if the case is homicidal. He is not bound to inform police in case of suicidal/accidental cases (but should inform all cases for his safety).

20. Half of the head/neck—4.5%; Top half of front torso—9%; Top half of back—9%; Full top half of right arm—4.5%; Half of front abdomen—4.5%.

    She should provide life-saving measures, document the injuries sustained, preserve the evidences (clothing, blood, hair sample), inform the police, record the information provided and take the informant's signature, if she is about to die, she can record the dying declaration without waiting for the Magistrate.

Appendix

Police Intimation Form

Ref. No.: _____   Date _____ 2000
                                                     Time _____
         The Sub-Inspector of Police/SHO   Hosp No. _____
              _____ Police Station   Inpatient No. _____

Sub: Intimation Regarding Medico-legal Case

Dear sir/madam,
Mr/Mrs/Miss _____aged about
_____ years said to be normally residing at the below mentioned address has come to the Emergency Medicine Department of this hospital with a history of _____
                         (as stated by the patient/attendant)

The Patient
- ☐ Does not require admission and so is being permitted to go home immediately/by _____ am/pm
- ☐ Is being admitted to the hospital in _____ ward _____ floor _____
- ☐ Is in a serious condition Please come and record the statement Immediately
- ☐ Has expired on _____ at _____
                         Date   Time
- ☐ Has absconded from the hospital on _____
                                              Date
- ☐ Is being discharged from the hospital on _____
                                              Date

Patient's residential address   Kindly do the needful
_____   Yours faithfully
_____   Signature
_____   Name
Site of accident if (any) known   Designation
Intimation received by the police on _____ at _____
                                                  (Date) _____ (Time)

Seal of Police

Brought Dead Cases

Ref. No.:   Place

                                                              Date:

                                                              Time:

To: The Sub-Inspector of Police/SHO

                 _____ Police Station

Sir,
This is to inform you that the below mentioned has been brought dead to the Casualty/Trauma Center of this Hospital on _____ at _____ AM/PM from _____

Name: _____

Age: _____ Sex: _____

S/O or D/O or W/O: _____

Address: _____
_____

Identification marks/Left thumb impression of the deceased are given below:

(i) _____

(ii) _____

The dead body is preserved in the hospital mortuary. Please communicate with the in-charge of the mortuary and do the needful.

                                              Signature:

Left thumb impression   Name:

(of the deceased)   Reg No.

                                              Designation:

                                              Address:

                                              Official Seal:

Copy to In-Charge Mortuary

Note: On receipt of this letter the Police will register the case and prepare First Information Report (FIR) and arrange for Police Inquest and send the body for Medico-legal Autopsy.

Medical History and Examination Form—Sexual Violence

1. GENERAL INFORMATION

First Name		Last Name	
Address			
Sex	Date of birth (dd/mm/yy)		Age
Date/time of examination	/	In the presence of	

In case of a child include: Name of school, name of parents or guardian

2. THE INCIDENT

Date of incident:			Time of incident:		
Description of incident (survivor's description)					
Physical violence	Yes	No	*Describe type and location on body*		
Type (beating, biting, pulling hair, etc.)					
Use of restraints					
Use of weapon(s)					
Drugs/alcohol involved					
Penetration	Yes	No	Not sure	*Describe (oral, vaginal, anal, type of object)*	
Penis					
Finger					
Other (describe)					
	Yes	No	Not sure	*Location (oral, vaginal, anal, other)*	
Ejaculation					
Condom used					

If the survivor is a child, also ask: Has this happened before? When was the first time? How long has it been happening? Who did it? Is the person still a threat? Also ask about bleeding from the vagina or the rectum, pain on walking, dysuria, pain on passing stool, signs of discharge, any other sign or symptom.

3. MEDICAL HISTORY

After the incident, did the survivor	Yes	No		Yes	No
Vomit?			Rinse mouth?		
Urinate?			Change clothing?		
Defecate?			Wash or bath?		
Brush teeth?			Use tampon or pad?		
Contraception use					
Pill			IUD	Sterilization	
Injectable			Condom	Other	
Menstrual/obstetric history					
Last menstrual period (dd/mm/yy)			Menstruation at time of event Yes ☐ No ☐		
Evidence of pregnancy Yes ☐ No ☐			Number of weeks pregnant .... weeks		
Obstetric history					
History of consenting intercourse (only if samples have been taken for DNA analysis)					
Last consenting intercourse within a week prior to the assault	Date (dd/mm/yy)		Name of individual:		
Existing health problems					
History of female genital mutilation, type					
Allergies					
Current medication					

Vaccination status	Vaccinated	Not vaccinated	Unknown	Comments
Tetanus				
Hepatitis B				
HIV/AIDS status			Unknown	

4. MEDICAL EXAMINATION

Appearance (clothing, hair, obvious physical or mental disability)			
Mental state (calm, crying, anxious, cooperative, depressed, other)			
Weight:	Height:	Pubertal stage (pre-pubertal, pubertal, mature):	
Pulse rate:	Blood pressure:	Respiratory rate:	Temperature:

Physical findings
Describe systematically, and draw on the attached body pictograms, the exact location of all wounds, bruises, petechia, marks, etc. Document type, size, color, form and other particulars. Be descriptive, do not interpret the findings.

Head and face	Mouth and nose
Eyes and ears	Neck
Chest	Back
Abdomen	Buttocks
Arms and hands	Legs and feet

5. GENITAL AND ANAL EXAMINATION

Vulva/scrotum	Introitus and hymen	Anus
Vagina/penis	Cervix	Bimanual/rectovaginal examination

Position of patient (supine, prone, knee-chest, lateral, mother's lap)	
For genital examination:	For anal examination:

6. INVESTIGATIONS DONE

Type and location	Examined/sent to laboratory	Result

7. EVIDENCE TAKEN

Type and location	Sent to.../stored	Collected by/date

8. TREATMENTS PRESCRIBED

Treatment	Yes	No	Type and Comments
STI prevention/treatment			
Emergency contraception			
Wound treatment			
Tetanus prophylaxis			
Hepatitis B vaccination			
Post-exposure prophylaxis for HIV			
Other			

9. COUNSELLING, REFERRALS, FOLLOW-UP

General psychological status
Survivor plans to report to police OR has already made report   Yes ☐   No ☐
Survivor has a safe place to go to   Yes ☐   No ☐   Has someone to accompany her/him Yes ☐ No ☐
Counseling provided:
Referrals
Follow-up required
Date of next visit

Name of health worker conducting examination/interview: _____

Title: _____ **Signature:** _____ **Date:** _____

Source: **WHO, UNFPA, UNHCR. 2004.** "Clinical Management of Rape Survivors: Developing Protocols for use with Refugees and Internally Displaced Persons—Revised Edition," pgs. 44-47.

Appendix

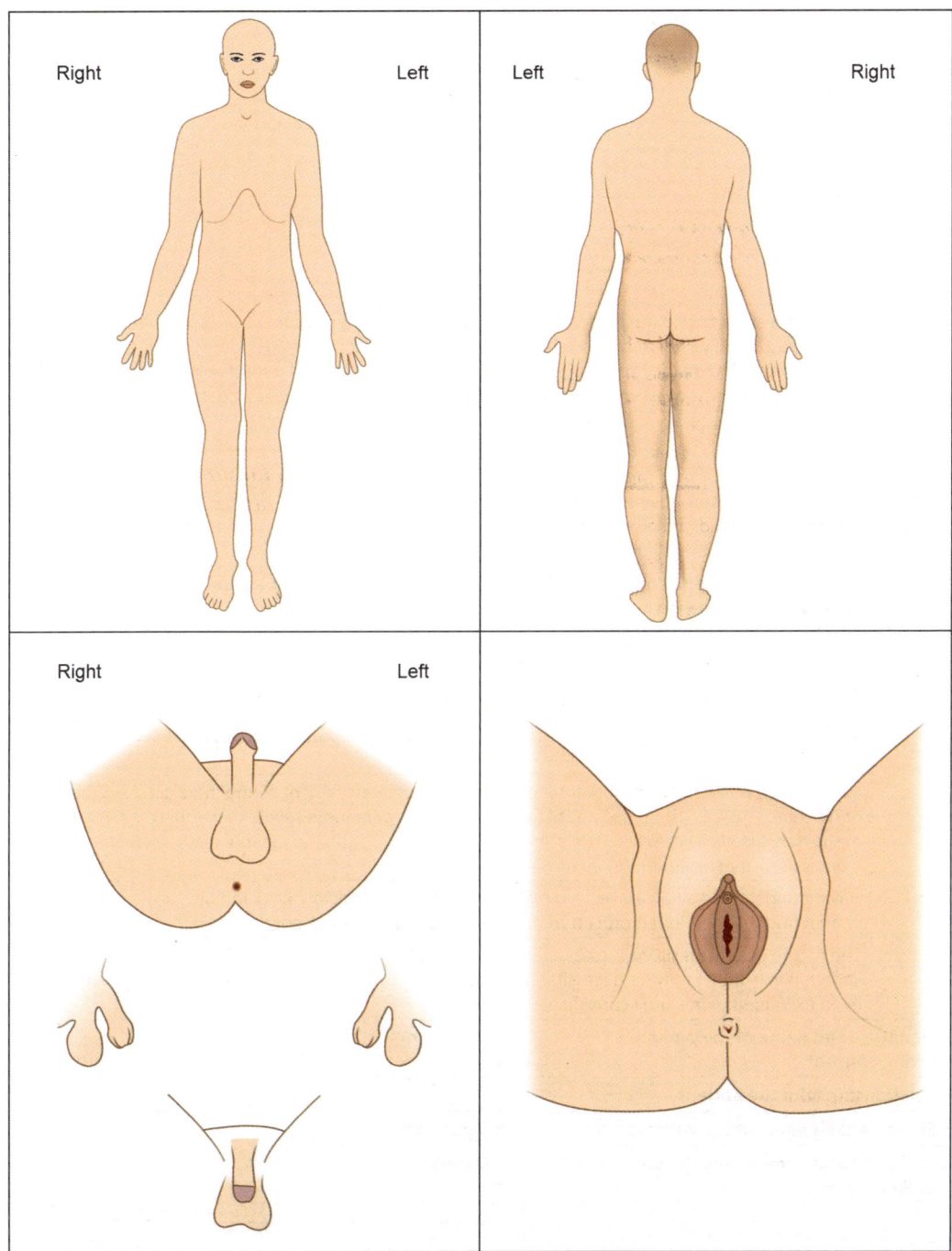

Informed Consent Form—General Surgery

Patient's name			UID	
Gender		Age	Ward/Bed No.	
Sl. No.	Description			

Sl. No.	Description
1.	I here by authorize Dr .... and those whom he may designate as associated or assistants, to perform upon .... (Myself or name of patients when the consent is being given by an authorized person), the following .... (Name of operation/procedure)
2.	It has been explained to me that during the operation/treatment/procedure, unforeseen condition may encountered which may necessitate surgical or other procedure in addition to or different from those contemplated I therefore further authorized the above named doctor and his designate to perform such additional surgical or other procedure as are deemed necessary by them
3.	Following has been fully explained to me and I have understood the same: 1. The nature and procedure at the operation and/or procedure 2. Expected outcome of this procedure/operation 3. The possible alternative to his method of treatment 4. The risk involved in the treatment and 5. The kinds and possibilities of complications
4.	It has been explained to me that risk at the operation/procedure in my case in high/low (..........%) because of the following factors: 1. .... 2. .... 3. ....
5.	I understand that if I need blood or blood products these carry risk of contracting HIV/AIDS, hepatitis or reactions, such as the symptoms of fever, chills, hives or in more severe reactions, the destruction of the transfused red cells (Hemolytic Transfusion Reaction), antibody stimulation, bacterial infections or, in rare situations, death.
6.	Having understood all of above, I am ready to lake the high risk involved and give my consent for conducting the mentioned procedure/operation upon me/my patient
7.	The nature of anesthesia viz .... (General/spinal/local/other), the possible variation in it, if that may be necessitated at the time of operation/procedure, and risk involved has been explained to me and I consent for the same
Signature and name of the person giving consent	Date/Time	
Relationship with the patient		
Signature and name of the witness	Date/Time	
Signature and name of the doctor taking consent	Date/Time	

References and Further Reading

1. Amar AF, Sekula LK. A practical guide to forensic nursing. Indianapolis: Sigma Theta Tau International; 2016.
2. Baxter Jr E. Complete crime scene investigation handbook. Boca Raton: CRC Press; 2015.
3. Bell S. A dictionary of forensic Science. Oxford University Press. New York 2012. Available from: https://www.google.co.in/books/edition/A_Dictionary_of_Forensic_Science/P1hEpzq-9HIC?hl=en&gbpv=1&dq=define+evidence+forensic&printsec=frontcover
4. Berishaj K, Boyland CM, Reinink K, Lynch V. Forensic nurse hospitalist: The comprehensive role of the forensic nurse in a hospital setting. J Emerg Nurs. 2020; 46:286-93.
5. Bhan A, Rohatgi M. Legal systems in India: overview. Available from: https://uk.practicallaw.thomsonreuters.com/w-017-5278?transitionType=Default&contextData=(sc.Default)&firstPage=true
6. Biswas G. Review of forensic medicine and toxicology. New Delhi: Jaypee Brothers Health Sciences Publishers; 2021.
7. Constantino RE, Crane PA. Young SE. Forensic nursing. Evidence-based principles and practice. Philadelphia: FA Davis Company; 2013.
8. Constitution of India. Available from: https://byjus.com/free-ias-prep/constitution-of-india-an-overview/
9. Darnell C, Michel C. Forensic notes. Philadelphia: FA Davis company; 2012.
10. Dash SK, Patel S, Chavali K. Forensic nursing—global scenario and Indian perspective. J Forensic Leg Med. 2016; 42:88-91.
11. Dougherty CM, Nursing. In: Siegel J, Knupfer G, Saukko PJ (Eds). Encyclopaedia of Forensic Sciences. London: Academic Press; 2000. p. 1123-28.
12. Ethical practice: NCLEX-RN. Available from: www.registrednursing.org
13. Finn C. Forensic nurses' experiences of receiving child abuse disclosures. J Spec Pediatr Nurs. 2011; 16:252-62.
14. Forensic nursing. Available from: https://forensicnursing.weebly.com/a-historical-perspective.html
15. Fundamental Rights. India Book 2020—A reference annual. Available from: https://knowindia.india.gov.in/profile/fundamental-rights.php#:~:text=Article%2012%20to%2035%20contained,opportunity%20in%20matters%20of%20employment.
16. Garg P, Das M, Goyal LD, Verma M. Trends and correlates of intimate partner violence experienced by ever-married women of India: results from National Family Health Survey round III and IV. BMC Public Health. 2012;21:2021. Available from: https://doi.org/10.1186/s12889-021-12028-5
17. Ghofrani KF, Manoochehri H, Mohtashami J, Kiani M. Consequences of presence of forensic nurses in health care system: A qualitative study. Iran J Nurs Midwifery Res. 2020; 25:195-201.

18. Gorea R, Lynch V. Forensic nursing—a boon to the society. JPAFMAT. 2003; 3:32-36.
19. Guidelines for forwarding crime exhibits. Forensic science laboratory. Govt. of NCT of Delhi. 2016. Available from: https://districts.ecourts.gov.in/sites/default/files/GUIDELINES%20FOR%20FORWARDING%20CRIME%20EXHIBITS%281%29_2.pdf
20. Harish D, Chavali KH. The medico-Legal case—Should we be afraid of it? Anil Aggrawal's Internet Journal of Forensic Medicine and Toxicology [serial online], 2007; Vol. 8, No. 1 (January - June 2007): [about 15 p]. Available from: http://anilaggrawal.com/ij/vol_008_no_001/others/pg/pg001.html. Published : May 11, 2007, (Accessed: April 03, 2023)
21. Haryana Medicolegal Manual 2012. Health dept Haryana. Available from: https://kaithal.haryanapolice.gov.in/writereaddata/Images/pdf/pkl96.pdf
22. Houck MM, Crispino F, McAdam T. The Forensic Team. In: The Science of Crime Scenes. Elsevier: Philadelphia. 2018; p. 71-84.
23. Houck MM, Siegel JA. Fundamentals of forensic science. 3rd ed. Oxford: Elsevier. 2015. https://main.mohfw.gov.in/sites/default/files/953522324.pdf
24. Indian Nursing Council (MSc in Forensic Nursing Program), Regulations; 2020.
25. Indian Nursing Council. The gazette of India Extraordinary part III—section 4 published by authority (to be gazetted). Available from: https://www.indiannursingcouncil.org/uploads/pdf/16467408926898102536227459cf3aa2.pdf
26. Johnson D. Forensic evidence preservation: the emergency nurses' role. Aust Emerg Nurs J. 1997;1:37-40.
27. Kaur S. Rights of accused persons. Legal Service India. E-Journal. Available from: https://www.legalserviceindia.com/legal/article-219-rights-of-accused-persons.html
28. Ladd M, Seda J. Sexual assault evidence collection. In: StatPearls. Treasure Island (FL): StatPearls Publishing; 2023.
29. Lawler MJ, Talbot EB. Child abuse. In: Ramachandran VS (Ed). Encyclopedia of human behavior. 2nd ed. London: Academic Press; 2012. p. 460-66.
30. Legg MJ. What is psychosocial care and how can nurses better provide it to adult oncology patients. AJAN. 2010; 28(3):61-67.
31. Lynch S, Varela R. Forensic evidence collection for nurses. AMN Healthcare Education Services; 2014.
32. Lynch VA, Duval JB. Forensic nursing science. 2nd ed. St Louis Missouri: Mosby; 2011.
33. Lynch VA, Maguire K. The foundation and future of forensic nursing science. Forensic nursing science: a global health initiative in developing and developed countries. In: Gorea RK. 2021
34. Mailhes J, Yarrarapu SNS, Callahan AL. Sexual assault clothing collection and documentation. In: StatPearls. Treasure Island (FL): StatPearls Publishing; 2022.
35. Mauro J. Role and responsibilities of forensic nursing. Glob J Nurs Forensic Stud. 2022; 6:183.
36. McMahon JR. Collection, packaging and submission of forensic evidence. Onondaga County Executive. Available from: http://www.ongov.net/health/forensic/documents/EvidenceCollectionSubmissionManual.pdf
37. Medicolegal Manual. Govt of Punjab 2018. Available from: https://health.punjab.gov.in/sites/default/files/Punjab%20Medicolegal%20Manual%20jan30.pdf
38. Ministry of Health & Family Welfare. Guidelines & protocols. Medico-legal care for survivors/victims of sexual violence. 2014. Available from:
39. National Human Rights Commission (NHRC). Available from: https://byjus.com/free-ias-prep/national-human-rights-commission/#:~:text=Functions%20%26%20Powers%20of%20NHRC&text=NHRC%20can%20investigate%20any%20complaints,of%20violation%20of%20Human%20Rights.

40. NSPCC. Sexual abuse. Available from: https://www.nspcc.org.uk/what-is-child-abuse/types-of-abuse/child-sexual-abuse/
41. Nursing jurisprudence. Available from: ictionary.thefreedictionary.com
42. Nursing jurisprudence. Available from: mpedia.com
43. Padmakumari SVL. A study to assess the knowledge regarding the need of forensic nursing in emergency department among the staff nurses in a selected hospital at Visakhapatnam, Andhra Pradesh. IJSR. 2022; 12: 217-31.
44. Patil MR. Fundamentals of forensic science. Bilaspur: Shashwat Publications. 2021.
45. Pavithra V, Muralidhar R. Victim rights in India: Is the focus of the criminal justice system shifting from the accused to the victim? IJLMH. 2021; 4 (2):774-81.
46. Peel M. Opportunities to preserve forensic evidence in emergency departments. Emerg Nurse. 2016; 24:20-26.
47. Personnel duties and responsibilities. Available from: https://www.crime-scene-investigator.net/respon2.html
48. Peter R, Sharma SK. National nursing and midwifery commission bill: hopes and challenges. J Med Evid. 2022; 3:55-59.
49. Professional misconduct. Available from: www.cno.org
50. Rahmqvist J. Forensic care for victims of violence and their family members in the emergency department. Linnaeus University press Växjö. Linnaeus University Dissertations No 337/2018
51. RAINN. Child sexual abuse. Available from: https://www.rainn.org/articles/child-sexual-abuse
52. Report submitted by UN human rights bodies, global-database.unwomen.org
53. Rutherford A, Zwi AB, Grove NJ, Butchart A. Violence: a glossary. J Epidemiol Community Health 2007; 61:676-80.
54. Scannell MJ. Fast facts about forensic nursing. What you need to know. New York: Springer; 2019.
55. Sekula LK. Forensic documentation and testimony. A practical guide to forensic nursing. In: Amar AF, Sekula Lk (Eds). Indianapolis: Sigma Theta Tau International; 2016. p. 285-302.
56. Shalini S. What are the rights of the accused person in India? Available from: https://www.myadvo.in/blog/rights-of-accused-in-india/
57. Sharma S, Joseph J. The paradigm of forensic nursing for nursing aspirants in India: Promises, caveats & future directions. J Forensic Legal Med. 2022; 86:1023-21.
58. Siegel JA. Crime scene investigation and examination: collection and chain of evidence. In: Siegel J, Knupfer G, Saukko PJ (Eds). Encyclopaedia of Forensic Sciences. London: Academic Press; 2000. p. 409-12.
59. Silva JOM, Santos LFS, Santos SMD, Silva DPD, Santos VS, Melo CMD. Preservation of forensic evidence by nurses in a prehospital emergency care service in Brazil. J Trauma Nurs. 2020; 58-62.
60. Silva RX, Ferreira CAA, Sá GGM, Souto RQ, Barros LM, Galindo-Neto NM. Preservation of forensic traces by nursing in emergency services: a scoping review. Rev Lat Am Enfermagem. 2022; 30: e3593.
61. Singh HN. Collection, preservation and transportation of biological evidence for forensic DNA analysis. IJARESM, 2021; 9:1123-30.
62. Sobti PC, Biswas G. Sexual abuse in children. In: Gupte S (ed). Recent Advances in Pediatrics. Vol 13; New Delhi: Jaypee Brothers. 2003; p. 406-25.
63. Subashini SP, Verma S, Kaur S. Forensic Nursing. Indian J Forensic Med Pathol. 2021; 14:237-39.
64. Suri S, Mona, Sarkar D. Domestic violence and women's health in India: Insights from NFHS-4. Observer Research Foundation. 2022. Available from: orfonline.org
65. The Gazette of India Extraordinary. The protection of children from sexual offences Act, 2012.

66. The Gazette of India Extraordinary. The protection of children from sexual offences (Amendment) Act, 2019. theory of forensic nursing care: A middle-range theory. J Forensic Nurs. 2020;16:188-98.
67. Topcu ET, Kazan EE. The opinions of senior nursing students about forensic nursing. Egypt J Forensic Sci. 2018:1-7.
68. Trace evidence recovery guidelines. Scientific working group on materials analysis (SWGMAT). Evidence Committee; 1998. Available from: https://www.nist.gov/system/files/documents/2016/09/22/trace_evidence_recovery_guidelines.pdf
69. United Nations Human rights. Declaration of Basic Principles of Justice for Victim of Crime and Abuse of Power; 1985.
70. Valentine JL. Evolution of forensic nursing theory—Introduction of the constructed
71. WHO: Injuries and violence. 19 Mar 2021. Available from: https://www.who.int/news-room/fact-sheets/detail/injuries-and-violence
72. Wikipedia. Forensic nursing. Available from: https://en.wikipedia.org/wiki/Forensic_nursing#Worldwide
73. Wikipedia: Violence. Available from: https://en.m.wikipedia.org/wiki/Violence
74. Yesodharan R, Shehata SA, Jose TT, Hagras AM, Nayak V. Medico-legal history taking from the victims of sexual assaults: the role of nurse examiners. Egypt J Forensic Sci. 2022; 12:24.
75. Yesodharan R, Shehata SA, Jose TT. Medico-legal history taking from the victims of sexual assaults: the role of nurse examiners. Egypt J Forensic Sci. 2022; 12:24.
76. Yukta K. Rights of victims in Indian criminal justice system. Legal Service India. E-Journal. Available from: https://www.legalserviceindia.com/legal/article-5591-rights-of-victims-in-indian-criminal-justice-system.html

Index

Page numbers followed by *b* refer to box, *f* refer to figure, *fc* refer to flowchart, and *t* refer to table.

A

Abdomen 142
    scar on 161*f*
Abdominal pain, severe 62
Abortion, unsafe 62
Abrasion 129, 130*f*, 131
    healing of 129
    imprint 129
    linear 129
    pressure 129
    types of 129
Abuse
    economic 20
    emotional 19, 20, 26
    in domestic violence, types of 20*f*
    physical 26
    psychological 20
    spouse 20
    types of 26
    verbal 26
Accidental marks 160
Accountability 38
Accused person 98*f*
    post-trial rights of 99
    pre-trial rights of 98
Act, salient features of 113*fc*
Active listening techniques 53
Additional swabs 87
Addressing survivor's emotional wellbeing 71
Admission and discharge 55
Adolescents survivors, dealing with 71
Advisory powers 37
Age, medico-legal importance of 157
Agoraphobia 168
Algor mortis 147, 152
Anal intercourse, victim of 165
Angina 191
Animal hair 160
Animation, suspended 143
Anthropology division 12
Antidotes, administration of 177
Apnea test 144
Artificial intelligence 13
Asphyxia 146
    cardinal signs of 171
    conditions 171
    positional 173
    signs of 172
    traumatic 172
Assault 43
    classification of 23
Assist forensic team 55
Attempted ligature strangulation 175
Attempted manual strangulation 175
Auditory hallucination 167
Autoerotic asphyxia 175
Autopsy
    pathological 140
    team, member of 50
Avulsion laceration 132

B

Bacterial action 151
Bail 109
Bailable offenses 109
Ballistic 11
    expert 49
Battered wife syndrome 21
Bed 82
Behavior signs 27
Behavioral characteristics 162
Biological evidence 79
Biological samples, forwarding of 91
Biological stains 83
Bite marks 86, 86*f*, 160
    self-inflicted 160

Black eye 131f
Bleeding per vaginum 191
Blood 14, 69, 83, 84, 163
    collection 83
    sample 83f, 85f
        drawing of 85f
    vessels 131
Bloodstain pattern analysts 49
Body
    chart 54
    packers 179
Bomb technician 49
Bone 156
    carpals 156
    clavicle 156
    femur 156
    fibula 156
    fragmented 155
    hip 156
    humerus 156
    ossification centers of 156t
    radius 156
    tibia 156
    ulna 156
Borrowed servant doctrine 124
Brain 152
    death, criteria of 144
    function of 147
    parts of 144f
Brainstem death
    certification 144
    diagnosis of 144
    Minnesota criteria of 144
Brainstem reflexes, absence of 144
Bruise 130, 131, 131f
    deep 130
    delayed 130
    ectopic 130
    patterned 130, 131f
    tire tread 135f
Buccal epithelial cells 83
Buccal swabs 83, 163
    collection of 84f
Buggery 24
Bullet 87, 88, 136f
    preservation of 88f
Burking 172
Burn 90, 137
    classification of 137, 138t
    injury 137f
    thermal 137
Burning micturition 62

C

Cadaveric spasm 149
Caffey-Kempe syndrome 26
Cameras and photography techniques 12
Carbon dot powders 13
Cardiovascular diseases 146
Caste 72
Central nervous system 146
Cephalic index 155
Charaka Samhita 7
Chelating agents 178
Chemical 88
    analysis, viscera preservation for 142
    antidotes 178
Chest 141
Chief complaints, history of 66
Child abuse 20, 26, 160
    reporting of suspected 26
Child for pornographic purposes, use of 112
Child sexual abuse 26
    identifying 27
    signs of 27f
    situations of 71
    symptoms of 27f
Child Welfare Committee 113
Choking 171
Civic benefit 43
Civil and criminal case 107
    procedures 106
Civil negligence 123
Clinical forensic medicine 31
Clinical forensic nurse specialist 32
Clipping 82
Clostridium perfringens 151
Clothing 82
Code of Criminal Procedure, trial under 109
Cognizable offense 108
Collection techniques 81
Coma 144, 146
Commit suicide, attempt to 108
Common and expert witness 56
Communication 40
    effective 53
    privileged 42
    skills 53
Complaints, presenting 21
Compulsion 168
Conduct money 121
Consent 73, 80, 124, 127
    absence of 73
    ages 125

expressed 125
implied 124
presumption of 74
reasons for 125
rules for 125
types of 124
Constitutes rape 73
Constitution and Composition of Council 36
Constitution of India 104
Constitution, salient features of 95f
Consumer Protection Act 126
Contact offenses 19
Contact pallor, areas of 150
Contact poison 177
Contributory negligence 123
Control swabs 83
Contusion 130
	estimation of age of 131
Cornea 147
	reflex, loss of 147
Coroner's inquest 120
Council proceedings and actions 44
Counselling 200
Court of Law 43
Court questions 122
Cranial sutures, closure of 157t
Crime
	against human body 107
	against property 107
	scene 48
		investigation 48
	suspected 43
	victims 55
Criminal and Civil Law 107fc
Criminal courts 105fc
Criminal negligence 123
Criminal Procedure Code 108
Cross-examination 122
Cultural and educational rights 96
Cultural and spiritual aspects 53, 72
Custody, chain of 90, 90f
Customary Law 104

D

Dactylography 162
Dead bodies 163
Dead cases, brought 196
Death 143
	apparent 143
	brain 144
	cause of 145
	certificate 145
	changes after 146
	description of manners of 145t
	determining
		cause of 159
		time of 160
	early changes 147
	fall of temperature after 148f
	homicidal 150
	immediate changes 146
	immediate signs of 147
	investigation team, member of 49
	investigators 49
	late changes 147
	legal concept of 144
	manner of 145, 145fc, 150, 172
	mechanism of 145
	mode of 146
	molecular 143
	moment of 143
	natural 145
	putrefactive changes after 151f
	scenes investigators 10
	somatic 143
	sudden 146, 150
	suicidal 150
	temperature after 148
	types of 143
	unnatural 145
Decomposition
	first external sign of 152
	first internal sign of 152
Defense wounds on palm 133f
Delusion 166
	types 166
Dentition, age estimation from 156t
Deoxyribonucleic acid 12, 83
	analysis, methods of 163
	division 10
	evidence 13
	fingerprinting 8, 163
		uses of 164
	identification 8
	profiling 8
	typing 8
Diaphoretics 178
Digital forensics 12
Diphtheroids 151
Dipsomania 168
Disciplinary action, procedure of 43
Disorganization, phase of 25
Doctor Contravening Provisions of Act 128

Documentary evidence, types of 121
Domestic violence, types of 20
Double jeopardy, right against 98
Drowning 172, 174
　atypical 174
　dry 174
　near 174
　shallow water 174
　types 174
Drug 88
　abuse 163
Drunkenness 179
　blood sample in case of 179
Dyes used 161
Dying declaration 120, 122
Dying deposition 122
Dyspareunia 62

E

E-filing of complaints 126
Elbow 157
Elder abuse 20
　types of 21f
Emergency cases 127
Endocrine causes 146
Enquiry 44
Erotomania 167
Ethics 35
　and professional conduct, prescribe code of 37
Evidence 111
　circumstantial 79, 154
　collecting 74
　collection 177
　　and preservation of 78, 81
　documentary 79, 111, 121
　documentation of 91
　hearsay 111
　labelling of 90
　observation of 81
　oral 111
　pathology 14
　primary 79
　procedure of recording of 122
　real 79, 79t
　recognition of 81
　recorder 48
　secondary 79
　types of 13, 79
Evidence collection
　and preservation 81f
　　purpose for 79b
　purpose of 79

Executive committee 36
Executive magistrates 106
Exhaled air 89
Exhibitionism 24
Exhumation 154, 154f
　purpose for 154
Expert witness 56, 74
Exploitation, right against 96
Ex-post facto law, right against 98
Eye
　after death, changes in 147, 147f
　changes in 152
Eyeball 147

F

Facial hair growth 154
Faded tattoos, identification of 161
Familial Alzheimer's 164
Family courts 105
Family Courts Act 105
Family violence 192
Family, friends and community, role of 71
Federal system 94
Feigned insanity 169, 170
Feticide, female 128
Fetishism 24
Fetus, miscarriage of existing 62
Fidelity 38
Filing complaint 44
Fingernail
　clippings 69
　scraping 84, 85f
Fingerprint 162, 162f
　analysis 8
　blood, hair 9
　classification of 162
　division 10
　recording of 162
　removal of 163
　types of 162
Fingertip bruising 174f
Firearm 87, 88
　division 11
　evidence, collection of 88b
　injury 135
　　documentation of 91b
Fixation, testing for 150
Footwear 82
Forced anal intercourse 165
Forced diuresis 178
Forehead 158
Foreign qualification, registration of 37

Forensic
　analyst 48
　anthropology 4
　ballistics 4
　biology 4
　chemistry 4
　correctional nurse 33
　entomology 4, 153
　evidence 4, 78
　genetics 10
　odontology 4
　pathology 4
　pediatric nurse examiner 33
　physics 4
　psychiatry 4, 166
　scientists, tools for 13f
　serology 4
　specialists 10
　team members 48
　toxicology 4, 176
Forensic medicine 3
　basic 117
　experts 10
Forensic nurse 34, 49, **50, 53,** 57
　code of ethics for 41, 41t
　death investigator 33
　documents 51
　examiner, role of 71
　expert witness 57
　hospitalist 34
　responsibilities of 34, 35
　role and responsibilities of 34
　role of 35f
Forensic nursing 30
　and Indian Laws 1
　care, comprehensive 61
　development of 31
　history of 4, 8, 31
　　development of 31t
　skills 42
Forensic psychiatric nurse 33
　role of 169
Forensic science 3, 4fc, 9, 13
　branches of 3
　careers 10
　development of 5
　history of 7f
　scope of 9
Forensic science laboratory 10, 11f
　collection of samples for 68
　divisions of 11fc
　equipments for 12t
　findings, negative 70
　functions of 13
　instrumental facilities in 12
Fresh body, best sample in 163
Frontal eminence 158
Frontonasal junction 158
Frotteurism 24
FTA card 83f, 84f
Fundamental rights 94, 95, 96f
　and constitution 95

G

Gag reflex 144
Gallbladder 142f
Gastric contents 89
Gastric lavage 178
　agents used for 178
　contraindications of 179
　tubes used for 178
Gastrointestinal system 146
Genital and anal examination 199
Genital and anal swabs 86
Genitalia, mutilated 62
Genitourinary system 146
Glabella 158
Grandiosity, delusion of 167
Graze abrasion 129
Gunshot injury 82
Gustatory hallucination 167

H

Hair 14, 69, 85, 160f
　and Fiber analysis 12
　blackening of 137f
　bulbs 131
　follicles with roots 84, 163
　sample, collected 84f
　singeing of 137f
Hallucination 167
　types 167
Hanging 171, 172, 173f, 175
　mark of 194
Headspace gas chromatography 10
Health response, basic elements of 74
Healthcare provider, legal duties of 177
Hearsay evidence 79
Heart 152
Hemodialysis 178
Hemoperfusion 178
Hemophilia 164
Hemorrhage 131

Henry and Galton system 162
Hesitation cuts 134
　usual sites of 134
Homicidal poisoning 177
Honor killings 19
Hostile witness 57
Human being, valuing 40
Human hair 160
Human rights and doctors, violation of 100
Human Rights Commission 94
Human rights watch 101
Humanitarian forensic nurse 33
Huntington's disease 164
Hyoid bone, fracture of 172
Hypochondriacal delusion 166

I

Identification 155
　absolute 155
　complete 155
　data of 155
　partial 155
　types 155
Iliac crest 157
Illusion 167
　personal 167
　types 167
　universal 167
Immersion syndrome 171
Impulse 167
Impulsive control disorder, diagnosis of 168
Incident 197
Incised wound 132
　over chest 133*f*
Indecent assault 24
Indian Constitution 94
Indian Evidence Act 110
Indian Judicial System 104, 105*fc*
Indian Judicial System and Laws 104
Indian nurses register, maintenance of 37
Indian Nursing Council 35
　functions of 36
Indian Penal Code 106
　debated provisions of 108
　structure of 107
　victim's rights under 97
Individual, determining
　sex of 157
　stature of 155
Infertility 62
　delusion of 166

Inflict injury, weapon used to 54
Influence, delusion of 167
Informed consent 52, 65, 125
　form, general surgery 202
Injury 129
　absence of 70
　classification of 129
　duration of 53, 54
　electrical 138
　extra-genital 69
　fabricated 135
　firearm 136
　lack of 70
　local 69
　manner of 133
　mechanical 129
　nature of 54, 129, 130
　particulars of 52
　patterned 134, 135*f*
　self-inflicted 135, 135*f*
　thermal 129
　type of 52
Innocence, presumption of 98
Inquest 119
　types of 119
Insane
　civil responsibility of 168
　criminal responsibility of 169
　delusions 169
Insanity 166
　true 170
Instruments, basic 12*t*
International Association of Forensic Nurses 31
International Sources of Law 104
Interpersonal relationships 40
Intestinal contents 154
Investigation 108
Ischial
　spines 159
　tuberosity 159

J

Joule burn 138, 139*f*
　characteristics of 139
Judge, powers of 106*t*
Judgement, error of 123
Judicial decisions 104
Justice 38
Juvenile Justice Act 74
Juvenile Justice Board 106

Index

K
Karl Pearson's formula 155
Kautilya's Arthashastra 7
Keratinocytes 163
Kevorkian sign 147
Kidney, half of each 142f
Kleptomania 168

L
Labor courts 105
Laceration 132f
    characteristics of 131f
Latent fingerprint 162
    expert 49
Laws and law-making powers, sources of 104
Legal aspects 54, 72, 176
Legal matters 30
Legal medicine 3
Legal procedures 119
LGBTQIA 72
Ligature mark 172, 173f
Lithotomy position 69f
Liver 152
    part of 142f
Locard's exchange principle 8, 80f
Love, delusion of 167
Low rectal temperature 148
Lucid interval 168, 169
Lungs 175

M
Magistrate
    courts 105
    inquest 119, 120
    powers of 106t
Mandible
    female 159
    male 159
Masochism 24
Mass spectrometers 12
Master-servant rule 124
Mastoid process 158
McNaughton's rule 169
Mediation 126
Medical certificates 121
Medical evidence 121
    types 121
Medical examination 199
Medical examiner system 120
Medical facility, duties of 22
Medical history 68, 198
    and examination form 197
Medical practitioner 98
Medical Termination of Pregnancy Act 127
Medicolegal autopsy 140
    objectives of 140
Medicolegal care, protocols of 63
Medicolegal case 54
    intimation regarding 195
Medicolegal certificates 122
Medicolegal interview 66
Medicolegal report 54
Menstrual disorders 62
Menstrual history 68
Mental abuse 26
Mental illness 166
Mental status, altered 175
Mentally-ill person 166, 169
Microorganisms 151
Migratory bruises 130
Misleading advertisement 126
Monozygotic twins and clones 8
Motor vehicle accidents 89
Muscles, involvement of 150
Mutilomania 168
Myocardial infarction 191

N
Nail scratches 174f
Nanotechnology 13
National Human Rights Commission 99
    composition of 100fc
    limitations of 100
    major issues to 100
National Nursing and Midwifery Commission 37
    Bill 37
Near hanging 174
    signs 174
    survivor of 174f
    symptoms 174
Neck 175
Neglect 26
Negligence
    defences against 123
    types of 123
Neurologic symptoms 175
Neurosis 166
Nightmares 25
Nihilistic delusion 166
Nonbailable offenses 109
Noncognizable offense 109

Noncontact offenses 19
Non-forensic emergency department nurses, role of 34
Nonliving inorganic matter 79
Non-maleficence 38
Notifiable clauses 43
Nuchal crest 158
Nurse
　code of ethics for 39
　code of professional conduct for 40, 40f
　coroner 33
　death investigators 49
　disciplinary action for 44fc
　ethical principles for 38, 38f
　witness, responsibilities of 56
Nursing
　ethics 35, 41
　jurisprudence 30, 35, 119
　practice, Acts related to 126
　promote research in 37
　qualifications, recognition of 36
Nysten's rule 149

O

Oath 122
Obsession 168
　compulsion 168
Obstetric history 68
Obturator foramen 159
Odontology division 12
Offenses
　against state 108
　and penalties 127
　and punishments 111
　unnatural 108
Offenses under Protection of Children from Sexual Offences Act 111fc
Olfactory hallucination 167
Oniomania 168
Oral evidence 79, 121
　types of 121
Oral swab 84
　collection 85f
Orbits 158
Othello syndrome 166

P

Palate 158
Panchnama 119
　preparation of 119

Paraphilia 24
Paraphilic disorder 193
Pedophilia 24
Pellets 88
Pelvic
　cavity 159
　inflammatory disease 62
　inlet 159
　outlet 159
Pelvis 159f
　female 159
　male 159
Penal erasure 123
Penalties 22, 126, 128
Penile swabs 87
Perineal swab 87, 87f
Perjury 122
Persecution, delusion of 167
Petechiae 175
Phobia 168
　simple 168
　social 168
　types 168
Photographer 48
Physical antidotes 178
Physical evidence 79
Physical examination 52, 68
Physical treatment 52
Physical violence 67
Physiological antidotes 178
Plastic print 162
Pluck hair 84, 163
　from roots 84f
PM staining
　color of 150
　fixation of 150
Poison 176
　by excretion, removal of 178
　case of 177
　classification of 176
　ingested 177
　inhaled 177
　injected 177
　removal of unabsorbed 177
　suspected case of 177
Police inquest 119
　purpose of 119
Police intimation form 195
Polymerase chain reaction 12, 163
　requirements for 163
Post-assault activities 67

Postmortem
 caloricity 148
 changes, time scale of 153t
 conducting 50
 staining, development of 150
Preauricular sulcus 159
Preconception and Prenatal Diagnostic Techniques Act 128
Pregnancy
 length of 127
 unwanted 62
Prenatal diagnostic techniques 128
 regulation of 128
Prevention of Sexual Harassment Act 25
Products liability 123
Professional misconduct 43, 43b, 124
Professional negligence 123, 124
 punishment for 123
Professional secrecy 42
Prostate 152
Protection of Children from Sexual Offences Act 111
Protection of Women from Domestic Violence Act 21
Protection officer, information to 22
Proteomes 13
Provisional opinion 70
Provisions for Victims Under Indian Laws 97
Psychosis 166
Psychosocial
 aspects 53
 care 71
Pubic hair 85
 collection of 86f
 preservation of 86f
Pubis body 159
Punishment 24, 42
Pupils 147
Putrefaction 153
Pyromania 168

Q

Quality nursing practice 40

R

Race 162
Rape 24, 126
 and sexual assault 191
 commit 72
 custodial 73
 establishing 64
 gang 73
 medicolegal examination of 65
 punishment of 73, 74
 survivor examination, guidelines for 65f
 trauma syndrome 25
 trial, cross-examination in 74
 victim, revealing identity of 74
Rat hole appearance 136f
Real life forensics 9
Recognition of nursing institutions, withdrawal of 37
Rectal temperature, high 148
Redressal agencies 126
Re-examination 122
Referral cases 55
Registered medical practitioner 63
Religion 72, 161
Reorganization, phase of 25
Reproductive system 146
Res Ipsa loquitur, doctrine of 124
Res judicata 123
Respiration, irreversible cessation of 147
Respiratory system 146
Retina 147
Right to appeal 99
Right to constitutional remedies 96
Right to cross-examination 99
Right to equality 95
Right to expeditious trial 98
Right to freedom 96
 of religion 96
Right to get copies of documents 99
Right to have bail 98
Right to humane treatment in prison 99
Right to legal aid 98
Right to present during trial 99
Right to privacy and protection against unlawful searches 98
Rights of accused 97
 during trial 99
 under constitution 97
Rights of arrested person 99
Rights of victim 96
Rigor mortis 149, 149f, 152
 breaking 149
 conditions simulating 149
 testing 149
Road traffic accident 10, 132f
Rule of 12 149, 149f
Rule of 9 138, 138f, 138t
Ryle's tube aspirate 90f

S

Sacroiliac joint surface 159
Sadism 24
Safe kit 63f
Saliva 14, 69
    stains of 172
Satellite pellet wounds 136f
Scalp 141
    hair 85, 89
    spilt laceration on 132f
Scar 160
    age of 160
Sciatic notch 159
Sclera 147
    opaque and sunken 147f
Scrapping 69, 82
Self-incrimination, right against 98
Semen 14
Seminal discharge 172
Serology 12
Sessions case 109
Sessions Court 105
Sex determination 163
Sex linked disorders 24
Sex selection, prohibition of 128
Sex worker 72
Sexual abuse 26
    perpetrator of 72
Sexual asphyxia 175
    methods of producing 175
Sexual assault 23, 61, 82, 112, 160
    breast of victim of 86f
    cases 68t
    examination of survivor of 66b
    forensic evidence kit 63, 63t
        contents of 64f
    health consequences of 61
    investigation team, member of 50
    long-term effects of 25
    nurse examiner 31, 32
    penetrative 111
    physical consequences of 62t
    psychological consequences of 62t
    survivor 61, 63fc
        comprehensive care of 62
Sexual attraction to animals 24
Sexual dysfunction 62
Sexual harassment 24
   at workplace 25f
   of child 112
   of Women at Workplace (Prevention, Prohibition And Redressal) Act 25
Sexual history 67
Sexual offenses 24
    classification of 23
Sexual perversions 24
Sexual violence 64, 197
    types of 23f
    victims of 63
Sexually transmitted infections 62
Shapiro's rule 149
Shot gun 136f
Shoulder 157
Sickle cell anemia 164
Single paper bag 90f
Skeletal remains, examination of 155
Sketch preparer 48
Skilled witness 56
Skin
    avulsion of 132f
    cells 14
    incisions 140
        I-shaped 140
        modified Y-shaped 140
        types of 140, 141f
    marbling of 152
Skull 141, 158f
    female 158
    male 158
Small intestines, upper part of 142f
Smothering 171
Sodomy 24
Somatic death 143
Specimen selection and preservation 163
Split laceration 132
Stab wound 133, 133f
    shapes of 133
    types of 133
Staphylococcus 151
State medicine 3
State Nurses and Midwives Council 37
State Nursing Council 37
Statutory rape 72, 73
Stomach contents 153
Strangulation 171, 172, 173f
    classification of 171
Streptococcus 151
Stretch laceration 132
Subcutaneous tissues 132f
Subpubic angle 159
Suffocation 171
Suicidal firearm wounds 137f
Suicide 133
    by firearm, features of 137

Summons 120
  case 109
Suprameatal crest 158
Supraorbital margins 158
Surgical history 68
Survivor 62
  particulars of 66
Suspension, degree of 171
Swabs 69
Sweat 14
Syncope 146

T

Tache noire 147, 147f
Tactile hallucination 167
Tattoo 136
  erasure of 161
  marks 161
  permanent 161
  upper arm 161f
  visibility of latent 161
Termination of pregnancy, doctors requirement for 127t
Testimony 58f
Thanatology 143
Therapeutic misadventure 123
Throttling 174
Thyroid cartilage, fracture of 172
Time since death 154f
  determination of 152
  estimation of 152t
Tissue bridges 131
Tongue, protrusion of 172
Touch 167
Toxicological analysis, sample preservation for 89t
Toxicology 12
  cases pertaining to 88
  division 10
  evidence 14
Trace evidence 14
  division 11
Transvestism 24
Trauma 51
Treatment and information to police 74
Trial procedure 110
Trolley sheets 82

U

Under criminal law 98
Urinary bladder, contents of 154

Urine 89
  alkalinization 178
  and feces, discharge of 172
  sample 89, 89f
Uterus 152

V

Vacuum sweeping 82
Vaginal smears 87f
Vaginal swab 87f
Vaginal washing 86
Venereal disease 43
Veracity 38
Vicarious liability 124
Victim 62
  and family, comprehensive care of 47, 51
  body 12
  caring of 53
  compensation to 97
  comprehensive care of 34f, 51fc
  impact statement 97
  perpetrator and environment, relation between 23f
  rights under code of criminal procedure 97
  rights under constitution 97
Violence 17, 22
  against women 19
  and sexual abuse 17
  categories of 19
  child maltreatment 20
  classification of 18fc
  collective 18
  community 18, 191
  death of victim of 55
  deprivation 19
  domestic 20, 192
  dowry-related 19
  family 18, 19, 20
  from crime, surveillance of 23
  gender-based 19
  interpersonal 18, 19
  intimate partner 20, 192
  nature of 19
  neglect 19
  physical 19
  psychological 19
  self-directed 18
  sexual 19, 23
  types 18
  workplace 22, 191
Viscera preservation 142, 142f

Visible print 162
Visual hallucination 167
Vitreous humor 147, 154
Vomitus and stomach contents 89
Voyeurism 24

W

Wallace rule of 9 138
Warrant case 110
Weapon
    determining type of 160
    used 131
Whole blood 89
Whole bowel irrigation 179
Witness
    box 57
    common 56
    ordinary 56
    percipient 56

Wound
    accidental 133
    chop 134, 134f, 193
    close shot firearm entry 136f
    direction of 52
    entry 135, 136, 136f, 137f
    exit 136, 137f
    homicidal 133
    lacerated 19f, 131
    location of 52
    superficial incised 135f
    types of lacerated 132
Wrist 157
    hesitation cuts over 134f

Z

Zygomatic arch 158